# Praise for *In My Life*

This is a book of striking life stories by youth AIDS activists in South Africa, crafted over the course of two decades, an entire generation. The collection's 12 narratives by young people of their lives from their teens to their thirties turn into evocative and reflective accounts of the unfolding of a self. In these, *In My Life* shares something delicate and important: how to create a way of knowing one another deeply in our country of distances and invisibility. Their stories of ordinary nearness, of friendship, risk, trust, hurt and trying again convey the vital possibilities of everyday realities in South Africa. Together these give the collection an almost breathtaking force. Through it, we are invited to wonder what it means to be *near* one another, in a multitude of ways. *In My Life*'s hard-won, jagged intimacies and depth of relation come from 20 years of practicing a radical, difficult, continual becoming and togetherness.

– Gabeba Baderoon, author of *Regarding Muslims: From Slavery to Post-Apartheid* and *The History of Intimacy*

*In My Life* tells the story of two decades of talking and walking in which boundaries blur and friendships are forged. It is a stunning exposition of ethnography-of-(e)motion as the South African transition dead-ends at the top and ignites from below.

– Ashwin Desai, author of *We are the Poors: Community Struggles in Post-Apartheid South Africa* and *Inside Indian Indenture*

This pathbreaking ethnography convincingly demonstrates that any genuine attempt at bridging the divide between research, activism and social justice must be based on intimate relationships, expressions of love and the capacity for empathy.
– Luke Sinwell, author of *The Spirit of Marikana: The Rise of Insurgent Trade Unionism in South Africa*

The twelve powerful narratives come at a time when we as a country need a strong reminder of the importance of active citizenry and the much-needed social disruption driven by young people. The stories draw attention to the high levels of violence we live under in South Africa, the journey of activism from adolescenthood to young adults, the turning points for becoming a role model and social justice activist, the real-life issues we all grapple with from body shaming, drugs, mental health, to stigma, surpassed by admirable strength, resilience and leadership. This book belongs on the shelves of the history of our modern times and a must-read for those working in the fields of youth advocacy, global health and HIV.

– Dr Shakira Choonara, 2017 Women of the Year in Health South Africa, Technical Specialist at the World Health Organization, UN Women Thematic Lead and former member of the African Union Youth Council

In a period where research, activism and resources on and for HIV & AIDS have dwindled, the book, *In My Life: Stories from young activists in South Africa 2002–2022* is not only timely, but also reminds us of our collective unfinished business of getting to zero HIV infections. Importantly, amidst calls for the voices of young people to be at the centre of research and programming, *In My Life* showcases both the longitudinal, youth-focused participatory methodology that enabled the young people's creative practices over two decades, and unearthed their engaging, thoughtful and generative stories of how they see themselves, and how they have located themselves in the context of AIDS activism in South Africa.

– Relebohile Moletsane, Professor and JL Dube Chair in Rural Education University of KwaZulu-Natal

# In My Life

## Stories from young activists in South Africa 2002–2022

Edited by *Shannon Walsh,*
*Claudia Mitchell & Mandla Oliphant*

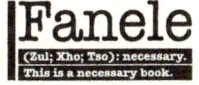

First published by Fanele, an imprint of Jacana Media (Pty) Ltd in 2022

10 Orange Street
Sunnyside
Auckland Park 2092
South Africa

© Shannon Walsh, Claudia Mitchell and Mandla Oliphant, 2022
Cover photo of Khayalethu Mofu by Neels Kleynhans: nkphotography.co.za

All rights reserved.

ISBN 978-1-77634-589-2

Also available as an e-book

Cover design by Maggie Davey and Aimèe Armstrong
Editing by Lara Jacob
Proofreading by Megan Mance
Indexing by Adrienne Pretorious
Set in Sabon 11/16pt
Printed and bound by Creda Communications
Job No. 003962

See a complete list of Jacana titles at www.jacana.co.za

# Contents

Acknowledgements . . . . . . . . . . . . . . . . . . . . . . . . . . . . . . . . . . vii

### PART ONE: Methods & Histories

1 Storytelling, friendship and activism. . . . . . . . . . . . . . . . . . . .3
2 Creative practices, young people and the AIDS pandemic . . .14
3 Overtime/over time . . . . . . . . . . . . . . . . . . . . . . . . . . . . . . . .19

### PART TWO: Narratives & Reflections

4 Background to the projects . . . . . . . . . . . . . . . . . . . . . . . . .37
5 Kaylene Schroeder . . . . . . . . . . . . . . . . . . . . . . . . . . . . . . .53
6 Khayalethu (KK) Mofu . . . . . . . . . . . . . . . . . . . . . . . . . . . . .89
7 Lindeka Cynthia Rwida Joka . . . . . . . . . . . . . . . . . . . . . . .115
8 Mathew Johannes . . . . . . . . . . . . . . . . . . . . . . . . . . . . . . .139
9 Ann Thembeka Dipa . . . . . . . . . . . . . . . . . . . . . . . . . . . . .175
10 Nosibusiso (Nosy) Mcunukeli . . . . . . . . . . . . . . . . . . . . . .197
11 Mphumzi Mphura Xokozela . . . . . . . . . . . . . . . . . . . . . . .211
12 Bridgette Magqaza . . . . . . . . . . . . . . . . . . . . . . . . . . . . . .227
13 Thozamile (Thozzi) Vanto . . . . . . . . . . . . . . . . . . . . . . . . .231
14 Danlia Wiener . . . . . . . . . . . . . . . . . . . . . . . . . . . . . . . . . .247

15  Chinomy Jacobs.................................255
16  Mandla Oliphant...............................263

## PART THREE: Endings?

17  This is not the last chapter........................293

### APPENDIX

Notes............................................. 302
Publications related to the project ...................... 310
Index............................................. 313

# Acknowledgements

MANY PEOPLE CONTRIBUTED TO THIS PROJECT over 20 years, from running workshops and sessions and sharing expertise, and creating art and writing. These early collaborators included our partner at the Centre for the Book, Elisabeth Anderson, organiser Dammon Rice and coordinator Thandi Lewin. The facilitators of workshop sessions and speakers included Anne Schuster who led the incredible youth writing and poetry workshops, and Abigail Dreyer who contributed multiple times over the years to facilitate discussions around HIV, gender and sexuality. The first workshops and symposium sessions in 2002 included rich presentations, spoken word, performance art, poetry, readings, live graffiti and artworks by Shaheen Ariefdien, K. Sello Duiker, Naila Keleta-Mae, Suzanne Leclerc-Madlala, Thabo Lehlongwa, Tebhoho Mahlatsi, Themba Malaza, Jerry Manganyi, Gcina Mhlophe, Zach Modirapula, Robin Rhode, Ann Smith, Kylie Thomas, Mara Verna and Sue Williamson.

We acknowledge the wonderful support of Relebohile Moletsane, Naydene De Lange and Jean Stuart who so enthusiastically promoted *Fire & Hope* and *In My Life* through the Centre for Visual Methodologies for Social Change at the University of KwaZulu-Natal. June Larkin was an early collaborator in our thinking and workshops on arts-based HIV prevention with young people through the GAAP project. Farah Malik, Jackie Kirk and Stephanie Garrow were collaborators on the AWID funded 'Girls Speak Out Project', which is discussed here. The principal and teachers at Atlantis Secondary School were very supportive of this work and supported sessions at the school through 2003–2005.

Special thanks for research assistance from Trish Everett, who significantly helped in bringing together all the materials and transcripts for each participant over the past twenty years. Lara Jacob, our editor at Jacana, deserves special thanks for her insight, enthusiasm and perseverance in making this book possible. Ann Smith provided early comments, Nesa Bandarchian Rashti helped in copy editing this manuscript, and Megan Mance at Jacana provided support around the images.

Linda Keiser filmed sessions in 2019, Kaveh Nabatian shot video, Drew Malamud did the sound and Gene Pendon created the hand-drawn poster for the short film *Fire & Hope* in 2003. Eugene Arries photographed sessions in 2018 and Faith Ilevbare edited video material and assisted in editing archives. Lan Yan designed the incredible Memory Books we used in 2019, Lizza Littlewort and Sarah-Anne Raynham created our original poster and cover artwork in 2003, featuring an image supplied by Robin Rhode of a session he did in our 2003 workshops.

We want to acknowledge some of the other young people who contributed significantly to this project over different phases: Aisha Pandor, Andrew Fischer, Barbara Matasane, Clinton Stemmel, Nadia Brown, Naseema Meeran, Nicolene Linnett, Nolubabalo Mkona, Nombulelo Moeti, Reyaan Mentoor, Ruth Allison Fillies, Thulani Hono and Wendy Tapleni.

We gratefully acknowledge the financial support of many funders over the years, including the Social Sciences Research Council of Canada (SSHRC), the Canadian Society of International Health's (CSIH) Small Grants Fund, the Canadian Bureau for International Education (CBIE), the Canadian International Development Agency (CIDA) Innovative Research Awards, the Fonds Quebecois de la recherche sur la société et la culture (FQRSC), the Peter Wall Institute for Advanced Studies (PWIAS) International Visiting Research Scholars Award, The Centre for the Book, the Gendering Adolescent AIDS Prevention project (GAAP), the National Research Foundation (NRF) of South Africa, Association for Women's Rights in Development (AWID), McGill University, UKZN, and the University of British Columbia Publication Fund.

# PART ONE

*Methods & Histories*

# 1

# Storytelling, friendship and activism

> The habit of looking at the spectacle has forced us to gloss over the nooks and crannies.
> — Njabulo S. Ndebele[1]

IN MY LIFE CONTAINS EXCERPTS and fragments of a project spanning 20 years that included creative writing, arts-based educational workshops and filmed documentary interviews. It began as an HIV prevention programme with a racially diverse group of young AIDS activists in South Africa, facilitated by South Africans and two Canadians. As time went on, the work together became another kind of journey. The stories in these pages are fragments of moments we took together and alone – as researchers, participants, artists, writers, creators, activists, teachers and many other things in-between and beyond.

We did not start out thinking we would stay together so long, or that our staying together would erupt into new kinds of meaning, but we did and it has. Much of what ties us together in these pages are intimacies formed and forged; friendships both ordinary and complicated, and born from new ways of seeing and collective struggles.[2] Along the way we also started to recognise what Njabulo Ndebele talks about, that the spectacle of violence in South Africa often turns focus away from where politics actually lives, in everyday life. He writes,

> The ordinary day-to-day lives of people should be the direct focus of political interest because they constitute the very content of the struggle, for the struggle involves people not

abstractions. If it is a new society we seek to bring about in South Africa, then that newness will be based on a direct concern with the way people actually live.[3]

Life stories, in all their contradictions and fragments, are the places where meaning is made, where we find reflections of truth, and ways towards hope and connection. It can be a space, too, for a radical living politics. Taking seriously lived experience is about allowing stories to exist as they are.

The early 2000s were a time of optimism and exuberance in newly democratic South Africa. There was an electricity in the air. Transformations were afoot, and there was a courageous desire for change, even with the stark realities of HIV and AIDS-related illnesses looming. Old ideas around race, class, gender and sexuality were all being contested. Yet, as the years slipped away, so did much of that enthusiasm. Stories were a place where one could hide, find solace or find ways to be connected again. As Stacy Hardy reflects on her own post-apartheid experiences after losing fellow writers Phaswane Mpe and K. Sello Duiker to violence and suicide:

> Faced with a growing sense of loss, at a loss as to how to address this loss, I lost myself in books. I soon discovered that I was not alone in my lostness or my aloneness. South African literature is full of loners, lost relations, and thwarted relationships. Friendship when it does figure is at best fleeting, tenuous. More often than not it fails us, or we fail it... And this lostness is really what saved me, I think, from a deep despair, and not just about the suicides and the deaths, but from the idea of death, and the ongoing poverty, deprivation, and violence that dogged our society despite the emergence of democracy, and a fundamental feeling of differentness or aloneness or separation from other people. Both literature and friendship extend the possibility of immersion in another consciousness. They're the forms in which we find the power, in language, to inhabit, perceive, and recreate a shared world. Aloneness that undermines aloneness; a portrait of loneliness that leaves us less alone.[4]

Stories can forge connection, empathy and understanding. Many South Africans' stories remain untold, many voices still buried. That aloneness can be fatal. The stories in this book offer portraits of people who have struggled through an incredible range of experiences, and remained authentic and honest about their journeys, offering life lines of connection in troubled waters. 'There is no unearned heroism here, there is the unproclaimed heroism of the ordinary person,' writes Ndebele.[5] Stories of everyday struggles remind us we are not alone. Ordinary stories of people's extraordinary lives help us remember what it is we are fighting for. And there is love, and friendship. While disappointing at times, troubling, and not nearly enough, loving can be a 'subversive gift, and a significant political act'.[6]

We thought a lot about how to present this work spanning two decades: how to synthesise it and what it might give to readers. What might these stories offer by reflecting on what has happened in the last twenty years in post-apartheid South Africa? The shadows of history are cast over our early encounters. At times, this can make ways of seeing murkier and, at other times, it clears our vision. We often got stuck in where our voices belonged as researchers; where they intersected and became entangled with participants; and where they became overbearing and unnecessary. Many discussions, over many years, circled around these questions. In the end we fell upon the idea to allow the stories to breathe and to have space and context all on their own. As Mandla implored,

> Now we are confronted with the question you need to answer from your perspective, not from someone else's perspective … you have to confront yourself. You have to talk about things from your perspective. Even as I was listening while Lindeka and Mphumzi were talking, I could hear that it hasn't registered to them yet.
> That it is not 'our' anymore. It is 'I'.
> As much as all of us were there, we have experienced the waters differently. We have been changed differently. We all drank from the same river, we drank the same water, but it has affected us differently. You can't speak from a second or third

person, you have to speak from the first person. From your first-hand experience. We have to do away with 'our'.

Toggling between 'we' and 'I', we have been together, alone. There has been true connection, and shared parts of a journey, but also distinctly separate roads; impossible friendships because of the expansive divides between us. In heeding Mandla's imperative to write from the first person, what follows in Part Two comes directly from the voices of participants themselves, with all its contradictions, ellipses and holes.

In many ways, this book in itself has become method. As Lindeka beautifully writes, 'This is a true story and I'm the narrator of this story.'

## ETHNOGRAPHY-IN-MOTION

Behind the desire to highlight the importance of everyday stories is an understanding that knowledge is power. Those who hold, create and maintain knowledge are often those who rule the world and maintain hegemony. Yet, power can be disrupted by looking at knowledge produced in everyday life from below. As the anti-colonial thinker Franz Fanon said, the 'problems of the colonized are deep and intricately connected with the racist gaze and the oppressive colonial state which is fully equipped with language, books, teachers, experts, and even the Bible, which it uses to oppress the colonised subjects.'[7] Fanon believed liberation could be set in motion through close observation of the everyday ways that colonialism was built and maintained, and through the retrieval of alternative forms of knowledge production.

Similarly, Steve Biko, founder of the Black Consciousness Movement, developed a type of activist ethnography during the struggle against apartheid, as a way to understand the oppressive environment in which he lived through the everyday realities of other Africans. Biko described research he and fellow activists Barney Pityana and Jerry Modisane undertook which involved,

> listening to ordinary people in ordinary situations, on buses,

> in sports fields and queues, even shebeens [where] ... acts of everyday rebellion are woven between the narratives and stories of black people retold in positive and creative ways, to produce a matrix that allows for the imagination of the black self positively and the production of communities that are able to resist and produce wor(l)ds against the exploitative and oppressive system of apartheid and capitalism.[8]

Through this approach, the Black Consciousness Movement allowed for the 'changing, lived experiences of people to shape and determine its evolution'.[9] Similarly, in South Asia the Subaltern Studies group considered dominant versions of history and power that may be disrupted through knowledge 'from below'.[10] Beyond everyday sites of learning, activist theorising also happens at meetings, on the streets, in late night discussions, with friends, at demonstrations and organised events. Activist spaces are important sites for intellectual development and crucial for the messy work of social transformation. Knowledge is learned by being part of movements and actively engaged in struggles, as the young AIDS activists in this book were.[11]

Throughout this journey we engaged with a method of ethnography in-motion.[12] Ethnography-in-motion is a research approach that brings together engaged educational practices, personal narratives, visual methods, learning from social movements and liberatory models of social transformation.[13] Ethnography, simply understood, is the close study of everyday life and practices of a particular community or people. A method developed by social anthropologists, others such as post-colonial, anti-racist, feminist and Indigenous scholars and activists have been drawn to ethnography as a politically engaged research practice. Many have argued that everyday practices and experiences can provide the essential knowledge needed to understand and challenge forms of oppression.

Ethnography-in-motion is 'in motion', then, by being participant-led, ever-changing and dynamic. As a research practice, it is organic and evolves with the people who are at its core. An ethnography-in-motion seeks to create a space of collaboration between researchers and participants, but also with readers, allowing the work to function

*Storytelling, friendship and activism*

as a prism that refracts and transforms as we view it from different angles. It is a process of seeing which does not omit points of view, but hopes to allow them to flourish. Ethnography-in-motion disrupts binaries of inside/outside and subjective/objective, to learn-while-walking together within the encounter.[14]

Our process of working together in this project involved multiple modes and methods: from everyday life experiences in relation to the AIDS pandemic and the post-apartheid context, as well as creative expression, storytelling, education and social engagement. At its heart were the crucial engagement, voices and stories of young people, so essential to curbing the tide of HIV infection, both then and now.

## THE RESEARCHER/PARTICIPANT DIVIDE

> Literature cannot give us lessons, but it can only provide a very compelling context for us to examine an infinite number of ethical issues which have a bearing on the sensitization of people towards the development of the entire range of culture.
> – Njabulo S. Ndebele[15]

With a project that unfolds over decades, the boundaries between researcher and participant blurred as the years passed, and we became friends and peers. Indeed, stark separations between participants and researchers can often hide more than they reveal. As anthropologist James Ferguson writes, an attachment to an imagined research 'field' creates a mythology that 'powerfully suggests two separate worlds, bridged only at the initiative of the intrepid anthropologist.[16] Participant-led research creates even more of a blurred landscape where fluid relationships must be handled with empathy and a keen sense of ethics. We are not apart from each other in this process. We all grow and change together, if in different ways.

Over the years, as relationships developed and grew, there were moments where friendship was an undeniable dynamic. Shannon and Mandla were both in their mid-twenties when they started as co-facilitators, and so the age difference was less remarkable than that of race, class, background and culture. We knew so much about the participants' lives and they had shared so much with us. Each of these people are participants in our life stories as much as we might be characters in theirs. We had genuine interest in one another. We'd watched them grow up, and we'd aged with them. We cared about each other, even if that care was complicated by the impossible distances created by a deeply divided society. There was no 'exit strategy' within these relationships. Did that mean the research was indelibly tainted? Is developing human relationships inherently a research flaw? Are we unable to care for each other and still learn from each other? Were the lines too blurred? What kinds of expectations emerge in the wake of such work?

In 2002, KK was an outspoken teen activist working with the Treatment Action Campaign around HIV prevention in Khayelitsha, and one of a dozen young people involved in the multi-year qualitative educational research project that forms the basis for this book, which included workshops, interviews, the production of literary texts, a documentary film and a series of creative art works. KK was an inspiration to everyone who met him; verbose, intelligent, funny and creative, he always made everyone around him engage more deeply with the issues at hand. Yet, over a decade later, he was still struggling to fulfil his dreams as the relentless poverty and racism around him took its toll, and he struggled to survive, while still helping build one of the first Xhosa language theatres in Cape Town.

By 2019, KK expressed his hurt and anger that we had not supported him further as an artist in his career, and it was heartbreaking. His pain and disappointment were real. Was there something we could have done differently that would have changed his feeling, or is such unease familiar to ways other researchers have talked about participants' feelings of abandonment, anger and dismay at the end of a research relationship?[17] It is impossible to compare.

The friendships also had other kinds of impacts and implications as relationships evolved. As Shannon wrote in her field notes in 2004,

> It's a sunny warm day and we are slow to get back to Atlantis after a long day of working with the group on *Fire & Hope* in Cape Town. Kaylene and I drop everyone at home and are left

alone together in the car. We have become really close over the last few years of working together. She has grown out of being a teenager and we seem to be connecting in a different way – as peers more than as researcher/subject or teacher/student, with all its inherent power dynamics.

We talk the whole drive back. Our conversation becomes more personal and she begins to explain the details of her sexual assault and her attempt to press charges against the rapist who was a part of her community. I pull over in a parking lot so I can give her my full attention. Her story is powerful and troubling. I am amazed again at her strength, honesty and conviction. At the same time, I feel confused. Has our relationship shifted? Is she telling me this story as a friend or as a researcher? We have been working together all day, but somehow this feels different, somehow outside the realm of my research. Could I use this story as a way to discuss the deeper impacts of sexual violence these girls face? Or would that be breaking her confidence? Am I worrying about this needlessly? When she first divulged her rape in an interview on camera, I stopped rolling to check in with her that she really wanted this recorded and possibly even used in the documentary. She agreed at the time, and had clearly thought about it before she divulged the story. Why do I now feel that she would not tell this to the Shannon wearing the 'researcher' hat, only to the Shannon who has become her friend? I err on the side of safety, and don't discuss our conversation in my writing, but the problem remains unresolved.

As these notes attest, engaged, participant-led research can trouble any clearly defined boundaries. We grow close, we care about one another, we have expectations and there are millions of little things said and unsaid that bring us close and keep us apart. Speaking of these blurred relationships, this beautiful passage from Laurent Dubois captures the painful contradictions that working together closely can evoke between friendship and research.

> I keep thinking about him, as I saw him last, drying out leaves for medicines in front of his hospital room, and I want to go back, and I want to learn more from him; and then, in part, I want him to keep his knowledge away from me. I don't know what I would do with it – I would write it down, I would make an article from it, I would take his picture – I would turn his friendship into something else; sometimes, I don't want to. Sometimes, I want to leave it alone, keep it there, stop asking so many questions, stop writing – just like he told me to – asking me: What are you writing? Stop writing and listen to me.[18]

These moments of convergence, recognition and empathy are important as we work, grow and learn together.[19] So too are the disappointments, the things we miss, the people we lost and the ways we could have served each other better. Much of what we have uncovered over this long span of time together has been about these shared relationships: the political importance of friendship and the power of holding space for each other's stories. Time was indeed a scale with which our intimacies flourished. Intimacies too are subversive and political acts.

At times, we delayed in writing up our research as we attempted to parse what to make of this journey. As time goes by, so too the story changes. Just when we think we can see one set of impacts, life takes a swerve and things change once again. We witnessed Mathew find his sexuality and gender identity, KK become an articulate director and performer in theatre arts, Kaylene become an advocate and activist in her community, Lindeka become a front-line worker around HIV and AIDS, Mphumzi become a husband and father and a student once again, Nosibusiso an advocate for workers' and women's rights, and many more changes. We also lost many people, including the death of Bridgette, and the falling away of many others along the way, like Danlia, Chinomy, Andrew, Ruth, Naseema… Then, we saw COVID, and a new kind of pandemic swept across the planet, with new kinds of impacts on South Africa.

Along the way we've struggled with the feeling that publishing these stories was either not enough or too much. What did we hope to get out of these relationships, beyond the frame of the research questions posed and answered? What we were taking versus what we were leaving; such tensions don't easily dissipate.

Equally important as the tensions are the deep levels of affection and friendship that have profoundly shaped us. Shannon writes in 2022,

> Revisiting Mandla's words of thanks in our interview in 2019 made me so uncomfortable I wanted to delete them from the transcript. The context was so impossible to transmit, and my equally felt thanks to him about the important role he'd played in my life felt inadequately expressed; the very real element of reciprocity and friendship that has been the undercurrent of how things unfolded between all of us over time; of the ways that we changed, and changed each other as much as any other element of impact we may have affected.
>
> I guess like Mandla says, he has had to pay the black tax, and I have also got the white rebate. The inequality of our lives is so much more deeply apparent the longer we work together and experience the unjust divisions in the trajectories of our lives in context. No one has changed me, impacted me, perhaps as much as Mandla. Except maybe Claudia, without whom I can't even imagine what my life might have been, and who impacted my life's path perhaps more than anyone in the world.
>
> As Lauren Berlant asked me when I was interviewing her some years ago, 'You haven't decided if you want to position your object in front of you, beside you, or behind you.' She reminded me that her preference, of course, would be in-relation, that she was not talking just to talk, she was talking to *me*. I should remain in the frame. My presence to what she was saying mattered.

The conversations and texts in this book also can't be seen outside of the relational. They are always between and amongst us. Our differences of place, age, location, race and class are what created the dynamics that allowed and deepened the kinds of insights and conversations that we had. That is not something that should be omitted or erased. It is the very bedrock of what was formed between us. In a very real way, this is a project of friendship, of meaning making through difference and time that happened because we stayed together.

If the relational is everything at the heart of this project, it is also the glue between all of the participants in the group that stuck together, and also between us as researchers, facilitators and writers. These relations seep out from the spaces between the words. As the interviews went on through the years, our tone changed and you can read the shift in the text itself.

# 2

# Creative practices, young people and the AIDS pandemic

THE EARLY 2000s WAS A TIME of hope, urgency and denial around the AIDS pandemic, as well as vital and vibrant activism. Much like the 1976 student movements under apartheid, and the #FeesMustFall uprisings in the last decade, it was a generational moment where the fight was intense to contain or halt the HIV pandemic in South Africa that was consuming so many lives. It was an exciting, and daunting, time in South Africa. Apartheid had ended, social movements were flourishing and there was real hope and dreams for a new South Africa.

At the same time, the end of apartheid had not brought economic equality, and the majority of South Africans were still living in poverty, housing was a critical issue, and the Mbeki government had embraced neoliberalism and was privatising everything. It was a galvanising moment for new social movements that had grown out of networks built during the anti-apartheid movement, and many were in the streets contesting privatisation and fighting for housing, access to electricity and water. There was still an optimism that things could continue to change; after all, ordinary South Africans had brought down a repressive regimen.

It was in this context that the Treatment Action Campaign (TAC) emerged, building grassroot networks fighting for an end to discrimination against HIV-positive people, and access to life-saving medications for all South Africans.[20] HIV infections were rising in epic proportions in South Africa in the 1990s. Given the intersecting issues of a crumbling and unequal healthcare system, many people living in extreme poverty in close quarters, and a government that denied the existence of the virus, things got worse quickly. Alarms were beginning to sound as the death toll rose. Young people had become one of the fastest growing groups of new infections. In 2000, the XIII International AIDS conference 'Breaking the Silence' was held in Durban. As Claudia recalls:

> It was late 1990s, leading up to the 'Breaking the Silence' International AIDS conference held in Durban in July 2000. At the time, I was leading a large Canadian-funded project with the National Department of Education. Amongst other components, it included developing the South African Schools Act, setting up the policies and practices which would guide the formation of School Governing Bodies, and establishing the Gender Equity Task Team to create the blueprint for the gender equity machinery within the education sector in South Africa. A key feature of this work, highlighted in numerous publications including an Amnesty report Unsafe at School, was a recognition that school leaders needed to be addressing high rates of sexual violence. Few educational leaders at the time were talking about gender-based violence and even fewer were talking about HIV and AIDS. It was not even clear whose responsibility it should be to address HIV and AIDS with youth. All this began to change, though, at the Durban conference. Although it would be another two years till the International AIDS conference in Barcelona where attendees would be carrying signs 'where are the youth?', the Durban conference was a key moment for everyone, including those in education, to wake up to the fact that young people were dying.

Leading up to the Durban conference, Claudia was also conducting a small-scale study of youth engagement with South African young adult literature in several schools in Gauteng.[21] While that project didn't specifically have a focus on HIV and AIDS, it did take a social change approach to working with young people in reading circles and focusing on social realism. Inevitably, some of the novels addressed HIV and AIDS. One of the participants in that project lamented that the steady stream of social realism in literature was infused with narratives about AIDS: 'AIDS, AIDS, AIDS, that's all we ever hear. We are sick of AIDS!' His statement could refer to young people literally being sick of AIDS – and there were already many young people sick with AIDS and dying – but it could also refer to being sick of hearing about AIDS. Both could be tragic. It was a catalyzing moment. Something different needed to be done that did not simply reinforce the dreary and moralistic Abstinence-Be-faithful-Condomize (ABCs) or the scare tactic messaging young people were hearing. Youth-centred approaches were direly needed.[22]

LoveLife was already going strong in South Africa, and as a national initiative it served to reinforce the significance of youth-focused, innovative and future-oriented approaches that would challenge the death sentence narratives that were all around.[23] Claudia seized upon the idea of addressing 'sick of AIDS' through the ongoing messages and approaches taken by groups like LoveLife, Steps for the Future, Bush Radio, Soul City, DramAide and others who were mobilising youth culture in relation to HIV prevention strategies. These initiatives aligned with the 'Breaking the Silence' theme of the Durban conference and the emerging activist agenda of those like the Treatment Action Campaign, along with the many calls to action to contest the AIDS denialism of President Mbeki. Bringing young people into the picture was essential.[24]

In 2002, we set about organising the first round of workshops and symposiums in Cape Town, which took an arts-based and educational approach to research with young people around HIV prevention (see chapter 4 for background on the projects). Creative workshops were facilitated by artists and writers and combined with training on gender, sexuality and HIV transmission, alongside roundtable discussion where young people were encouraged to share their thoughts and experiences as peers. While this was meant as a one-off research project, we were overwhelmed by the avid interest in young people's voices and, in turn, the hunger with which young people wanted to speak about their experience, perceptions, curiosities and fears about

AIDS. In those days, only a scattering of young people were present at major events focused on HIV and youth. Much to our dismay, when they were invited, the articulate and powerful young people who had so much to say about their own sexuality, their agency and the struggles they faced on a daily basis were typically asked to perform song and dance numbers for visiting dignitaries and adult experts. Now and then they would be slotted five minutes in a plenary to read a canned message 'from the youth'. After the lights came up, we'd often have a chance to speak to those same youth in the corridors or over lunches and, not surprisingly, again and again they expressed their feelings of marginalisation – a sense of being tokenised, unheard.

At one level there was no shortage of writing about young people and HIV and AIDS in South Africa – in medical and educational journals, grey literature reports by NGOs, clinical data and obituary columns, novels, short stories and television scripts. Yet, the voices of young people, when they were sought out, were often mediated, interpreted, tokenised or qualified by adult experts. As the years have gone by, there still remains very little book-length literature that gives voice to the experiences and realities of young people themselves in relation to HIV and AIDS.[25] Bringing youth voices and youth culture into the conversation around sexual health was a crucial part of the context for the work we began in the early 2000s.

Artistic expression was also critical to this era of AIDS activism globally. Art was a key element in the fight against stigma and discrimination around AIDS in the 1980s onwards, as well as a way to collectively deal with the enormous levels of mourning and loss.[26] Groups like ACT UP in North America sparked a range of cultural production, including performance art, posters, paintings and video, creating a community of people who felt implicated in the fight against AIDS.[27] Later, people would reflect on how this cultural and intellectual work literally sustained, changed and saved lives.[28] AIDS cultural activism challenged the 'assumption that issues of representation or discourse are secondary to the problem of finding a medical cure or changing government policies'.[29]

From urban queer communities in North America and Europe

in the 1980s to postapartheid South Africa in the 1990s, AIDS activism was forcefully buttressed by influential and imaginative cultural programs ... communities of activists, critics, and artists seized the virus as a strategic model and a contagious metaphor for intervening in public space, and for creating new spaces ... in order to fight the many forms of harm it unleashed on local, national, and global scales.[30]

In South Africa, artistic expression and representation were ever-present in early activism around prevention, treatment and an end to discrimination. From the 1990s onwards, major artistic exhibitions and interventions were happening in South Africa. Notable in these was Gideon Mendel's photojournalistic account of AIDS in Africa at the South African National Gallery, the Memory Box projects, the Bambanani Women's Group 'Long Life: Positive HIV stories', beadwork projects, and the work of major artists like Sue Williamson, Sam Nhlengethwa, Senzeni Marasela, Penelope Siopis and David Goldblatt, Clive van den Berg, among many others. Any history of the AIDS movement in South Africa or globally must include the many stories born from our collective and creative undertakings as people grappled with the impacts of the pandemic and attempted by all means necessary to slow down the rates of infection, illness and death.

Today we see the legacy of these important artistic and civil society wins and interventions in public space and discourse, as treatment has become mainstream, even while infection rates continue to grow.[31]

It was in this context that we began the first iteration of this creative research project with teen activists in Cape Town.

# 3

# Overtime/over time

Time is a complex and endlessly fascinating phenomenon, not simply the medium through which we do research, but an important topic of enquiry in its own right.[32]

WHEN THE THREE OF US STARTED working on *Soft Cover* in 2002, we never imagined that we would be still working together two decades later on more or less the same project. Or that we would be working with the same youth activists, first as 16- to 18-year-olds, into their early twenties, and then periodically as they moved well into their thirties. 'Overtime/over time' feels like a fitting term for a chapter about a project that goes on and on. It also helps to draw attention to time as method (the 'how' of conducting work over 20 years), time in relation to longitudinal work with youth (as they grow older), and time in the life of researchers (as we grow older) – and, of course, time in relation to critical themes and issues such as race, class, work, sexuality, mental health and the transition to adulthood. Some of the issues that are time sensitive with young people also include sexual health in the age of AIDS and political activism across the life course. What happens to empowered young people when they are no longer young?

We have an extensive collection of field notes, photographs, emails, video footage, participant writing and various publications and co-produced pieces. We can look back at the photographs taken in 2002 at the 'Getting the Word Out' symposium of very passionate secondary school students presenting their findings on the situation of HIV and AIDS in their communities [See photographs in picture section] or re-watch the short film *Fire & Hope* we created with participants in 2004 [See photograph in picture section]. We can fast forward to pictures from 2018 around the table at the Centre for the Book or further to 2019 where participants, juggling the responsibilities of children, families and work, gather with us at a rented house in Simon's Town to spend a weekend engaged in looking back/looking forward and engaging with Memory Books [See photograph in picture section].

This research was not originally envisioned as a longitudinal study, but, as our approach to an ethnography-in-motion evolved over time, our appreciation grew for qualitative longitudinal research[33] and 'reflexive revisiting' studies, as Julian Sefton-Greene and Jennifer Rowsell term the work of returning to a research site.[34] We found further inspiration around documenting the regular return to participants over time through the work of Michael Apted's highly acclaimed television series *Seven Up*.[35]

The Up series dates back to 1964, and was meant to study the ways in which class in particular might contribute to the life chances of youth in a society that had been highly class-based in the UK. Apted has followed fourteen youth who were aged seven in 1964 at regular seven-year intervals, resulting in the original Seven Up, followed by *14 Up, 21 Up, 28 Up, 35 Up,* and so on. The most recent, *63 Up,* was released in 2019. Michael Apted died in early 2021, igniting questions about whether another film would be made, and whether the glue that bound that group together would melt away.[36] The Up series turned participants into well-known characters in the UK, making it very different from a research study. At the same time, we think there are some important overlaps between the series and the stories that are gathered in this book. Perhaps most important is the idea of continuity over time and within groups, and a focus on hearing directly from participants about what is happening in their lives. Although Apted met participants regularly at planned seven-year intervals and our meetings were more random, based on availabilities and circumstances, in both instances, the participants had a sense of themselves as a group, and that their lives were being documented over time. In the beginning, Apted went into *Seven Up* as a documentarian with no intention to continue. It was only after proposing a second visit seven years later that the idea for studying change over time became solidified, particularly how time might be a method to make visible issues around class, family and work. As such, the questions posed every seven years had a sameness to them: Where are you now? What has happened since our last interview? In *42 Up* Apted also included questions about what difference being part of the series had made on the participants' lives.

## WHAT DIFFERENCE DOES IT MAKE?

For us, the question of impact was our North Star in the first few years after the intensive creative and educational work of the early projects had passed. We posed many questions to our participants around what difference this work had made in their lives, often specifically around their behaviour in the context of the high rates of HIV and AIDS: practising safer sex, getting tested, knowing your status. Attempting to be responsible researchers and educators, we wanted to find ways to evaluate such a qualitative project as it unfolded over time.

Starting from a premise that arts-based work with youth on HIV and AIDS could make a real difference in behavioural change, we wanted to track impact over time. This was an urgent undertaking. After all, HIV and AIDS were life and death issues. Young people were dying and being infected at epic proportions. At least two young teens in our small projects had already tested positive before coming to work with us. Additionally, we were hearing from young people that information-heavy messages in Life Skills classes were exacerbating the 'sick of AIDS' messages and they were feeling exhausted by the negative messaging. Nonetheless, we worried that perhaps the focus on arts-based productions and youth engagement was overly celebratory and not much else. In 2004, we produced an evaluative report for the initial funder, but, beyond having to produce a report, we were forever seeking to do check-ins and follow-ups because this work was precisely what we were trying to replicate with youth in other parts of South Africa, Swaziland, Canada and beyond.

At the outset, our interrelated questions had considered the following: What difference does social research make, in this case, social research in relation HIV prevention? Did sexual behaviour change? Did the messages transform young people's vulnerabilities? In this case, what were some of the other unforeseen impacts the research was having due to its emphasis on participation, personal empowerment, writing and creativity? The question of what difference projects like this make is one that often lingers in projects that attempt to make positive changes in participants' lives. As Claudia points out,

> one of the challenges of social research relates to isolating the features or factors that make a difference (if at all) in an interventionist project. If we attempt to evaluate the influence or impact, the short time frames of many interventionist studies make it likely we fall into the potential trap of making exaggerated claims, or miss significant outcomes simply because we stopped too soon.[37]

Ironically, our preoccupation with wanting to track the behavioural impacts of arts-based prevention projects perhaps skewed the direction of our early conversations. Yet, their responses were surprising, and started to reveal things we had not been looking for, which we have discussed here and elsewhere. Even allowing for the contested nature of terms such as 'empowerment' and 'agency' so frequently associated with projects with youth, we had such a sense of ways they were talking about their lives and what they could do, along with the support of deepening friendships, especially between and among people of diverse racial backgrounds.

Yet, from the moment of making the film *Fire & Hope* and becoming engaged in the daily lives of participants through meeting with them in their own homes and communities, something had already begun to shift. What we describe in chapter 1 as an ethnography-in-motion had begun to emerge. This organic process adapted and changed over time, in a dynamic with participants. Nonetheless, we were still frequently drawn towards the question of 'what difference did it make' to be part of HIV prevention projects as young people, when what we also wanted to know was what was happening in life, now.

The responses to our questions were so often framed by the events happening in each person's life at that moment, and moved us from trying to study impact towards a recognition of the significance of context and variability in each person's life. We only fully comprehended this when we tried to wrap up the project in 2006, two years after any official funding had ended, and realised that depending on what point we declared 'the end' would mean a different ending. The structural barriers at play for each individual were transforming any perceived impacts as adulthood set in.

The underlying assumption of the initial Soft Cover project was that developing capacity in young people towards peer-to-peer interventions was a vital resource in transmitting HIV-prevention messages. That was indeed the case while the participants were going to school and running various AIDS awareness activities and initiatives. Many of the participants not only became local peer educators, but were invited to participate in national and international youth forums, and carry the voices and concerns of young people forward. There was powerful evidence of impact. Many of the participants from Khayelitsha in particular talked about achieving local fame for their stories and poetry circulating locally as part of the *In My Life* book. Initiatives in schools, talks and workshops were happening in Atlantis and Khayelitsha. First it was with *In My Life* and *Fire & Hope*, then continuing with the participant-led writing workshops and films like *Facing the Truth*, *Street Fear* and *Voices from Atlantis*.

If we counted the last months of doing activist work in schools as the final part of the 'data set' on impact, we would end on a celebratory high. But much changed. KK didn't get to finish his matric and ended up having his education disrupted. Mathew went off to first-year university, but after being on such a roll in terms of success, he was confronted with tragedy after the death of two close family members, and with all that had happened, he could no longer attend university at all. Ann was living through a violent situation at home, and her brother had been shot and killed. Claudia offers her fieldnotes from a cold and wet day in Khayelitsha in 2006 where she and Shannon realise that so many of the youth are available to have check-ins and interviews in the afternoon because they are not going to school or finding work.[38]

It is a cold, wet, windy and thoroughly miserable Cape Town winter day in July of 2006. As my colleague, Shannon, and I make our way on foot through section R of Khayelitsha with Mandla, the former youth worker who helped us to convene the Soft Cover project, a school-based literacy and creative arts-focused HIV&AIDS awareness initiative several years earlier, we wonder who will actually show up for the interviews we plan to conduct with former participants in the project. It is just over three years since the launch of their publication, *In My Life: Youth Stories and Poems on HIV/AIDS* and the release of a short documentary *Fire & Hope* that Shannon has directed and that includes many of the participants from the project speaking about how they see their role as youth activists in addressing HIV&AIDS. We decide that it would be fascinating to find out what various members of our project are now doing. In the context of a country that is hard hit by HIV and in the context of working with a group of young people who are (or were the last time we had seen them) committed to social activism in relation to HIV prevention and access to treatment, it is no insignificant question to want to know what they are doing even a few years later…

We aren't quite sure who will still be around, especially in the middle of a weekday afternoon when you would think that most 19- or 20-year-olds would probably be in university or training or at work. This day there are four of the original group who show up at the house of Thozzi, one of the group members. They are not at work, they are not studying or in training, and really it turns out that mid-afternoon is a perfect time to meet because they are doing nothing that afternoon or most weekday afternoons. We gather in the small two-room house, which closely resembles all the other small two-room houses of section R of Khayelitsha. We hear many things that afternoon. Some, like KK, the one whose peers would have voted most likely to succeed in 2003, hasn't actually been able to complete his matric, even though three years ago he was on the verge of writing his final exams.

Lindeka feels discouraged. She is still talking about the piece she wrote for *In My Life*, but now that she has part-time work as a cashier in Checkers, a supermarket chain, she can't figure out how she can do any more writing, the one activity that has given her some personal satisfaction.

Mphumzi is working on a building site quite close to KK's and we go to visit him on his break, but even there we hear the frustration in his voice about having a low-paying, unskilled job and uncertain hours, and then working out in the rain and wind and cold on this Cape Town winter day. KK would like to get something going in drama and performance in the community. In the intervening years he has had a chance to participate in an arts-based workshop in Europe, for which he has received funding but is not sure how to go about getting some local activity off the ground.

As we saw through this work, time was a significant component in making visible underlying inequalities and issues like race, class and health status. All the education in the world could not rectify some of the historic and structural factors that came to play out in the lives of this group of young people. When we met KK, he was 18 years old and an outspoken young activist working with Treat Action Campaign (TAC) around HIV prevention in Khayelitsha. Through the work he had already been doing, and the creative work he was involved with within this project, he became a well-known youth spokesperson, and flew to conferences around the world teaching young people about HIV prevention and speaking on health-related issues. As he moved from his teen years into adulthood, he became a recognised theatre performer and director. But structural forces had an impact too, as the extremely unequal playing field in South Africa made every upwards move challenging, and violence, alcohol, economic hardship and other factors took their toll. Time made evident how structural factors impacted the activism and creative work he was part of in his teen years.

While we were able to draw some important recommendations from working over time, such as an understanding that projects with young people should never stop at exactly the moment when they are in transition to adulthood, our reflections also highlighted several other points worth noting. First, there is a need for work with young people that acknowledges the on-going nature of life. Life doesn't stop at some pre-determined moment, or when the camera or researcher stops watching. Second, this work has shown us that there is a need for more academic humility, and a danger of exaggerated claims around the success of a project – typically found at the end of an article or report to the funder. Finally, there is an under-studied component of the relationships that develops in research carried out over time, along with all the adjacent ethical considerations that come with them. As noted in Shannon's field notes in the previous chapter about the blurring of lines between participant/friend, sticking to a script in longitudinal qualitative research over time is challenging.

## ON METHOD

Methods and approaches in qualitative longitudinal research vary. As we write in chapter 1, we developed and adapted a type of ethnography-in-motion, but, as years went on, we came to understand the longitudinal nature of what we were doing as posing another set of issues and imperatives. Bren Neale talks about a variety of frameworks for longitudinal work, including looking forward and looking back, and offers suggestions around a number of different tools, such as life-maps, diaries, and essay writing about the future as ways of addressing longitudinality.[39] In Apted's Up series, there were standard questions that included, 'How has your life changed since the last time we spoke?' In the **63 Up** film however, we learn that at least one of the women participating noted that Apted seemed to ask men more questions about economics and women more questions about personal relationships. We cannot claim standard interview questions throughout, and, as noted above, at a certain point in our questioning we tried to move participants away from primarily commenting on the creative projects we'd done in the past to focus more on the present.

Some of the interviews, including the discussion in our final chapter, come from group interviews being video recorded. This is something we think is worth highlighting since Shannon is also a filmmaker, and video making was a key method used throughout our projects with these young people. Being 'on-camera' does create a dynamic different than notes on pen and paper. There are a range of implications around video recording that we don't have space to get into here, but it is worth noting that video as a research method over time offers a space of public testimonial that can elicit deep and thoughtful responses from participants. There was also an interesting alignment with the 'Up' series, or Robert Linklater's *Boyhood*, which created a space for 'life-recording' that became as important to participants as it was to filmmakers/researchers. Similar to the 'Up' series, we also viewed *Fire & Hope* in both small group and public screenings together, and in the final group interview at the end of 2019, everyone viewed it together again.

To engage in this 'over time' project with the participants, we did not go back in an explicit way to the transcripts and creative productions from the original educational project. We note this because we recognise that, unlike many longitudinal studies including the 'Up' series where the 'over time' interviews are the point, our original project was an intense educational intervention carried out over several years. The interviews came later. We have, however, been able to go back to the many narratives and poems written by the participants from the *In My Life* book published in 2003, as have the participants. That collection offered an interesting 'prospective' on their world when it was published in 2003; in later work it has served as a 'retrospective' on 'this is what I thought then'. This prospective/retrospective is critical, we think, in work on youth sexuality and HIV and AIDS, although we have not done a full discourse analysis of how participants talked about sex then (before widespread access to ARVs in South Africa) and 20 years later where there is much greater access but still major health inequities. Worth considering too is what difference it makes to talk about the issues as secondary school students versus talking about sexuality as a parent, as is the case for several of the participants.

The core material for Part 2 of this book are the edited transcripts based on the extensive interviews and group discussions conducted over time. All participants had a chance to read the edited transcripts, and comment on how the transcripts had been put together, but also to create a framework where participants could choose if there were elements of the material that should be omitted, or if there were additions that needed to be added. These are very personal stories, expressing many emotions and experiences between 2003 and the present and we wanted to make sure that participants would have the final say. As Raissadat[40] notes in her own project of working with transcripts in a participatory way with participants, there are numerous methodological concerns, starting with the question of how to do justice to this personal material that has been offered, when to leave out something; what to do in relation to grammatical structures and conversational idiosyncrasies; what to do with the voice of the interviewer; how and when to link quotes or signal time change as part of producing a text for readers that is comprehensible; when are these chunks of text from a person's life are an excerpt or quote and when are they, as we decided in Part 2, meant to be read as individual authored stories with each participant named as the author. Shannon, who had conducted all of the interviews in the first place, worked and re-worked these transcript-stories and we collaborated over time with each of the participants. Were they okay with what we have selected and how it is put together? And as an addition to the 'over time' of this project, when participants received the edited transcripts in 2021 and 2022, many then proceeded to add an update or another reflection, thereby adding to the 'without end' revisiting process.

Like Neale, we created a tool specific to the longitudinal field work. For us this tool was in the form of Memory Books [See photograph in picture section]. The idea of Memory Books provides a 'looking back' lens and is complementary to the extensive body of work on Memory Boxes within the context of AIDS.[41] Drawing on photos, writings and transcripts, we created a Memory Book as a personal workbook for each participant. As with much of the work on participatory analysis, creating the Memory Books brought a level of researcher subjectivity on our part as we worked with a research assistant to create 'longitudinal moments' dating back to some of the early interviews, writings from *In My Life*, excerpts from the *Fire & Hope* film, and excerpts from video and transcripts of interviews dating from 2006 onwards.[42] The Memory Books ensured that no one got lost in the middle of a group discussion, and offered something of the 'nooks and crannies' of individual stories. We of course wondered later if we had really captured the right memory moments (the excerpts may have been more on what stood out for us and not the participant). We also had much more transcript data for some participants than others simply because of who was able to attend interview sessions over the years. Aside from these limitations, the Memory Books served as a different kind of evidence for the participants who had not been privy to what interview data looks like and, perhaps, if we are not to be too celebratory, powerful evidence from their earlier lives.

## THE RELATIONAL CONTEXT FOR LONGITUDINAL RESEARCH

We would be remiss if we did not say anything about the shifting of our own positionings throughout the 20 years, including our relationships to the participants and to each other. Time had built more than a lens through which to view our work; it also provided us with a fabric of relation and knowing that would not have been developed otherwise. As Shannon noted in our 2019 group discussions,

> I think the trust that we developed had a lot to do with time. Time is critical. We didn't start out with the intention that the project would unfold over so much time, but if it hadn't happened over time, I don't think we would have developed the trust or intimacy we have.

That too is part of the 'over time' of qualitative longitudinal research, although it is an area that is understudied, or perhaps just underreported, in publications. Researchers might write about some of the challenges to exiting a longitudinal study, or some of their own personal dilemmas in relation to confidentiality or anonymity,[43] but we have not found extensive attention to researcher positionality in longitudinal work and, in some cases, it is conspicuously missing.[44] It may be that although a study is identified as longitudinal it may be that the length is five to eight years (still counting as longitudinal) but perhaps not what might be identified as 'generational'. A generation typically refers to a timespan of twenty to thirty years, although the discussions around Millennials, GenZ and so on suggest shorter time frames for defining generations.

In the previous chapter, Shannon comments on age/time and what it meant to be the same age as Mandla and also how relationships changed over time with the participants becoming friends and the significance of friendship in activism. Claudia has reflected on her own positioning in her research as central to navigating a tension between 'what is the point?' of social research to 'what difference might this make?'; the significance of research over time and the role of autoethnographic reflexivity in this work.[45] Mandla offers a comment on his own changing positioning at the 2011 symposium at Salt Rock, when he highlights a shifting sense of where he sees himself:

> I mean the reality of the matter is that I need money to live on. And activism is not going to give me this. I mean, not now. Like, here we are fighting for the future, but I'm hungry now, I'm starving now. So, I kind of needed a solution to that. So, I think for me the change started to happen there, is like, now I'm empowered enough, I understand things and I understand the vigour that I had to change things, that was not going to happen overnight. It was kind of defeating really when you actually see what you have been working hard for. It didn't make any difference. I mean, just a very small difference, but you would have hoped that people would have understood things the way that you do, and changed things the way you want things to change for all of us. So, it's kind of defeating to see, actually, things are getting worse. So, all the knowledge, all the education, the workshops, kind of went to waste. It was a drop in the ocean.[46]

Interestingly, this take from Mandla is somewhat frozen in time back in 2011. In 2019, he had a different sense of what change meant to him. As Mandla remarks eight years later:

> You don't get to see the impact immediately. It's only after a while, when you look back, and you kind of say, oh, that actually had an impact. I think that's what activism does. It's hard work. And you are up against people who don't care about what you're trying to do. In fact, they're doing everything in their power to make sure that your voice is drowned out, and that no one hears you. We have had to go through all of that. Even at the end, still people don't see it.
>
> We fought. We joined the Treatment Action Campaign to fight HIV, create awareness, fight stigma. We did that for six years. Did it make a difference? Was it worth it? I mean, shouldn't we have just spent our time doing something else? What we know for a fact in life is, if we didn't do anything, then it would be worse. These things may not be better, but they are certainly not worse. There would be no treatment to talk about. There would be no prevention to talk about. There would still be a whole lot of people who died, and those got killed simply because someone suspected that they had HIV and AIDS. So, things would have been worse.
>
> With activism, because the results are not immediate it can be harder to see. It would be a nice thing if it was as impactful as other things. Like you do something now and people change right now. It would be very nice. But unfortunately, activism is a lifelong journey.[47]

## WE GREW AS WE GREW

The stories that follow in Part 2, we hope, speak for themselves. Rather than pointing to each line of the transcript and imploring the reader where to focus, we hope that you can find your own way through the text, your own connections and resonances.

Unlike some other work in this genre, we are aware that the act of revisiting is in itself part of this project. For participants, having foreign white women come back year after year to ask participants to reflect on their lives actually changed the way a number of people said they thought about their lives. The emphasis on the idea that what you had to say was valuable changed the significance of how they viewed themselves, the reflections about the previous year and their own personal growth.

While not part of our initial plans, self-reflection became an essential element of the project for some participants. Periodic space for self-expression and stocktaking from the teen years through into the thirties engendered beliefs, thoughts and ideas that impacted their life journey. What does a life observed tell us about the reflective process? How does self-reflection transform personal growth? As Mathew memorably remarked, 'We grew as we grew.'

Researchers are asked to report on the impacts of research, and yet it is extremely rare to have a long-term perspective on what (if any) impacts remain in participants' lives years after projects are completed. As Mandla notes above, positive impacts over time can be hard to quantify. In the case of life and death issues such as HIV infection, it seems critical to be able to assess the strategies and goals of educational projects. Education around sexual health is a difficult and complex terrain. Many innovative educational approaches using visual methods have been adopted to combat rising HIV infection rates amongst young people globally. Yet, there have been very few studies that have followed the effects of visual methodologies over time. As participatory visual methodologies gain popularity with researchers and community-based facilitators involving teachers, learners and health care professionals, a critical investigation into potential pitfalls, and lasting impacts, of such qualitative work can provide guidance towards shaping future initiatives.[48]

We have had the rare opportunity of having followed and interviewed this small group of research participants over these past 20 years. In the case of this work, many of the young people involved here have continued to make huge impacts in their schools, communities and environments. From training other young people and speaking in schools, to doing creative and front-line community work around social issues, we've found that there is a disproportionately high level of engagement within this group.

Through this time, we have watched the changing material and social conditions in their lives, but we have also watched an incredible group of young South Africans grow into amazing adults. Their stories have inspired us and have taught us more than could ever be captured in these pages.

We hope, through their honest, inspiring stories, you get a glimpse of the story of South Africa over that same period and, with it, hope for the future to come.

# PART TWO

*Narratives & Reflections*

# 4

# Background to the projects

IN 2002, THE CANADIAN Society for International Health Initiative funded our first initiative, in partnership with the Centre for the Book in Cape Town, to organize a symposium and then create a series of workshops with a small group of youth from the Western Cape.[49] The project was concerned with ensuring gender-sensitive and participatory approaches to HIV prevention with young people. The initial project was not a big one and not a long one, and certainly not something that would cover two decades of work.

Over a period of 13 months, we worked with a group of 15 young people from several diverse high schools in Cape Town as part of an arts-informed international health project that we called Soft Cover. In February and March 2002, the first phase of the project began with a symposium titled 'Getting the Word Out: Young people and HIV prevention' followed by a series of arts-based educational workshops called 'Soft Cover'. A group of 15 young people from different racial and class backgrounds around Cape Town were recruited from local school Student Representative Councils (SRC), and HIV activist networks, especially the Treatment Action Campaign (TAC). Claudia Mitchell was the lead project investigator, and Shannon Walsh was the coordinator from the Canadian side, and the key organisers included Mandla Oliphant, Abigail Dreyer, Thandi Lewin and Dammon Rice.

Soft Cover used a youth-led participatory approach to AIDS prevention, bringing young people together in hands-on visual and literary arts project to provide a youth-to-youth vehicle for addressing issues of sexuality and AIDS. The project explored what we referred to as a youth action space approach to HIV prevention. In mapping out the project in those early days, we were concerned with a variety of factors, including the particular vulnerability of youth to HIV and AIDS and, at the same time, the information-overload among young people who were already saying we are 'sick of AIDS', a phrase that would come to be the catalyst for innovative approaches to education.[50] At the time, AIDS education apathy was an emergent reaction to prevention campaigns, an over-saturation of messages, and in some cases, the changing landscape created by drug availability.[51]

In these early days, we were interested in situating two interlinking dimensions of working with young people. The first related to the significance of the arts and creativity in AIDS activism and youth culture. Art activism had been a critical response to the AIDS pandemic worldwide. Probably no area of public health had been more the subject of the arts than HIV and AIDS. Some of the cultural touchstones included the Names Memorial Quilt Project, a vast array of mainstream and experimental film works, Mapplethorpe photography in the United States, and ranged from Femi Kuti songs emerging in Nigeria, to the inclusion of major art exhibitions at the large AIDS conferences such as those held in Durban, Barcelona, Paris and beyond in the 2000s.

Central to this early work was the necessity of seeing how to re-position young people themselves at the centre of cultural production and as the producers of messages related to HIV and AIDS. Youth culture is a rich artistic space for arts activism, and the types of images and messages that exist in that terrain define, supplant and inform the way that young people's social networks function. This was a time before the pervasive use of smart phones and social media, and youth culture was still being defined on the streets. Sites of visual cultural production included graphic novels, hip hop, street fashion, music videos, animé and graffiti. In the early days of this project, Facebook was still a few years from emerging, and it would be close to a decade before it had saturated the youth social networks in South Africa. Youth culture was local, often underground, and crossed multiple sites and modes. The idea that young people need to define for themselves the prevention messages that made sense to them was central to our early thinking in this project.

To do this, we first brought together young people already active in their communities with a cross-section of inspiring and talented writers, artists, graffiti writers, musicians, activists, filmmakers, and entertainers. The symposium provided a wonderful launching place to what would become a series of facilitated hands-on workshops to engage these same young people in producing their own writing, art and messaging.

The young people were bussed into the Centre for the Book and provided time and preparation to actively participate in the symposium as experts on their own lives as young people targeted by HIV prevention messages. The two-day symposium brought together a range of luminous figures from the era, including writer K. Sello Duiker, academic Suzanne Leclerc-Madlala, filmmaker Teboho Mahlatsi, writer Robin Malan, artist Robin Rhode, poet Thabo Lehlongwa, cultural activist Gcina Mhlophe, and many other notable artists, activists and academics.

The same 15 young people who participated in the symposium came together over seven weeks to participate in a practical hands-on implementation of some of the ideas that surfaced during the symposium. In this phase, creative workshops focused on how HIV and AIDS messages could work together through visual images, poetry and narrative writing, cumulating in hand-made books. Each of the sessions dealt with issues around gender, health and prevention issues, sexuality, message making and the social and political context of AIDS. The young participants worked with AIDS activists, community workers, local illustrators, visual artists, poets, hand-made bookmakers and authors on their books and prevention messages.

Amongst the workshop facilitators were HIV-positive women from the Memory Box project who taught handmade book-making techniques to the participants. The Memory Box project engaged people living with HIV and AIDS to create a box full of artworks, stories and memorabilia from their lives. Abigail Dreyer, a gender facilitator from the School of Public Health at the University of Western Cape, also led an intensive session around gender, consent and gender-based violence.

In May 2002, there was a launch for the hand-made books, and participants presented to over a hundred attendees – family, friends, community workers, facilitators and AIDS activists. Four buses brought people in from Khayelitsha. Appetizers and drinks were served and a dance troupe performed. Later in May, four participants flew to Midrand as youth delegates for the 'Conference on HIV/AIDS and the Education Sector: An Education Coalition Against HIV/AIDS' hosted by the Department of Education. There they took part in a pre-conference workshop with 15 other youth from around South Africa in preparation for a Youth Declaration on HIV/AIDS. In July 2002, the Centre for the Book and Kwela Books held an event called 'Celebration of Youth Creativity' where the Soft Cover participants participated with other youth groups. Several months later the group also presented their work in their schools with public readings that drew on the individual action plans of the youth participants.

## IN MY LIFE: WRITING WORKSHOPS

Based on the enthusiastic response of the young people to the writing they did in the bookmaking phase of Soft Cover, in 2003 we convened a series of workshops on writing about HIV and AIDS, led by well-known local writing facilitator Anne Schuster and facilitator Abigail Dreyer. Anne Schuster was an author and experienced creative writing facilitator. Her approach to writing workshops used games, drawing, free writing and other techniques to create a non-threatening, spontaneous and productive space for writing. Abigail Dreyer was a gender, sexual violence and AIDS facilitator and at that time worked through the University of Western Cape's Public Health Unit. Abigail also worked with us as a facilitator during the first series of Soft Cover workshops.

Many original participants from the Soft Cover project joined these workshops, but there were also a number of new participants from nearby communities in Retreat, Gugulethu and Khayelitsha. At this stage, we had already lost a few of the original participants from Rhondebosch and Athlone.

The short self-published anthology that emerged from these workshops was called *In My Life: Youth Stories and Poems about HIV and AIDS*. *In My Life* investigated how HIV and AIDS played out in the personal lives and communities of the participants. The workshop not only generated writing from the young people themselves, but it also served as a catalyst for discussion and debate about issues around AIDS more broadly. A number of participants commented that they felt that they were able to express things that they had never discussed before. One young woman disclosed her HIV-positive status, which allowed for some serious reflection and discussion in the group. As Clinton wrote in his journal after telling the story of his father's death:

> I could not believe it was true. It felt as if my heart was going to stand still. It felt as if I was going to die. But my friends were there to comfort me and support me through the loss. And now I feel even better because I am writing about how it felt, and this makes me feel good inside

The process of writing served many different functions for the youth in the group. For some it was a way to ask questions about AIDS that they had not been able to before; others felt they could discuss AIDS more openly in their communities, since they were assigned the topic to investigate when back in their neighbourhoods. Others felt that there was a 'safe space' provided in the workshops to divulge sensitive and personal information with the group; some felt that they learned that their experiences were also shared by people from different backgrounds and communities. All of the young people in the project reported that, regardless of what they had to say about the issue, they felt they all had been affected by HIV and AIDS.

The anthology was widely circulated in South Africa and even brought some acclaim to particular writers who were published there. By 2005 *In My Life* was on its third reprint. The enthusiastic response to the collection of writing by educators, young people, HIV and AIDS organisations and NGOs reinforced for us the need for youth-authored and -produced materials to take centre stage in creating viable and engaged prevention strategies.

The strategy of working with, rather than working for, young people had the added advantage of ensuring that both the medium and the message are localised and personalised. At the time we frequently discussed how one of the limitations of many HIV and AIDS campaigns had been the idea of one-size fits all. This ignored the gendered aspect of HIV and AIDS, and differing social contexts; raced, gendered and sexual identities. By working with young people directly and in localised settings, there is greater possibility of ensuring the centrality of the personal in beliefs, attitudes, behaviour and activism itself.

As Claudia reports in her field notes in 2003:

> When I visit Ann's school several months after the launch of the book of poetry that she has written, Ann speaks before a school assembly of 1700 students about her involvement in the project and of the importance of taking HIV-prevention work seriously. She confidently reads several poems that she has written as part of the project. The thunderous applause from the audience is only one aspect of her activism. She is also now involved in a journalism project on Saturdays and she has decided that she wants to be a writer when she finishes school. While we are not sure what action the principal and teachers in the school will take, we can see by their expressions at the assembly and afterward that they are impressed by Ann's dedication. In a follow-up English class that we participate in, some of her classmates want to know if they too can write poetry about AIDS and whether it can be published.

The creative practices in the Soft Cover project demonstrated the significance of crossing boundaries between research and activism, and encouraging participants to lead in how they wanted to take action in their own lives.

### *FIRE & HOPE*: THE DOCUMENTARY

Starting in early 2004, we began work on a documentary film with many of the Soft Cover participants, which included new interviews, this time in their homes and communities. During the filming of *Fire & Hope*, participants opened up more personal information about their lives and their relationships to HIV than they had in the workshop and focus group context. At this point, we had been working with this group of young people close to a year, and the participants had developed a relationship with the interviewer, Shannon. Most of the interviews were also filmed in the young people's homes or neighbourhoods. *Fire & Hope* emphasised the need to end gender- and gang-based violence, to provide practical solutions to HIV prevention, to provide treatment and medication for those already living with HIV/AIDS, and to empower young people to take action in their own lives. Young viewers responded during screenings of *Fire & Hope*:

> It was interesting to see real, everyday- teenagers sharing their experiences with AIDS, crime and violence in their communities and how they have managed to stay away from these dangerous activities. Hopefully they can teach other South African teenagers to do the same ... youth will identify with the issues raised and will not feel as if they are being bombarded with AIDS information from teachers and other adults which, after a while, can be extremely boring. – Atang Moletsane, age 18

> We are hardly ever shown how people living 'around' the virus feel about it...
> [In *Fire & Hope*] we are introduced to four young people living in the Cape, and we hear their views about the virus ... it's something we are not used to seeing in AIDS documentaries.'
> – Kethabille Mhlongo, age 19

These first major phases would be followed by participant-led creative projects in Khayelitsha and Atlantis, including the videos *Facing the Truth (FATT)* and *Street Fear* and the workshops and writing project Voices from Atlantis. The following notes give some background and context for some of the interview and writing excerpts found in this book and provide brief outlines of various phases of how we worked together between 2002 and 2022.

2002 Facilitated group and panel discussions as part of the Soft Cover workshops

This was our first point of meeting, and there are some limited excerpts from workshop transcripts. The Soft Cover project was an intensive multi-week workshop, with HIV prevention and gender education, creative activities, hand-made bookmaking, facilitated discussions, a symposium 'Getting the Word Out' on HIV and AIDS prevention in March 2002, and a book launch at the Centre for the Book in Cape Town and various secondary schools. We have written about this project elsewhere in various articles and book chapters (see Appendix for a detailed list of these).

2003 *In My Life: Youth Stories and Poems about HIV and AIDS*, writing project

The poems and short writing that begins many chapters in this book comes from a writing workshop that was self-published as a small book and circulated widely in South Africa. The workshop was facilitated by Anne Schuster at the Centre for the Book, born from a research project by Claudia Mitchell and coordinated by Shannon Walsh. In June, we held a book launch at the Centre for the Book for the publication, attended by friends, family, learners, community workers, educators, government officials and activists. Award ceremony presentations and public readings by authors happened at Atlantis Secondary School in Atlantis and Manyano High School, Joe Slovo Comprehensive High School, Zola Senior Secondary School and Thembelihle High School in Khayelitsha.

2003 *Fire & Hope*, short documentary and interviews

In January 2003, we began the production of *Fire & Hope*. For a three-week period, project participants came together in individual and group settings. We used a question protocol developed for individual one-on-one interviews with each of the project participants and made transcripts of all the data collected over this time period. These interviews provided the basis for the documentary *Fire & Hope*. We travelled to their homes to do the interviews and met parents, family, community members and friends. Through this 'big picture' view of our participants, we were able to go back to the original focus group work and workshop transcripts and add in additional and more complete information. A rough cut of the film was presented at the conference 'Sex and Secrecy' in Johannesburg in June.[52] The film and facilitator's guide were completed and screened extensively from 2004.

2003 **Muizenburg gathering**
Later in 2003, we organised a one-day event in Muizenberg that brought all the project participants together. Organised as a fun activity at the beach, it also provided an opportunity for everyone to reconnect with each other and to do some informal evaluation of the project thus far. While there was lots of laughing, swimming and playing soccer going on, there was also some more personal discussions about lives, and HIV and AIDS in their lives. We documented this process through video and photographs.

2004 *Facing the Truth (FATT)*, **short documentary**
Over a few weeks of discussions and writing, members from the Khayelitsha group created a detailed, participant-led proposal around making a documentary called *Facing the Truth (FATT)*, which included interviews with learners in two private schools, one inner-city school and two public township schools. Facilitated primarily by Shannon and Mandla, this video was conceptualised and created entirely by the participants. They interviewed 15 learners at these five schools with the aim of confronting invisible social and political realities of AIDS, especially around race, with an intended audience of other young people in their community. The final video and interviews were conceived of and filmed by Lindeka, KK, Mphumzi, Nosibusiso and Thozzi, with

support from Shannon and Mandla.[53]

2004    **Voices from Atlantis, workshops in Atlantis Secondary School**
Inspired by the Soft Cover project, in 2004, Mathew, Kaylene, Chinomy and Danlia conducted and developed three days of intensive HIV-prevention workshops called 'Healing Words' in their high school. They worked with students aged 14 to 17, with support from Shannon. Sessions included a full-day writing session on issues of AIDS in the learners' lives, a painting and drawing workshop based on the writing and prevention messages, and a full day of learning and discussion around gender, sexuality and prevention. The work concluded with a bound book of poems and stories from the students titled *Voices from Atlantis*.

2004    *Street Fear,* **video and facilitated workshops**
In January 2004, Shannon ran video workshops for a mixed group of eight girls as part of a small grant from the Association for Women's Rights in Development (AWID). The video and workshops were part of a larger research project led by Shannon Walsh, Farah Malik, Jackie Kirk and Stephanie Garrow. The group included Lindeka, Nosibusiso, Kaylene and Chinomy, as well as a few girls from private schools in Cape Town, and included isiXhosa, Afrikaans and English speakers. Through a facilitated workshop, the girls decided on issues most important to their lives and storyboarded ideas for a video, then shot and created it. They chose the topic of sexual violence, and the final video made by the group of girls with support from Shannon was titled, Street Fear.

2006    **Individual interviews**
In July 2006, Claudia and Shannon visited a number of people at their homes and did individual video interviews and updates.

2008 **Cape Town gathering**
Shannon and Claudia organised an informal gathering and dinner in Cape Town, resulting in conversations with Mathew, Kaylene, Mphumzi, KK and Mandla.

2011 **Salt Rock conference: 'What difference does this make? The arts, youth and HIV and AIDS'**
This conference – organised through the Centre for Visual Methodologies at the University of KwaZulu-Natal, the HIV and AIDS unit in the Faculty of Education, Nelson Mandela University and the Participatory Cultures Lab at McGill University – involved a panel discussion and multi-day retreat in Salt Rock Hotel. The Soft Cover participants spoke to academics and educators on a panel titled 'Ten Years Later: Memory, Pedagogy and Social Change in Cape Town', and also did individual interviews with Shannon on video at that time. Present were KK, Mathew/Eva, Kaylene, Chinomy, Mandla, Claudia and Shannon.

2015 **Informal gathering, Lansdowne, Cape Town**
A number of members of the initial group gathered informally to connect with Shannon in Cape Town at Chukka Road Sports Club in June.

2018 **Centre for the Book facilitated gathering**
In 2018, a group gathered at the Centre for the Book in Cape Town for a focus group facilitated by Abigail Dreyer. Dreyer had done gender and sexuality workshops with the same group back in 2002. Present around the table that day were Lindeka, KK, Nosibusiso, Mathew, Kaylene and Bridgette. Also present were Mandla and Shannon.

2018 **Individual videotaped interviews**
Shannon held a series of individual interviews with people in their homes and workplaces in August.

*Background to the projects*     47

2019     Simon's Town, retreat, reunion and revisiting
In December 2019 we gathered for a weekend to look over the Memory Books we had created with excerpts from early writing and discussed the past and present. We watched *Fire & Hope* as a group and also did a recorded group discussion and one-on-one videotaped interviews. Present were Mathew, Lindeka, Nosibusiso, KK, Mphumzi, Mandla, Shannon and Claudia.

2021–2022     COVID-era communications
From March 2020 onwards, COVID prevented the group from meeting, but we collected some writing and testimonies to add updates to everyone's stories by email, texts and voice messages.

## A NOTE ON THE PARTICIPANTS' CHAPTERS

Each of the authors' chapters contain some of their own writing, done as part of the *In My Life* writing workshops, as well as transcripts from interviews that were part of facilitated group discussions and workshops, public panel discussions and one-on-one interviews. Many of these interviews were video recorded. We have written about this work elsewhere in articles and chapters with further detail about the context and specific goals of the project. We have omitted that kind of detail here in order to allow the stories to flow without interjections from us.

The process of creating the material for this section was complex, as anyone who has worked with 18 years of transcript material knows. It ranged from the actual transcription, through to developing a structure, selecting which material, and preparing it in a way that would work for the authors and for the reader. At one point we had considered thematic structures but, in the end, we opted for individually authored chapters each arranged longitudinally. We have edited the transcripts for readability and flow. The authors have reviewed these edited transcripts and have given their permission to have them published in this format in this book. Many, upon reviewing the transcripts, offered additional insights, reflections and updates, further adding to the material.

We acknowledge the potential confusion between the title of this book *In My Life: Stories from Young AIDS Activists* and the volume of poetry and stories published in 2003 called *In My Life: Youth Stories and Poems about HIV and AIDS*. When the participants mention *In My Life* in their narratives and reflections, they are referring to the 2003 publication.

## CONTENT WARNING

The first-person stories in this book may contain distressing material for some readers. The stories contain some strong language and frank discussions of sensitive issues such as gang violence, sexual violence, child abuse, parental and family members' deaths, substance abuse, mental health issues, suicide, self-harm and trauma. Reader discretion is advised.

## ATLANTIS

The thing I fear most in Atlantis is
The high crime
The gang-related wars
Atlantis has a lot of talent
All that we need is a good system and
More people to look up to in our community
People who can show our children
There are much greater things in life to do than
Increase our crime rate.

– Quinton, *Voices from Atlantis*


In some neighbourhoods
not much strange things happen
but on one specific day
something you have
nightmares about
happens and you are involved
and almost pay with your life.

You ask yourself 'where is the love'?
and some people just tell you
shut up
shut up
shut up

– Creswell, *Voices from Atlantis*

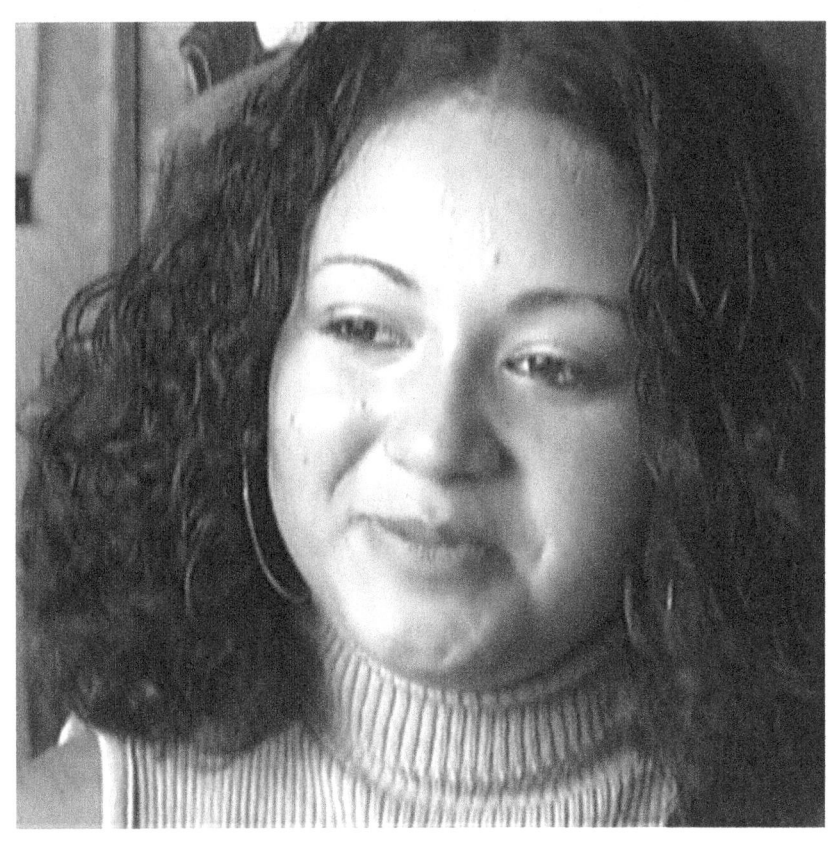

*Video still from* Fire & Hope, 2004

# 5

# Kaylene Schroeder

AT 16 YEARS OF AGE, KAYLENE *was already extremely wise and questioned much around her. She was the centre of any discussion and had a way of bringing the conversation into deeper waters, touching on emotional and personal issues with a rare thoughtfulness. She was involved with every phase of the projects we did together, including participation in the short documentary* Fire & Hope. *She grew up in Atlantis and faced many issues as a young person, including a sexual assault – something she talked about openly. Kaylene felt that young people didn't have a lot of options growing up in Atlantis, and she knew from early on that it was there that she wanted to make a difference.*

*She used her intelligence and her early experiences as a peer educator in HIV prevention to pursue social change. Kaylene scraped together what money she could to go to university where she studied social work. She showed again and again her intense commitment to making a difference in the lives of others. Over the years, she faced not only the problems stemming from the violence and poverty that surrounded her as she grew up, but also her own struggle with mental health issues. Now with a child of her own, she works with the government as a social worker and navigates the complicated environment in which she grew up.*

*Kaylene is a committed life-long activist who has faced many challenges and whose journey has taken different forms. She walks the talk. In our early workshops, we said, 'Each One, Teach One', and Kaylene has done just that.*

# 2003

*Kaylene at 16*
Interview for *Fire & Hope*
Atlantis

The gangsterism in Atlantis is everywhere. It's in our school, it's in our community – it's a part of us. And for me as a youth, not to become involved, is like a challenge, you know, 'I won't do that. I won't give in. I will stay away from that.'

The gangsterism, it effects everybody. For instance, this one girl was [opening our] shop, the other morning and I was on my way to school, and this guy molested her, right here. And that was quite [terrifying] because I walk that way to school every morning, and it totally freaked me out.

I've realised that I can't change the past, but I can change the future and I can help other people change their mindsets, I think I did that in some way. You know just talking to people about these things, about AIDS and stuff like that, it makes a difference. Even if you can just convince one person that, you know, it's out there, watch out, then that is enough for me.

Before I started working on the project, I had never met anybody with AIDS. I remember the white guy that came in and he spoke to us and I was like, 'Oh my god, he is gorgeous!' And then when he said he has AIDS, it was like, wow, it can happen to you too? I mean, that's the way I thought back then. But I don't think that way anymore. You know, I've realised that this can happen to anybody.

The message that I would like to send out to parents: Teenagers are having sex and they should accept that. So, they shouldn't have this perception that, 'Oh, my sweet darling angel, she won't do that' and all that nonsense. Instead of doing that, educate them rather.

I think it's very important that we talk about stuff like this so that it's out in the open and we break all the myths and the stigmas attached to it.

# 2003

**Kaylene at 16**
Focus Group
Cape Town

Some women are emotionally incapable of standing up for themselves. Maybe there is a baby in the house and the woman doesn't want to scare the kids. She'll feel guilty. She will feel, 'Ok, I owe him that. I owe him sex. I have to do it. I have no other choice. I can't stand up to him, he is the father of my children and he provides for my household ... so I must give him sex.' That's her mindset. But I mean, emotionally she'll think this is wrong, 'I don't want to do this, why do I have to do this?' but there's nothing she can do about it because she gets beaten up and then she'll go and fetch her family, then it's a whole ordeal, and then he'll go and fetch his family, and then it's a family clash. So, a lady always thinks of those things. Keep the peace rather; just do what he wants her to.

The movies present sex as though there is no risk involved, I mean, no pregnancy, there's no AIDS, there's no STDs; it's just free and out there, you know, and anybody can have it anytime with anybody!! You won't get anything; you don't have to worry about it. There should be – maybe there is in some teen movies – a girl who falls pregnant, but then there are her friends who are even bigger 'sluts' [she uses air quotes] than she is, and it doesn't happen to them. But everybody is at risk of getting pregnant – except the guys [laughs] – and contracting AIDS and STDs and they must highlight that in the movies.

# 2004

*Kaylene at 17*
At home in Atlantis

*Kaylene's bedroom is covered in magazine pinups of the latest rock and hip-hop stars. The room is small and overflowing with pictures of her friends, mementos and stuffed toys. She has collaged photos on the walls. A crucifix hangs on her mirror beside a beaded AIDS ribbon. Out her window is a back alley where gangsters gather at night, get drunk, curse, sing, carry on and even sometimes shoot their guns. She points over hte bars on her windoq to the dusty sunlit spot on the street where they'll be when night falls.*

We girls talk about how to protect ourselves. We are nervous about it ... gangsterism in Atlantis is everywhere ... Choose your friends carefully. It's difficult to trust people unfortunately.

Most girls will be with any guy at any time. Mainly because they just want to be loved. Especially in Atlantis. Most of girls come out of broken homes, so they have no mothers, no fathers, or their parents are alcoholic. So, they think this guy is wonderful and all they want is to be accepted and loved.

Ok, I'm going to be a little personal here. If I should talk to them, I'll tell my experience. I live in Atlantis and I was raped. It was a very traumatic experience for me. I'm still going through it. Stuff like that. I want to educate them about it and tell them not to trust anybody. Not to be so impulsive.

Because the reason why it happens to people, or why it happened to me was because the people you think are your friends are not your friends. It just doesn't work that way. So just be careful and watch out.

# 2006

*Kaylene at 20*
At home in Atlantis

I think I might be talking for everyone because we've all matured now, we're out of that teenage kind of thing, so we have a great clarity of purpose in life now. Everything that we are saying right now or everything I know I'm saying as absolute, you know, I know it was, what eventually I want at the end of the day, it's just throwing it all together, it's like how do I keep it all together. You know, it's all the little things basically. I'll worry about that when I get there, as long as I have the grand scheme of things that I want.

I think I was 16 or 17 when we first worked together. What the workshops did for me was they shaped me, they shaped my mind, they shaped me, you know, as an individual character. I think I'm still carrying it with me, I mean that is my major inspiration, was my major inspiration, for what I'm doing right now. Also, because it's not so different than what we did then, compared to what I'm doing now. Really, it's not that different, you know.

I would say that it definitely gave me confidence, an enormous amount of confidence doing the workshops. As a woman, it gave me some kind of empowerment. Right now, I'm at that place where I'm struggling, you know. When I'm thinking about relationships and stuff like that. I don't know, I don't want to end up being vulnerable, being oppressed when I am in a relationship. I mean, you know right now, we're at that age and dating and stuff like that, you meet all these guys and they have a certain frame of mind, 'You're a woman, this is the way it's supposed to be.' I'm somebody, I've always been this kind of person, I love to challenge you. So, if you're going to say that, then I'm going to say something completely in the opposite direction. If you can't handle it, then it's just your problem. There's the door, bye! I think as a woman it empowered me so much you know, I've become so comfortable with my sexuality and developing my womanhood basically, you know, being sort of like a strong womanly figure.

Me and Mathew we went to get tested on World AIDS Day. We

made this plan that we want to go get HIV/AIDS tests on World AIDS Day. It was at the kid's hospital. It was so awkward or whatever because they ask personal questions and like, I think it takes a minute or so, and it was the longest minute of my life! I'm looking like, ok, one line, two lines, oh my god, what's happening here, and the nurse is like, 'Oh no, you're fine you can go.' I'm like, 'That's it?! I went through all that for this? Really?'

# 2006

*Kaylene at 20*
Interview at home in Atlantis

At the moment, I'm 20 years old. I'm currently studying social work in Wellington. I'm in my second year now. Half way through. I'm finishing in 2008.

At the end of August, I quit my job. I got another one, but I only worked there for like three days. It was an office job. I hated it so much. I thought this is just not me, this is not what I want to do. This is completely nothing that I had planned for myself. I was so unhappy. And I don't know, somehow things sort of ... just worked out. After the three-day job, I worked in a pet shop.

I went to Oudtshoorn. It wasn't far but it was a nice little retreat for myself. Just to get myself organised and figure out where I'm going, what I want to do with my life. You know? I just have a dream, but you have to plan if you want to get that. Plan what you are going to do to get there.

For the holidays, I was at home and I didn't do anything the whole of January. It was the night before school started, and my mom and I were still struggling to get enough money together. We needed about five thousand rand, and we were just stressed. I figured we just needed to get the registration fee. The whole year was like that, just scraping money together. Coins we had in the house. It was so weird, because we had to even look in weird places for money that might be lying around. Eventually, we made up some money, and I went.

It was the first day of university. It was so overwhelming because my father dropped me off at this lady's place we were staying. Only after I moved in, I realised, oh my goodness, why did I decide to live with this woman? She was an older woman and told me that it would be just me and her and her grandson, but when I moved in there were like eleven of us living there. It was just so horrible. At least I had my own room, but it became a problem, and before March she kicked me out!

I never did anything. She started complaining about the stupidest things like, I mustn't take so many baths, but I would like bath in the mornings. And I couldn't wash my hair that often and my hair is long. She said I had to cut my hair because it was too long. She was a religious woman and she was preaching to me about religion. It came to a point where I told her my relationship with god is my business, it's got nothing to do with you. That pissed her off, and I couldn't care less. I kept quiet and I kept quiet the whole time and then one day I just snapped and I gave her a piece of my mind. She totally freaked out. I was thinking 'oh my goodness', all these challenges. It was never clear cut what is going to happen.

The minute that lady told me you have to get out of my house, I packed up all my stuff within an hour, and I was out. I was sitting on the stoep and waiting for my dad to come fetch me. It was eleven at night. I remember it was so cold that evening, I felt like I was having a nervous breakdown. It was just weird.

So, I was back at home. I really didn't want to stay at a hostel, I didn't like hostels, but I moved in and actually it was quite nice. At that moment, I believed god knows what you need and fulfills it. That's what happened to me. I moved into the hostel and where I stayed the section was completely cordoned off with the three rooms with a bathroom and the kitchen. It was nice, so my first year was nice. I did really well.

I'm so proud of myself 'cause this semester I got two distinctions for my two majors. It was so nice because at the beginning of the year when I started, I was thinking how the hell am I going to pull this off? I got assigned to the work with the college group. I thought: How am I going to help the students adapt to their first year at college and whatever? When we started out, there were some problems but everything went so fine, it was so much fun. A lot of what we did in our group sessions for Soft Cover, I used with them, which was really nice. I just applied the skills that were taught to me at college again, like listening skills and talking, being confident and all of that stuff.

I'm not saying it was easy, it's just that for some reason, I believe it's my vocation. It's something that I'm supposed to do. I love what I'm doing. It feels so natural. It doesn't feel like I'm studying at all. It's so interesting to me that I can just pick up something and read through it and completely understand it. It's weird because I was never a strong student in high school, and to be that strong at college, it's so amazing. It's a wonderful feeling. It's really working out for me.

Last year my parents paid for my fees. This year I actually got a bursary from the college but it was very little, so I got a loan at the bank and so that will help sustain me for the next two and a half years. It is always food, pocket money and clothes. It's not cheap living there.

We have almost a three-month break, so I worked at Shoprite last year, it was a lot of fun. I enjoyed it. The first few weeks were horrible because I had to stand all day long and I wasn't used to it but eventually I got to know everybody.

I wanted to get out and be in Atlantis in the community again. After I did my practicum in Atlantis I wanted to be out there. I wanted to get to know the community because it is there that I'm going to be working. I want to get to know the people and I want to know what their problems and concerns are, what we can do.

I figured the best place to work would be at Shoprite because everybody goes to Shoprite. You get to know everybody there, and you know everybody's business when you are in Shoprite. So yeah, I worked at Shoprite and the manager was really great. Unfortunately, I couldn't continue working there because I couldn't juggle coming home every weekend and going back to Wellington. It would cost more in petrol money than I'd make, so it didn't work out, but I learnt a lot and I got to know the people. Now when I'm there, the costumers come complaining to me! Which is funny, but it's also nice 'cause I like talking to them.

I like hearing their concerns, you know, because I feel for them. I empathise with them. It's not nice doing a mundane job, you know. People don't have respect for you. They look down on you as if you're a piece of nothing, so when I'm there I always try to uplift them, encourage them, and speak to them. It's frustrating, I mean, all of us have a dream. All of us have goals, you know. We want to strive, have a fancy life, but it doesn't always work out that way.

When I'm at Shoprite and I speak to them, their issues are often things that we take for granted. Like having food on the table, having the rent paid, having electricity in your house. Having a phone is a luxury for some of them, where some of us regard it as a necessity. It's those little things. What else can we do to help you? Just give you a little bit of happiness, you know. That is what I'm trying to figure out. What I'm going to do after my studies, I don't know yet, I'm still trying to think of a master plan, but I know I'll get there. I'll figure something out.

I definitely want to stay in Atlantis. Even if I go away, maybe to go and study in other places, I will come back here. I will come back. My roots are here and I want to be here. It's just a small quaint little place, and I like being here.

When I did my practicum in Atlantis, I thought to myself, 'How could I live for 19 years in such a bubble?' I never knew that people here live in absolute poverty. It's sickening. I don't know, for some reason I completely blinded myself. It was such an eye-opening experience. I worked with a social worker, and we drove in an area of Atlantis I usually don't go, even though it's right next to here.

People are so poor, using one teabag twice, just those little things. Having no sugar in your coffee or your tea, these things I take for granted. These are things you are supposed to have. They are your basic needs. You are supposed to have a roof over your head. You're supposed to have food on your table. You're supposed to be loved when you're a child. So how can you not have these things? Why are they not there? And why are we who can have, not trying to help you get it? You know? Even though we live in the same place, but some of us are better off than others. Why are we closing ourselves up? It's like we're looking down on these people, yet we live in the same community.

It was so sad for me. I met this girl who was a teenage prostitute when I had my practical here. There are young teenage prostitutes who were taken off the streets and brought to this place where people are trying to just invent programmes to just keep them there. These girls are making 8000 rand a night. To them it's money, it's food on the table, and it pays for whatever they want. Leaving that for doing a few workshops where people are trying to tell you how to live your life? They're thinking, 'Wow, how can I give up this money for nothing?' What they try to do is teach them skills. There was a lady who was an aesthetician, so she did manicures and massages and stuff like that and taught them how to do it. That's basically what I try to look at: skills development. What kind of skills are you lacking, and how can we teach people, and how they can use it to their advantage ultimately?

I did a report about it all afterwards, and I thought to myself, it's so amazing that I didn't get caught up in that whole whirlwind. They live not even ten minutes away from where I live. Why didn't I get involved in any of those things they got involved in? Why didn't I get into drugs and alcohol and all of those other things that are going around in a place like this.

I had a good parental influence but that eventually dies out when you're at school. That's the reality. No matter how strict your parents, or how great your values are, it's different when you're faced with a bag of marijuana in front of you to say no to. It got me thinking a lot about why I didn't get involved in that.

I've proven to myself that I'm responsible. I clearly know what I want, where I'm going. I have a value system. When I'm away from home I know not to go out and do drugs, or drink myself silly. It's not what I want to be doing. I'm supposed to be doing everything except for that. I don't have an urge to do that. I was thinking a lot about why they're ending up in those places. As cold as I might sound, and it's not hundred per cent the answer, but I think ultimately all of us have choices, you know. Life is about choices. It's a stupid thing to say when you're angry 'oh life is about choices,' but still, you can choose to stay in school. It's all about choices, and some of us, we make the right choices and others make the wrong choices.

I was faced with drugs and all of that nonsense and yes, I smoked some pot ... now and again when I was in high school, but the thing is, I tried and it is not for me. I didn't like the person that I became when I was drunk, when I used to drink. It made me so ugly and it made me feel ugly, and after the fact I realised that nothing had really changed, you know? I'm depressed, and even more depressed than I was before I started. The workshops that we did together really helped a lot in keeping me out of trouble and thinking about my life and where I wanted to go.

Apart from that, it was the influence of school. I had really strong, good teachers. They are guides along the way. These are things that are there for you, if you just open up your eyes and see. Not to constantly look only at your problems, but to look for the solutions around you which are there. When you are in a bad predicament, when you live in poverty, it's difficult to turn away from these things. But if you really want something for yourself, if you really want a life for yourself, you can always make the choices that, no, I don't want this. I'd rather go sit in a church for a Friday evening if that's what's going to keep you straight. If that's what's going to keep you off the street, and keep you away from drugs and prostitution and all of these things. People can think and say about me whatever they want, it's fine.

I think a lot of kids here in Atlantis are abused in their homes; sexually and physically. It breaks my heart.

While I was working at Shoprite, I was sitting around the back dumpster smoking, and two little boys came to me. One was four, the other one was six years old. They wanted money and whatever. I didn't give them money but I started talking and joking with them. They asked who I was and I said I was a lady that is on a popular TV show, just visiting Atlantis. Eventually they realised that I was talking nonsense and we all laughed. I asked them, why are you running around? Where is your mother? Where is your father? It's cold, why aren't you at home? Why aren't you wearing shoes? The little boy said, 'My mom is probably at home, drunk.' I thought it was a joke, you know, trying to play on my emotions. Even when they're young, they're not stupid. I thought his mother was probably somewhere in the shop or something. The little boy said, 'No, last night I had to sleep on the lawn, and it was raining, because my mother was drunk. When my mother gets drunk, she kicks me out of the house', and then the 6-year-old said, 'Yeah and sometimes they come sleep with us before they get drunk.' They were so open, and they were talking about these horrible things. I'm thinking, 'How can people do this? How can you do this to a child; a four-year-old child?' The child had to sleep all alone at night. It's not natural, it's inhumane, you don't do stuff like that!

I gave them money. I only had a limited amount of money to get food myself, and I gave them my last ten rand note. I know it's something I shouldn't have done because people would say that you are encouraging them, but I thought, actually it was just the two of them so they go and buy ice cream or whatever. It might just make their day, make them happy even if it's just for a second. I gave my money to them. I didn't eat that day, it was fine! I lost weight. It was fine because I wasn't giving to receive something. It was just a gift to make them happy, just for that moment. You know?

It's those little things that always bring such great happiness to those people's lives, those people that are poor, people that live in severe poverty and stuff. That really hit my heart bad.

They were so open to talk about it. They talked about it as if it's what's supposed to be happening. They didn't speak about it in a way that implied I should be helping them. They spoke about it like it's the way it's supposed to be.

These are our future men. These boys will grow up and become men. What kind of vicious cycle are they going to end up in? The next strongest influence that they're supposed to have is their mother, because the father is probably not around. Most of them come from single-parent households. If she's treating them this way, naturally that is the way they're going to end up treating women one day. He's going to have this resentment inside of him. He is going to think, 'All women are the same, I might as well slap you around, beat you, rape you' whatever. They won't have any regard for people. It's going to be this vicious circle.

I saw a glimpse of his future at that moment, and it made me so sad, you know? I prayed in that moment. I thought, dear god, give them some way out, something to hold on to.

At first, I wanted to become a psychologist, but I don't want to get caught up in an office all alone talking to people about their problems. I'm not coming down on psychologists in any way, the work they do is super important, but I want to be active and pro-active. I want to be out there and know what's happening. What can I do? Where can I do something?

I do think about great plans for this place. I'm sure we can do really, really great things here. We can put up shelter houses and start feeding children. The little things. I think for me it will come in time because I first need to find my field and feel secure. Once I can do that, I can go out and I can start materialising those things that I've planned.

I don't believe that we can't change this place around us. It's not so bad, you know. At the end of the day, we're all people, we all want things out of life. None of us were born to end up being absolutely nothing. I don't believe that for one second.

You know, it's Atlantis for me, and for Mandla it's Khayelitsha. It's a starting point. Eventually you can go out to other areas, which are even worse. Mitchell's Plain and Manenberg and Nova Park and Grassy Park, one of these places. This is great practice.

> We can put up shelter houses and start feeding children.

You know, Shannon, I was thinking, if it wasn't for you, I would've never ended up like this, you realise that? I know that. I don't think, I know. I just wanted to say thank you Shannon. Thank you for opening up this door, this world of possibilities, changing my mind around and sort of giving me a new outlook on life because, when I think back on our workshops, a lot of what we did is exactly what I'm doing now. You know, we also videotaped our activities, and yes so, it's like wow, you know. Since I was in school till now, in my mind sometimes I'm like why am I going to college to get this degree, this piece of paper to prove that I can do it, when I know I can already do it.: So, thank you, thank you very much.

You've inspired me to work harder, to get to college, to stay here,

Kaylene Schroeder    65

to want to be in my community. And I do think you are using a great medium. You know, using documentary, through the work that you're doing I think it's a great medium to give voices to concerns people have and give a face to it. Lots of people see it around them but they don't really see it, you know what I mean. It's like you see these little kids running in front of you driving your car, thinking 'Get out of the flipping way' but you don't think 'Does this poor child have food tonight? Is this child being abused in their home?' You don't think… So I think television is a great medium for portraying those things.

I've learnt to reflect daily. I think where am I at, and where do I want to go? I don't just stand still thinking, I have this, so what now. I do reflect a lot. I think about a lot of issues.

Being part of the Soft Cover project changed my sexual behaviour for sure. I'm very far from promiscuous. I know a lot of people who are into the casual sex scene, which is just freaking me out. People that I know, close friends, talk about how they went to a club and they met this guy and they ended up sleeping with him. And I'm like 'so what's his name?' and they can't even answer, I'm like 'wow, did you at least use a condom', 'oh yeah, yeah'. Like it's not important. It's scary, it's so scary. Nothing has really changed from when I was in high school amongst my peers, my close and personal friends. People still have this carefree attitude which is so shocking. I don't think that the reality of AIDS has really sunk in. Personally, I'm not promiscuous. I'm not into the whole casual sex friend scene. I don't want to say I don't believe in sex outside a marriage, but I do believe in sex within a relationship where you know you have stability and security.

About the AIDS workshops that we did, it's like people hear the word AIDS and it's like 'ooooh' you know? Ultimately, it's not just about sex – a penis going into a vagina and then you're having sex – actually it's got absolutely nothing to do with it. It's a small portion of it. What it all goes down to is your lifestyle, and the decisions that you make. We must equip teenagers in our community to live a proper lifestyle, and to make informed decisions about exactly what it is they want. To get them to a point where they can say, 'This is not what I want for my life, this is not the direction I want to go, so I'm going to say no.' In other words, give them confidence. I would really like to get involved again with the schools, but I don't have time right now. HIV and AIDS affects us all.

Another thing that I've learnt from our workshops is I think all of us have a certain way of thinking, an approach to life if I could say. There isn't just one right answer to all of this and all of us have an opinion that matters. I notice that now, some people are thinking similar to the way I do.

# 2011

*Kaylene at 24*
Individual interview
Salt Rock

I am 24 now, and I am working for the Department of Social Development. I'm currently working at the local office in Atlantis. Our office consists of eight people, social workers actually, and I'm one of the social workers and we use other administration staff. I'm doing community work, group work and individual work, where I actually have cases of families that I work with. And secondly, management and research. After Atlantis I stayed in Wellington. I lived there for about three-and-a-half years. And I worked in Bellville so I moved to Kells River and lived there for a time, and after that I was back in Atlantis for a month or two and then I moved to Freedenberg and I got a job there and I worked there. I was there for about a year and then I returned back to Atlantis for about two months. That was the longest I could survive. I had to go, I needed to get out. And now I have a cute little apartment on the beach in Aserfontaine, which is on the West Coast, and I love living there. Not because it is on the beach but because it is my haven – my little space that I've created for myself. I share it with a Jack Russell, 'Princess'. She's my baby and my everything.

I think I've always personally been an open person and I judge a person by their personality, not by your colour or your pigment, or whatever the case may be. I just think that this socialising of a group when it comes to being with other people, taking us out of that little small town that we were so used to, and exposing us to better things, or greater things in the world, that we wouldn't necessarily have known of at all. I mean, if it wasn't for that action, we would probably still be stuck in Atlantis. I would never have gone on to become a social worker and be motivated to work in my own community and try to help other youths and families over there. Mathew would have never reached his full potential in the kinds of activism he is doing right now. Because we would never have known that this exists, we would never have known that we were able to do that. I don't know if it makes sense, or if you can imagine, but if you've been so isolated, you're not really used to other things that that's quite a big thing for us.

When I think back, a great method that we used was group work. A big part of social work is group work. You know, sitting down, having groups with youth, families, mothers, whatever the topic may be, and, I mean, my exposure to group work was at the Centre for the Book and Soft Cover was a really good start, and where I found out, ok, I like this. I like the growth phases that take place in a group and going on to studying that and now doing it in my profession. I love group work, I love the sharing and the phases that we go through and the group growing. I think maybe more that part [stays with me], but not the painting and the writing, even though, should I want to incorporate it, I would make use of an outside or external source to do that work for me.

I think being part of the project dramatically impacted my life, because it showed me a different world, or a different way of seeing things and exploring things, and also it made me more aware of what's happening in the world and sort of freed me from the isolation that I was experiencing at the time. It was a great atmosphere to get together with other people from the same ages and to see how different or how alike our lives are, and even if it was different, we could still get along and we could still communicate.

I'm just thinking from a professional viewpoint, I think such a project like we did together would really be beneficial in the community that I am in. And I wish that I would, or could, be able to sort of implement it in my work. If I were to be a part of it now, I would try to involve other people who I know would benefit from it. But I think it came at the right time, and like I said earlier, it came at a time when your development was critical, you know? The way your mind is forming, establishing your identity and things like that. I think it came at a really critical time in our lives and also what Mathew said, it's not so much what we did, but it's about the process that was followed, which wasn't a big structural process. It was just how each one of us had the opportunity to grow at a very critical time in our lives.

Some of the things that stand out for me the most were the discussions that we were having and the good advice that I received and carry through with me in my life. Also, some of the processes, the theoretical processes which I now incorporate, and work with, as much for the creative side of it, writing, filming, I'm not so involved with that. But I think I said back there at the symposium, my father always told me my mouth is my biggest weapon, and I still carry that with me, so…

It was never my plan to do social work, even when I was at school. During the time I was in Grade 11 and Grade 12 my academics weren't very good. But being part of the Soft Cover project sort of made up for that in a way because, yes, I wasn't getting straight As at school, but my knowledge was so big. I could share that with class members and write about it in essays, and that part really strengthened my writing skills and vocal abilities, the way I think and express myself. So, I think that from being part of that project, yes, I didn't go into a field where I work a lot with numbers or what I wanted to do initially after school; I wanted to study horticulture, or something to do with animals, I still have a very big love for animals. I was so confused, I didn't know, I honestly didn't know. 'Do I want to work with animals? Do I want to work with things? Do I want to work with people?' I ended up working as a cashier. I was so miserable. For about six months I worked there. I was extremely miserable.

One day I just decided I am going to quit my job and I just did it. I quit my job. Social work was my second option. I started to research it to see what it is that really happens in social work, what job a social worker does and what other fields they go into. And I started to see a big co-relation between that and what we were busy doing and I figured, ok, I really liked what we were busy doing, that made me feel free, it made me feel like … I didn't feel so claustrophobic and so tied up, because my personality is one where I don't like to feel tied up and things. And so, I decided I would go and study. I needed to study this.

> it made me feel free … I didn't feel so claustrophobic and so tied up

No money, no job. My parents didn't have money. Ok, we had the shop and we were doing our own thing, but it was really just to put food on the table. I started to work at it and, I think I told Mathew, I suffered at the time from bipolar disorder. I think at the time I was in a manic phase, because I was completely on my game. I wanted something and I was relentless in pursuing it. I applied and I was accepted. I didn't make my final, my fourth subject for matriculation exemption, but they accepted me on a conditional exemption. And they told me, 'Okay, you can come and you can do those three subjects and we will let you do a course and if you pass that course you can continue your four-year degree in social work.'

I'll never forget the first day I went to college; my mother had this big can and she filled a lot of five rand coins from the time I told her I wanted to go study till that time. It made up more or less my registration money, and I figured, 'This is all I need, I don't need anything else.'

I lived with this woman that I didn't know. I'd heard of her and I phoned her and said, 'Can you please help me out, I really need a place to stay.' I stayed with her, and that ended terribly. Financially, it was just taking it step by step working my way through college. My parents paid for it out of their own pocket. I had nothing to contribute. It was really, really tough from the first go. But it was the best time of my life. I mean that is the time I really grew, and where I could figure out who I am, and what I want to do with myself. I felt free, whereas I never felt that when I was at home, and because I wasn't exposed to so many things. Going to college and completing my degree was a very big achievement for me. Especially since everyone in my life at the time thought that I would end up not doing that. You know, I'd just be one of those normal, mediocre people who work at the shop. I am proud of myself for achieving that. That was a big achievement for me.

It was a great example for me of where I have achieved a goal. When I look back and I look at when I was about 16, just when we started the Soft Cover project, I wrote down 10 goals in my life that I wanted to achieve. There are only two goals left on the list. I still have the list. I have achieved eight of those goals. So, to me it is a big thing. It shows me that I have within myself the potential to do that, the theoretical part and the work experiences are two completely different fields.

What I was taught is not what is happening. And this is really where my creativity comes in because you can't do things by the book, as much as you want to. In social work we are taught processes for helping people, but processes don't really work. You need to go with the client where they are, and try to help them on their level, and not what you think they need. I think that because you have AIDS you need to go and get your medication, but rather, you know, you are in this predicament right now, so what are we going to do from here? Just that difference in the way of doing things, it isn't a structure. It is one of the reasons I like my job. I like the flexibility it gives me. I plan and structure my own work. I do my own thing. I plan my own projects. I decide which intervention will be necessary.

Working in Atlantis is a big challenge. When I worked in Freedenberg, my office was on the beach and the community was so small and I mean I could sit on the stoep and have an interview with a client and that wasn't unethical, that was the norm because that was the way the community related to me. I had to morph myself and be part of their community to allow them to accept me. Or we'd go down to the beach and sit on the sand and have an interview, which fits perfectly with my personality because I don't see myself sitting behind an office desk working 8 to 5 doing that kind of thing.

I also did some group work with teenagers. It was very successful. Mainly life skills. After that I went on because the town is so small and lacking resources – one of the things they didn't have was a social worker in an office, or a place where they could go to a social worker, so I created an office. I found a space and created an office, and the people knew where to access our services and it was a big thing for our office, just mobilising that resource for the community. The office is still there and it is running successfully and there's two more social workers at the office. Even though I'm not there, it's nice for me to know that it is still going on.

After that I worked in Malmesbury. It's also close to Atlantis. I worked in the black community. And I can't speak Xhosa or Zulu, but I learned, and I adapted. I worked in a one-man office. Basically, I ran the show. I did everything. Answering the phones, doing the intake screening, doing the counselling, doing group work, community work and mentoring students. I was alone at that office and it actually suited me quite nicely. I enjoyed it. I think I was very successful, given that there was this notion to only put black social workers, because in that community, here I am, and they see me as a white person, but they really accepted me and they made me a part of the community. They would know really how to treat me with respect when I came into the community and sort of help me. It was a very, very great experience for me.

I spoke to my supervisor the other day and she said, 'No other social worker can do what you did here. Everyone here is still asking for you.' Then I came to Atlantis, and Atlantis is totally different from what I was used to in Freedenburg and Malmesbury where my work was appreciated, and my presence was appreciated.

When it came to Atlantis, it's like, the community itself, I think, because of its history, and I don't want to make excuses for it, but I think because of the history of Atlantis the people have become so isolated and that isolation has bred this really ill attitude that they have towards authority. There is very little respect for the police or whoever you are. And the challenge then comes in winning that respect from people. Not forcing it upon them: 'I'm a social worker and you'll do as I say', but more sitting down and saying, 'Ok, so what are your challenges right now. It sounds like you are going through a tough time. Because your son is using drugs and you are struggling with a baby. How can we make this a little easier on you?' More in that light. Making it softer. Saying, yes, let's just acknowledge that this is happening. We don't pretend you have this perfect and ideal life, but can you not abuse other people in the process while you are doing this.

I had a very interesting week last week. One of the very big drug lords in the community, I removed his child, because the child had inhaled crystal meth, or I suspected they had. The mother is breastfeeding the baby so obviously there is transference that had happened, and then I had to do a toxicology screening. I couldn't have the child be in that environment. The next thing I know he is on my doorstep; he is sitting there. And I'm like ... eish ... let's just relax. I called him into the office and I'm like, ok, can we talk about this? So, we were speaking, but we could sit down and relate to each other, whether he is a drug dealer and I am a social worker. I told him, 'I know what you are busy doing, it's not my place to tell other people about it, it's not my place to inform authorities about it. It is not your focus for being here. We are here because you are concerned about your child and because I am concerned about your child, so let's talk on that basis, and we can sort of work towards something, we could work towards something eventually. We could work towards something.' I just love THAT part of my job.

The part that I don't love, and this is the biggest part I think that is putting me off the most, is the politics, the bureaucracy, all the red tape. I cannot handle it. It makes your work so much more difficult. It loses the essence and really it takes away what you do for the community.

The government really takes for granted the work that social workers do in the communities and also, they don't mobilise us like we can be mobilised, because social workers are amongst the most highly skilled individuals. For example, when I did the one-man office thing, I was the receptionist, I was the administration clerk, I was a counsellor, I was a therapist, I was a project coordinator, I was all of that. I was a group facilitator, all of that in one. Even on some levels a manager, you know, because I had to give permission, you can do this here. I was a mentor to the students. I really think and feel that it is not being acknowledged. Whereas you can have one of them, one government official, who doesn't have the background we do, and their background is in administration and they have no way of knowing how to deal with people or how they function or anything like that and they are at top level structuring things. And you think to yourself, how did that person get there? Their thinking is so anal … it just has to be like that… So that is the part that I don't like.

The second part is that it is also very stressful. I mean, I always say, 'you only see your clients when they are at their worst', and you are an angel to them, because they depend so heavily on you, you know. They are so vulnerable at that time. They are in crisis. Whether it be an abusive relationship, whether it will be coping and finding out they are HIV positive, or teenage pregnancy, or rape, or child molestation or … you know, any crisis they are dealing with in their life, you are their biggest source of help at that time, and the only person sticking by them, riding out that process, basically.

What becomes challenging is switching off. That has been hard for me. There have been times where I've gone home and cried. There's been times where it has become too much. Even today's talk, you know making that … it's very difficult to switch off the emotional connection. And all of the negative energy and transference … so to me it is very important that my environment is right. That's one of the reasons why I've moved. My biggest joy is coming home from work and walking along the beach for two hours. That is my escape. Coming back. Taking a nice hot bath, getting into bed and falling asleep. I know it sounds so boring, but it is because my work is so busy that it's not boring to me. That is fine. That is acceptable.

There was last year a time when it became really bad for me… I removed a child. It was the time when they wanted to take me to the media, because this lady in the community said I wasn't doing my work properly. She wasn't even a client; she claims to be a community worker, but she has no qualifications. You have these people who just want to get involved and they shouldn't be involved.

She was threatening to take me to the media, and at the same time, I removed these children from their mother, a crystal meth addict. She was really bad. And she was going insane in desperation. Swearing at me and going on and whatever. She would come every day, and even though I would tell her you can't just walk in here and expect to see me, you need to make an appointment, and then see me ... you know, she would be demanding, 'I need to see her now, I want to see her now', and the front desk staff would often let her see me because they want to get rid of her. She came to me one day and told me, 'I'm going to kill myself if you don't give me my kids back.' I told her, you know, 'If that's what you feel will help the situation, then you need to do that and I will phone the police to check up on you, but that's not going to be a solution to the situation', and she actually went and hung herself from the ceiling. Luckily, the police got there. So, they actually responded. But that was a heavy time for me. It was really hard.

And at the same time, I was busy doing some community work. Community work is also hectic because it is a whole process that you have to go through. And I thought, no, I need to debrief, and I actually saw a psychologist at that time who charged me R900 or something for a session, but it was helpful, you know. Now what helps me is I have my boyfriend, and I have Mathew. My friendship with Mathew/Eva (for the last two years Eva has also been a part of our lives), has really helped, tremendously. Really. Just being able to talk about this stuff. My colleagues at work are a fantastic support network. We are really there for each other, but it's not always as easy as you would want it to be. I do try my best to guard my mental health. We actually see a shrink at work through this lady that comes up. She speaks to us. She talks a lot to us about using our energy. Switching off. Those kinds of things.

What we did with Soft Cover was excellent. The work we did was excellent. Like I said, I don't remember much now, in fact I don't remember the poems that I wrote, or anything like that but I will always remember the discussions we had, which were intense. You know, it helped us at that time because I don't think we had anybody that related to us, at that time in our lives, so it really helped us get through that. I don't think if we had to go back ten years earlier that I would change anything. And these last ten years flew by so quickly. Like I said, just being a part of the project changed my life dramatically. In a way that I would never have planned. So, maybe it was my destiny to be part of the project.

When I look at the short clip from *Fire & Hope* that we did, it's really a self-fulfilling prophecy. I mean, back then I didn't know what social work was, I didn't know it was something I would enjoy going into, or, you know, helping people or helping the community. Assisting people and helping them get through their lives and their daily challenges, I would have never thought that this is where I'd end up right now, even though looking forward I don't think social work is what I will be doing five or ten years from now. I will move on. But just getting this grassroots experience, this raw, very raw, social work at the bottom. It has made me so strong, such a strong person, and I learned so much from other people every single day.

There is never a day when I meet a client and I have this attitude of 'I know it all, I know all the answers, I know what we are going to do', I always have this notion of 'I know that you know what you want in life so let's speak about that a little, let's try to explore that and see how to make that a reality. That's what I want for you.' That's what I tell all my clients as well. I don't go home with you in the evenings, I leave. I don't know what it's like, I don't know what it's like to live with a husband who beats you every day. I don't know what it's like to go to bed hungry. I don't know what it's like to not have money in my pockets. Even though I do come from Atlantis, I can't say I could walk the walk. My parents always provided for me. They went out on a limb to do that for me. So, I don't know what it is like to go to bed and have a mother tell me, you know, 'My son couldn't go to school today because there was no food last night in the house and he was too hungry this morning and I didn't send him to school because...' I mean, I don't know what that's like. I can imagine it must be so hard, you know. Your pride, your self-esteem, your obvious feeling of hunger, I can imagine, I can let myself into that.

Atlantis is also not where I am going to stay. It's been nice to be there for this short time. In fact, last month I celebrated my year anniversary there and I grew dramatically while I was there.

I always have in the back of my mind that, were I not a part of the Soft Cover project I would never been able to have done this. So, I owe it to myself because I know I should do better now. Especially in my way of treating people. When it comes to policies, structuring, developing, those kinds of things, keeping it in mind, people, their circumstances, themselves, it is so important. That is really the essence, because from the project that is really what I got. I, as an individual, developed myself in the project. Not vice versa.

# 2018

*Kaylene at 31*
Group discussion
Centre for the Book

I am still Kaylene from Atlantis. Nothing has changed there.

I think one thing that I've always maintained over the years when we would meet up in groups, like when we were in Durban and whenever we would meet up with one another, is that coming to the Centre for the Book and being involved with the project really expanded my world. Made me realise that there is a bigger world outside of the little world that we knew as youngsters. I would like to think it made a profound impact on me as a teenager. Just knowing 'Ok, but there's other issues in the world, apart from what I'm dealing with right now'. It offered a very, very good perspective from negative things to focusing on positive things. Developing your creative side a bit more, you know, seeing what you have inside of you that you never thought could be tapped into. That is one thing that has always stuck with me throughout the years. I'm always curious to think how my life would have ended up when I was in Grade 10 and I met Abigail Dreyer for the first time, and opening up that world to arts, and a different life. Thinking back now, there was so much pressure on us as young people to perform academically when there was such a different world out there that could be explored, but wasn't entertained at the time.

What do I do now? I'm apparently a social worker. Working generic social work, so that means I do a bit of everything. I've never actually been a part of the HIV group at work. I've mainly focused my attention on mediation, and divorce, substance abuse, victim empowerment programmes and those kinds of things, because that sort of tickled my interest. So, being a part of this group really expanded my world. You know it showed me a completely different side of things.

I think also for us, there was a sense of belonging, you know, and escape. I don't know what other word to use: a positive escape from what we were accustomed to in the communities we came from, with issues like HIV and drug abuse and, I mean, that was life. And so, to come here and have another perspective on life was a beautiful thing to experience for me. I think that's all I have to say. I really enjoyed the arts and crafts and making of the books. And the travelling was nice. I enjoyed those things. And even after it all, today, you know, it's still techniques that you can apply in your life.

Those things that you've never really lost. In my office, I have the wall of creativity where I've got blackboard paint on one side and whatever you're feeling you can just come there and doodle and do whatever you want to do. It's great for the kids because they always come there with the chalk and they doodle and write things. The social worker in me will be analysing, 'ok, this is a house, this is a car, ok...' It's something that I have learned here, and 15 years later, would I still have had the ability to do that? I doubt I would have. I maintain my point that being a part of the project has really opened a whole new world for me.

> To come here and have another perspective on life was a beautiful thing to experience for me.

For me, work has been really challenging over the years. Firstly, working in government is absolutely horrible. I don't know why people always say they want to work in government...

Your resources are not there, the money isn't there, despite the fact that the image is portrayed that it's supposed to be. Also, just the kind of work that I do, having the opportunity to be an influence on other people, positively, especially the youth. Sometimes I wish in my line of work when I sit down with young people that there were more programmes like what we attended when we were teenagers. Like I said earlier, I found it to be a really great escape for me from what was going on and I think a lot of you also said that in a way, you know? And when I look at the youth today, there's just negativity all around and nothing positive to bring them out of that and to make them see there is another side to this world. Apart from being involved with the gangs, or falling pregnant young, or doing drugs or all of those kinds of things, you know?

Making them fall in love with school and what it can offer. Work has been a very big challenge for me over the years and I don't think I'm quite where I want to be, but I don't think that's the end of it either, so that's definitely an area that I want to build much more. I don't think I want to really be a social worker. I like the field. What's nice about it is there are so many options that you can do with it. There's definitely something for me to explore over the next 10, 20, 30, 40 years!

It doesn't matter who your parent is, a child is a child, and your child will always love you. To just take a child away from her parent is one of the most difficult things to do. So yeah, one of my core businesses is child protection, obviously, but I work more specialised now in foster care and there's a whole lot of things happening in foster care. We want to get rid of the whole foster care system, you know, where granny comes to apply for your child, and you get work in the Eastern Cape and now granny's sitting there. It just puts the child deeper into the system so there's like a whole [scam] going on. Also working with people who are not adequately trained or have no proper compassion for what they are doing, later on, you do become jaded.

It's like I'm just doing the same thing over and over and I'm falling into a bottomless pit. So that is why maybe in the next 10, 20 years, there's other stuff that I could possibly tap into and develop my skills into that direction. So that is me, when it comes to work. We have very little resources. People at non-governmental organisations actually have way more resources than we have. And department social workers and nurses and medical staff and wherever else, we really have to be so creative and even approaching NGOs to help us out, which is so insane, you know? Because what's the government doing with your taxes if we have to approach other organisations.

It is challenging being at work right now, but at the same time, it has grown me in more ways that I have to say. I don't think I would be the person that I am, had it not been for work. I don't think I would have developed the compassion, understanding and patience that I have. And the wealth of knowledge. It's really been a two-sided street.

# 2022

*Kaylene at 35*
Video interview online

It's really interesting to study the writing over time, and the way it unfolds. I was reading through it and I thought, okay, it's not as bad as I thought things were at the time. I was actually so much wiser when I was younger, without realising it. It was interesting to read about where I was, and all the way I came, till now.

I'm still not where I want to be, but at least I'm not where I was.

At the start of COVID, all of us were very afraid firstly. Firstly, COVID lockdown started at the time when I was on maternity leave. By the time I went back to work, it was about late May/June and we couldn't be a lot of people at the office. We only went to work every second week.

In December 2020, Elijah got COVID. He was 12 months old.

I'll never forget, it happened on the ninth of December. He co-slept with us and I always kept him in a sleeping bag. And then Elijah decided when I don't feel like sleeping in the sleeping bag and he was screaming, crying. And so, I told myself he is a year old already, and I can take him out of the sleeping bag since he's sleeping in bed with us. It so happened that one morning my husband was getting ready to go to work, and I got up to go to the loo. I just heard this loud thud. It's a sound that you won't be able to get out of your head, Shannon. He fell. I picked him up and inspected him. He looked okay to me. The days following he become so ill. He had a swollen head, problems of fever, vomiting so I took him to the emergency room. They said they had to do a scan to see if there's any damage to his brain. They admitted him, because they couldn't control the fever. I don't like this hospital. It's a private hospital but they have wards that are actually rooms. There is a yellow ward and the red ward. The red is where the COVID patients are and yellow was where they don't know what your status is yet. Elijah was in the yellow ward. The way it is setup is really silly because you can't really avoid people there. So, we were there and then the nurse told us that the child opposite was positive for COVID. Gosh man, I didn't think it would happen to him. He was discharged from hospital and my child just got so, so sick. I couldn't understand it. I took him back to the pediatrician, and it was COVID.

I also got it through someone who was infected at work. At that time, we only went out for emergencies if there was a serious crisis and a child was being severely endangered, or like beaten to death. Some of my colleagues responded to a case like that. My one colleague became infected, and she infected the other one and me, because we sit all together. It was the worst experience of my life. I've never felt that sick.

I was sick exactly nine days. On the tenth day I woke up and I was like, was I really sick? It was so perplexing the way like, just a few days ago I was in so much pain. I even didn't smoke through that time, can you believe it? I'm a chain smoker! I couldn't even smoke. It felt like there was a fire lit inside my chest. It was not a nice experience.

I've been diagnosed as bipolar. So, I'm on chronic medication.

When I take my meds it really knocks me out. I'm on antipsychotics, mood stabilisers and anxiety medication. It's enough to knock out a horse! But it helps.

The depression was there. In my 20s I think it really started to spike. After 23, by the time I was 24/25, somewhere around there, I was having more and more of these depressive episodes. I met a therapist, Marie, and she said she thought I should consider antidepressants. I went to the doctor and I was prescribed medication and it worked beautifully. I was doing so well. It was a three-month course. After that I was ok for a while, and then I just went into a dip again. And so, it went on, until I just decided to get help and was admitted to hospital.

I was hospitalised the first time in 2017, and that's when I was diagnosed. My first diagnosis was depression with psychotic features. Then, that doctor emigrated. I got a new doctor and I felt like he was just pumping me with meds. I felt overmedicated. I went through a stint thinking I wanted to get off his business as fast as possible, and I flushed all my meds down the toilet. That was the worst experience of my life. That didn't go well, because there were withdrawals. They aren't just psychological. I ended up back in the clinic again. I moved over to a new doctor while I was in hospital. I didn't want to go back to that same doctor.

The psychologist I have now, she's absolutely wonderful and I don't feel like I'm overmedicated. I feel like it keeps me rather stable, but I do still experience episodes of hypomania and depression. Bipolar is more depressive episodes than mania. I fought the diagnosis for a long time, Shannon, because I have seen crazy people with BPD, and I thought, I can't be one of those. My psychiatrist took me through what bipolar is, and explained it to me. It took me quite a bit to accept it, to understand what it is, and that, ok, I might possibly be on medication for the rest of my life. So that's how my diagnosis came about.

I'm feeling good though. I had a depressive episode recently where I couldn't work. I was just in bed. So, I just rode it out. It's all you can do. She said, you know yourself now, you know how to get yourself out of this. It's just recently, as of this weekend, that I'm feeling a bit better.

I'm still working in social work, doing the same work. I always say, thank god I've got medical aid, because there's no way I would have been able to afford the level of care that I get. When I look at some of our clients who have those same conditions as I do, and the level of care that they get, I think it is so sad. They slip through the cracks. You know, they don't get the help that they really should, and then it manifests into social problems. When you look at it, it's like, it's not social problems. It's psychiatric problems.

I'm also going through a divorce right now. I was married for 13 beautiful months. It's not like everything came crashing down, there was a lot of things that just happened.

To briefly summarise it, I was struggling psychologically long before. We did marriage counselling. I recently had a session with that therapist, because I've been going through a lot of dips. And it was so powerful, Shannon, for me to get the validation from someone outside of my life to validate that, yes, what you saw I saw too. You did not imagine it yourself. She even said to me, 'I was thinking in my head, this isn't going to go very far because you're not the kind of person who's going to stand for this.' I think that's the great thing of having someone in your life for so long is that, they know you. Obviously at that time, she wouldn't have said you need to get rid of this guy. It was a powerful moment, just last week, it's like wow, it's already so difficult to question your own reality, and then other people start questioning your reality. And then you are like, okay, so what is? Who's the crazy one here?

I've got very, very strict boundaries in place. And I've had to develop that in order for me to not lose my mind and for him to not take advantage. I'm over the guilt and the shame now of getting married and divorced so quickly. I would rather do that than be stuck in a marriage that was going absolutely nowhere. I was a single mother and a single woman in a marriage. And that's no life for anybody to live.

When I was pondering about the divorce I was thinking back. I always felt my father is a narcissist. He has been really abusive, not physically. My mother's still with him, she's just sticking it out. Firstly, she's never at home. She's by either one of us, because she wants to avoid him as much as possible. She's forever saying, what's the use of leaving him now? We've been married for more than 40 years. I remember this one time I was cooking in the kitchen and my mommy was here because she was helping me with Elijah. I sat in the kitchen one Sunday morning, and I asked my mommy, will god punish me if I get divorced? And then she said to me, 'Get out while your child is still young.' That just struck me. I'm sounding very dramatic, but this is a woman who knows what she's talking about. She went on to say to me, 'I couldn't leave because I didn't have the resources. I didn't have family to turn to and I had five children. Where was I supposed to go? But you don't have that. You have the resources, you have a house, you have a car, you have a job, you have your baby, you can put food on the table, you can buy clothes.' She was saying, 'I couldn't do that. Whether you leave now, or 10 years later, eventually you are going to get fed up, then rather leave now, instead of your child being exposed to all of this toxicity.' I was just like, wow, I didn't expect that from her. I honestly did not. She blew my mind. It really informed my decision to leave. It did. It was only when I brought it up that she gave her honest and frank opinion.

My son Elijah is two-and-a-half years old. He's turning three on the second of December. Elijah is an absolutely beautiful human being. I'm not just saying that because he is my child. I always used to joke and say, he's got his daddy's personality, because his father is so charming and social and whatever, and I'm not. After he left, Elijah was still like that. I said to myself, Elijah is not like that because of his father, it is because of you. He mirrors what he sees. That is why he's always feeling upbeat, or in a good mood, or whatever the case may be. He is amazing for such a tiny little human being. And I enjoy watching him unfold. And he's growing!

These last two years, it's been something different. When COVID started, they would stick with us with these lockdown rules and implementing this, implementing that. This is a global pandemic and people are dying. Ironically enough, I thought to myself, AIDS was a global pandemic, and yet you didn't institute a lockdown for that. People were dying left, right and centre. Why now?

I was feeling for the people around me, what are you afraid of? There are worse things out there like AIDS. It was interesting for me to see how our governments reacted. Why was HIV and AIDS not really a big concern or problem? When we still have maybe many people dying from it, maybe not as bad as before, and living with it? What I see now is that I think that they get a better quality of life, and medication seems to be more accessible to them. There are also more support groups. I was just thinking how different it was from how AIDS was handled.

I was talking to a teenage girl and using COVID as an example. I was giving her counselling and I said to her, the goal for us in life is not to stop all the bad problems, but to become resilient. Like during COVID. It is still here and it's going to be around for a long time. We had to do certain things to ensure our safety, like wearing a mask, sanitising our hands, maintaining a distance, not socialising.

I was using that analogy to explain to her that with your life, you also need to apply certain skills to help you get through the difficult times. COVID is a good way to explain that to people. I suppose what we did in terms of HIV and AIDS was like that too. It's not that you want to take it away completely, because it's not going to go away. But there are better ways of making your life more comfortable and making yourself more equipped to deal with the challenges that you're facing.

When I read through the phases of my life and what, what you recorded, you know, it reminds me that it's just the way that your mind tells you that things are not good.

When I read back, and I can see there was hope for me. I ended up not doing so bad with the trajectory of my life. I could see, yes, the challenges were definitely there, but somehow, I managed to get through all of that. I don't know how. I can only thank god for that. And I found my inner strength. My support system was big. I've got a very good support system.

Compared to what Mathew, Danlia and I went through, at this time things are bad in Atlantis. The youth are really getting lost. The situation feels hopeless. That is from a social worker's opinion. You always want to have hope for your clients, but how? How do you have hope? We were lucky because we had a Shannon in our lives. Shannon took us out of our isolation. I mentioned that, when I read through, in one of my stories, about the impact of being part of your project had on my world.

I was thinking a lot about if only we had that resource for our children to have a kind of outlet where they can see that the world is bigger. I always say to the children I see, 'Do you know the world is bigger than Atlantis?' They get caught up in the way they are living. They have no clue what it's like to live in other parts of the very same province we live in.

When I read that I thought, wow, I wish someone would come in and work more intensively with our youth. In terms of self-expression and self-confidence. We need a project like what we were part of with you. I often think if I didn't have that exposure, how would things have turned out for me? My mind would still be in Atlantis.

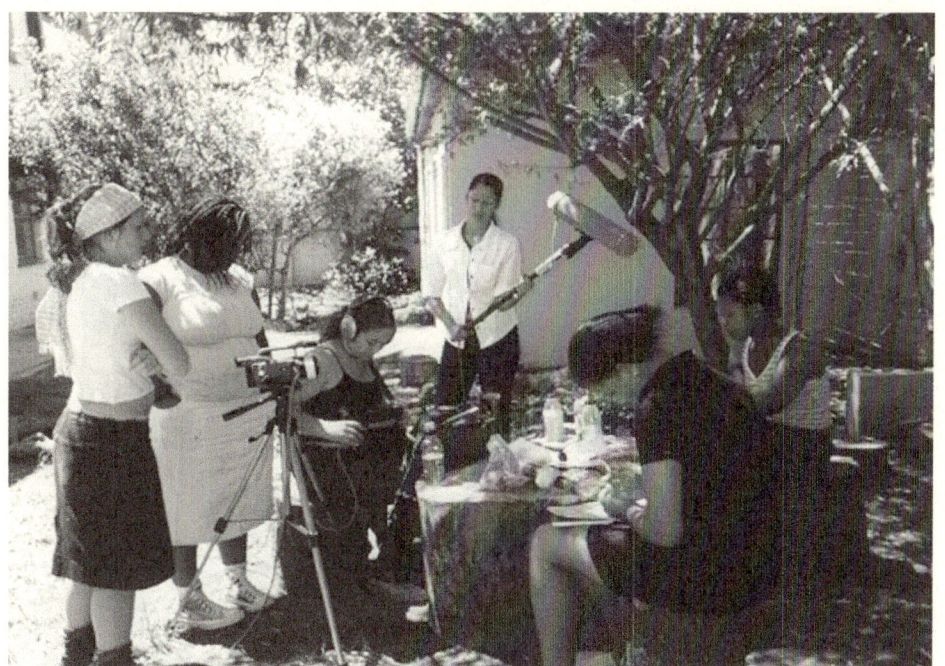

*Filming 'Street Fear' 2004 (L-R: Nadia, Lindeka, Kaylene, Chinomy, Ann, Wendy)*

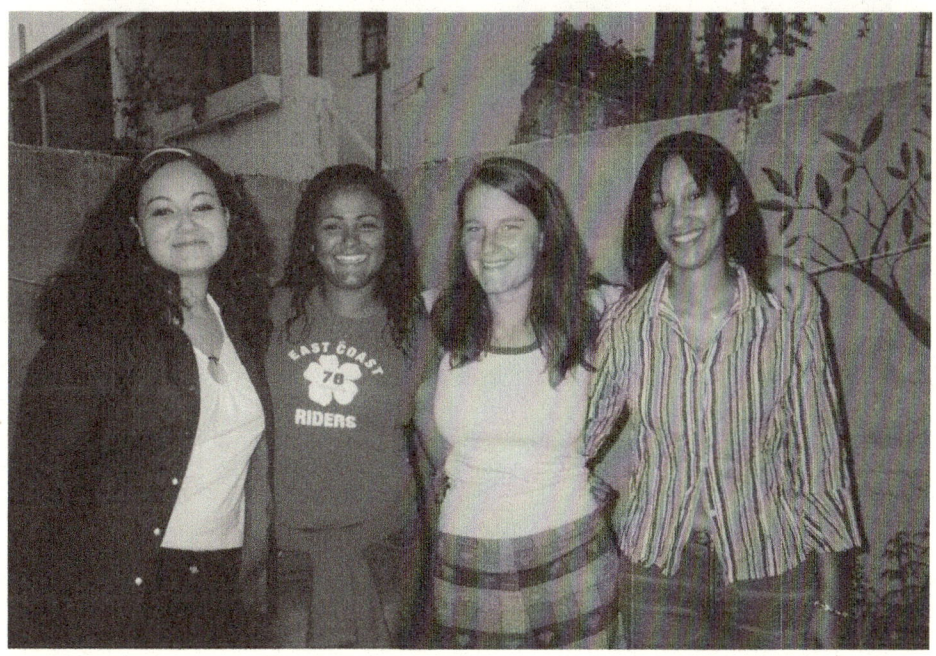

*Cape Town meet up, 2005 (L-R: Kaylene, Danlia, Shannon, Chinomy)*

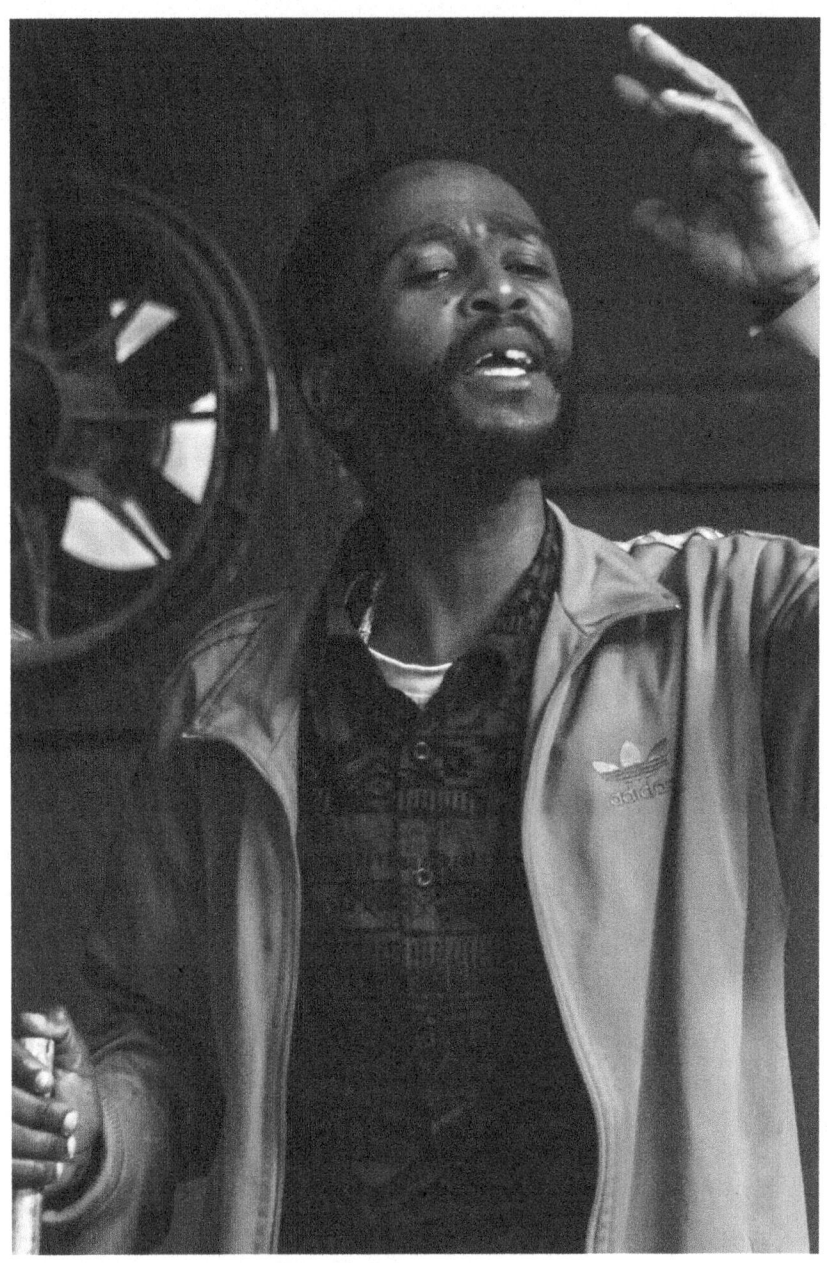

Photographer: Neels Kleynhans

# 6

# Khayalethu (KK) Mofu

KHAYALETHU, KNOWN IN OUR group as KK, was already an astonishingly creative and intelligent young man at 18 years of age. He is small in stature, but his presence always looms large. Wherever KK is, you know he is there. Everyone in the room will be laughing out loud or will be transfixed in silence listening to him.

A great public speaker and performer, he has the ability to command a room and bring people together to listen to his stories that he carried into the workshops and creative activities we did together. KK always had something to say, and a vision around how to say it. It was no surprise when, later on, he won awards and became an actor and theatrical director.

While KK the performer was forever present, he always took the AIDS pandemic seriously and was committed to do what he could to make a difference. KK was a star in the group of activists in Khayelitsha who came up through the Treatment Action Campaign. As a teenager, he travelled internationally speaking about HIV prevention and the AIDS pandemic. Among our group, he was highly creative, often reciting poems or doing improvised raps on social issues as featured in the documentary *Fire & Hope*. He was the instigator of the *Facing the Truth* video project that sought to use video to provoke conversations with white private school students about their perceptions of HIV and AIDS, and that specifically confronted racial inequality.

As KK grew into adulthood in Khayelitsha, the structural inequalities of township life for black South Africans took their toll. As the sparkle of youth faded, the speaking engagements changed, too. The support that was there for him as a young person withered as he became an adult, something he discusses in his own writing.

Social justice is never far from his sight, although the form and content of his advocacy has changed alongside the changing South Africa. He has had his share of intense hardships and setbacks along the way of achieving his goals, yet KK continues to fight for social justice. KK was one of the founders of the first isiXhosa shack theatre space in Cape Town, the Makhukhanye Art Room. He also directed or starred in plays such as *They Died Singing, The Champion, Night and Day*, and others. He continues to be an artist and activist to watch.

# 2003

*KK at 18*
Interview for *Fire & Hope*
Khayelitsha

My name is Khayalethu Mofu, but I go by the name KK. I am 18 years old. I live in Khayelitsha and attend Joe Slovo Comprehensive High School. I love listening to revolutionary music. I love speaking with people. I love acting – acting is my life! I am an artist who believes in the artistic life. I love writing poems, to express what I believe. I hate people who hurt other people's hearts and feelings, and what I especially hate is people who think they know me, though they don't. My life is not always happy, because other people are dying out there. Because of AIDS even my smile is not always a happy one.

My message to my lovely beautiful readers: Life is the journey, not a destination and there is no success without sacrifice. Do not make too many mistakes in life, because there is sometimes no second chance.

When I passed Grade 8, I started to change. I don't know why. I said that I wanted to be something. So, if maybe I would keep on going with these [gangsters]... About six of them died.

So, I said, 'Not me. I'm not ready to die. I said, Ok, I must change, and I changed.

Every day, even as we're talking right now someone is getting infected, which maybe my aunt, maybe my relative ... I don't know.

We'll see. Which means there's a lot to be done. The government must also support us as young people.

We've got a future, and we want the future.

Some people, they will say abstain, but I'm not saying abstain to people. What I'm saying is that they must make sure that whatever they do, they are safe. Abstinence is between two people. So, I cannot say people must abstain. They must make sure that whatever they do, they must make sure that they've got a future, they've got priorities that they want to achieve one day. So, they must make sure that they are safe.

### Rap in isiXhosa for *Fire & Hope*

*Children don't listen.*
*A girl of 15 leaves home*
*she comes back with HIV/AIDS*
*She has a big tummy*
*they say she's pregnant*
*that she needs AZTs.*

*that she needs a social grant*
*she is dying of hunger*
*I don't blame her*
*People must look after themselves*
*and avoid hunger*

*We got to the spot*
*saw them doing their thing*
*I didn't want to join them.*
*'Cause now I know, it's HIV*
*that's killing this country.*
*This country we live in.*
*BOOM!*

# 2003

*KK at 18*
Excerpts from *In My life*

## IN MY NEIGHBOURHOOD

I wake up in the morning. I fix up my things and go outside to get fresh air, listening to gunshots, dogs barking. Some crew of guys walking along my streets wearing dirty clothes and going to buy drugs to smoke. I speak to my dog and ask 'How was the night?' He doesn't respond because he can't talk Xhosa! I go and visit a friend of mine just to talk about stupid human beings, sometimes we just plan how to be successful.

At night I watch television or listen to my revolutionary music. I always hear approximately 12 gunshots after 8 o'clock. I speak with my father and we discuss international affairs, because he likes politics. I do my homework and study. At about 10 o'clock, I go outside, just to stand on the corner with friends in my community and discuss with them about life issues. Sometimes I fight with them when they think they are clever, though they're not.

Taverns are playing music all night.

On Sundays I wake up late. I wash myself then I eat my breakfast. Most Sundays I just stay home and wash my clothes and put the music on to a maximum volume and see some people walking past wearing their church uniforms. Sometimes I wake up early to go to the funeral services. I come back and write my poems and articles, then I think about myself and the future and also rehearse in the house alone. I go to buy some food for supper and I cook. I am a Perfect Man when it comes to cooking! Then I iron my school clothes for Monday and polish my shoes, making sure that everything is in a perfect manner. I watch TV until the middle of the night on Sundays.

In the street, people are always going up and down, busy with their own issues. Some of them drink alcohol from Monday to Sunday. Some young boys get involved with gangsterism and smoking heavy drugs and after they smoke they go around the place robbing people.

There was one young boy who was killed by his friends for smoking alone instead of calling them to come and smoke. There's another guy in my neighbourhood who now is mentally disturbed because of the dagga that he smoked every minute and hour. This guy has a matric certificate. Each and every day I will always see people fighting over nothing. Sometimes young boys play with guns on the corner.

But also in my section, there are many young people involved in youth organisations and that makes me happy. There are groups of young people doing drama; these days in my community drama is a very popular thing.

Then there is another guy who lives down in my street. You will notice this guy by his daily enthusiasm, always greeting people, especially young people. He always wears an HIV positive T-shirt and also a red ribbon, because his twin had AIDS and died last year. He now works in a support centre for People Living with AIDS. When he passes us boys he always says, 'Boys, don't forget to condomise.' There are people who are dying of AIDS in my community some of them have spoken to me about their status and I speak to them positively.

### Take off these chains

*People crying*
*death increasing*
*this is about the pain.*
*HIV and AIDS is killing us can't we see?*
*the daily deaths of HIV*

*Heal this suffering*
*whether you are infected or affected*
*turn this world into a conscious world*
*where there is no stigma,*
*or discrimination or denial*

*The young ones Nkosi Johnson*
*and Sibongile Mazeka*
*died of AIDS in the early stage of life.*

*and we have discrimination that lead*
*Gugu Dlamini to die*
*our minds can change this tragedy*

*Heal this suffering*
*for the sake of our brothers and sisters*
*mothers and fathers*
*who are no longer with us*

## AN UNFORGETTABLE MOMENT IN MY LIFE

One day, I was playing soccer outside the house with my friends. As we were playing, the day was getting later and later. Then we stopped playing and went inside the house to watch television. After a few minutes my aunt entered the house. I saw something was wrong. She told me to go to another house because my cousin had passed away.

When I went to the house, I heard people singing inside the house. I still didn't believe what I was told, but then I stepped up to the door and opened it slowly, and saw many people in the house. As I entered the house, I saw my cousin on the bed and her body was covered with the blanket. I still couldn't believe it, even though I did see her. And then I was crying. I realized that she was really dead, and remembered all the things she had done for me, and now she was gone.

My cousin had been sick for a long time, but we didn't see it as serious. She was drinking alcohol but still she was always a friend to everyone in the family and her friends, and in her school where she was a principal. Children were always treating her like their mother and also me. By 2002 she became much sicker than before and I had to take her to the doctor. The doctor told me that she had shingles, and prescribed medication. A few months later she couldn't even recognise me. Soon after that was when my aunts told me that my cousin was dead. That was a big unforgettable moment in my life.

After then I started telling myself that I will fight against HIV and AIDS in my own way and I will make sure that people are aware of HIV and related issues.

## We can conquer

*Pointing fingers at one another won't help us*
*we live in a world of sorrow*
*a world of painful circumstances*
*a world of HIV where our youth is not safe*
*our life is a mythful one*
*a confusing one*
*like flesh to flesh*
*that has spread HIV*
*that has caused fatality of HIV*

*I talk of HIV the killer*
*it has changed the many things in our nation*
*it has brought discrimination*
*it has stopped people from expressing themselves*
*Action must be taken*
*the mission is obvious*
*if we do that,*
*we can conquer*

## Chained souls

*There are hearts full of tears*
*there are eyes full of tears*
*there are souls with no joy*
*there are faces without happiness*
*there are humans who are still waiting*
*who blame themselves for no reasons*
*there are bodies who feel empty inside*
*who feel inferior*
*there are slaved hearts*
*there are chained souls*
*societies who lack love*
*people who create fear*
*because of their small understandings*

Khayalethu (KK) Mofu

*who only care for the beginning*
*giving no care for the ending*
*where people joke,*
*though the issues are serious*
*thinking that they are hilarious*
*when they become scared*
*then they bring back the consciousness*
*that's where they start to realise*
*they are chained souls.*

## 2006

### KK at 21
Interview with Shannon & Claudia
Khayelitsha Site B

*Shannon and Claudia met and interviewed KK at home in Site B, Khayelitsha.*

Right now, what's happening in my life? I don't know. I'm out of school now. I'm looking forward to going back to school next year, so I'm just here in the township, going around, having fun. That's it.

With school, it was unfortunate. I did my matric, but it was not good. I did get a passing grade, but for me, it wasn't satisfying. It wasn't satisfying my wishes, like what I wanted to do, so I went back to a finishing school in Langa. I go there and pay, everything. Recently they said I must attend a night school which is very far away from here. They say that I must pay 90 rand weekly for transport. I said, 'No, you suck. I can't afford 90 rand weekly you see.' I had to fight, so I'm not looking forward to go back again. One thing for sure is I must finish it. That's my plan, that's my plan, that's my plan...

I think things have changed since 2002 when we were first together. At the same time, I cannot say things have changed, because of one thing: When I look at the statistics, the problem is that those statistics, they do not decrease. They just increase. Of which in Khayelitsha West has the highest HIV and AIDS infections. I can say it is something like a home for this virus, because most people are from Khayelitsha who are having this virus. I'm not saying that in some other areas people haven't got this sickness, I'm not saying that. But Khayelitsha is rated as the township with the most people infected with this sickness, so... For me, I believe in one thing, if one person listens, and changes, it makes a difference. You cannot change a hundred people. If one person out of a hundred did take away something from what you are saying, you have done your job.

Recently, I also went to Amsterdam. I was at the Arts and Media Centre (Amec), I was doing photo journalism there as a high school learner and they were going to select people to attend [a conference in Amsterdam]. I think five of us were selected out of 70 applicants, of which I was one of the five. We were interviewed by two ladies and a guy. They asked us about issues affecting our society, HIV/AIDS, those kinds of things and of which for me it was a soft platform for me to talk. They were just asking questions, and I told them this and that. After they phoned and told me I'd won the interview, I must prepare myself for the trip. I told them about the project *Fire & Hope*, and the writing in *In My Life*, and I brought one videocassette that I was going to showcase.

I still remember when it was my turn to present at the conference, the whole room was full. I was one of the youngest ones there; most of the people there were old. Most people were like, 'Oh let's go see this young boy from South Africa', then I showed them the cassette of *Fire & Hope*. Afterwards, they wanted me to leave the cassette. A lady who worked for a TV station there in Holland said I must send the cassette. Everyone was like [impressed]. There was this guy from Ghana, I think he's the son of the president of Ghana, who was also there. Everyone was like flabbergasted at what this young boy can do from South Africa.

Being involved with these projects has also impacted my sexual behaviours for sure. For sure, it has had an impact. I mean as someone who has seen these things happening with HIV and AIDS before I could [become sexually active]. Now I know what to do. I mean now, in terms of relationships, I know how things work. I know in terms of the usage of a condom for instance, each and every time. When I got the chance, one thing for sure, I must not forget, I do not take risks.

⁂

I'm also involved with a programme called Men in Partners. Men in Partners, it's from Love Life. They focus on what men do; what men think like in society in terms of particular issues. It's for men only and we discuss issues that affect us as men. We discuss things around traditional perspectives and also looking at things from a Western tradition perspective, you see. There was this big topic whereby we were discussing the issue of being men, like really, really what does it mean for us? Not just to be 25 years old, but there's a stage and a certain path you should walk towards, you see, that now you're a man. That's what we were talking about. Ideas like how men should be: men should be aggressive, men should smoke, men should drink, men should fight you see, men should not be gay you see, things like that. That's what we were discussing. Men being parents. It was good for me 'cause I did learn a few things. Most of the issues, see, they started from HIV, STDs all kinds of stuff; the political perspective, economical perspective. It was the things that I knew but I couldn't say to them, no, it's more this way, you see. So, I just pretended to act like I knew nothing.

I'm still involved with them. They phone and say we are going to do a workshop focusing on this thing, and this and that. We just wait for them and then when they phone for us, they say we organised the event so that they can come. It is also to mobilise those guys who were involved before, to encourage other people to come and be part of this thing, but it is hard, it is difficult.

I'm actually still focusing on this platform of being an activist, but as a person, you grow sometimes, so you learn to take things differently. You see? For me, I can say I'm still an activist.

I'm also doing drama. In most cases I get the chance through drama. Like if maybe I direct a play, then we go with a play that showcases issues in our community, you see. For me, if people are watching [the play], so they get informed through stage acting. That's another way of getting the word out, you see, for me.

Currently I'm directing plays, and that is what I want to do. I mean that's the plan. For me even if I can to do it every day, I have no problem, you see. I have no problem with that. Because it's something I love. I just combined my passion and what is affecting, so through what I love I can be able to deliver and share.

# 2011

*KK at 25*
Conference panel
Salt Rock

*The group gathered together in 2011 at a hotel in Salt Rock, where everyone got to socialise and share experiences of the last number of years on a panel attended by educators, healthcare workers and academics. This excerpt is from a recording of KK speaking on the panel.*

We were all from different backgrounds, and different locations and Shannon came to all of this.

There was some sort of segregation in South Africa, yeah. Black people are normally in a city of theirs, and coloured people are in a city of theirs, and white in a city of theirs, so there is that distance in between us. And we've got our own ways of thinking and doing things, not knowing how others do things, and how others do things.

When I met these guys, I was actually already a member of the Treatment Action Campaign with Mandla by then. I remember the day Mandla told me, 'There's a symposium for a week to go and attend in Cape Town at the Centre for the Book,' and I said, 'Is it about drugs?', and he said, 'No it's about young people, sharing ideas around the issue of HIV and AIDS.' When I got there, it was like, eish, I've NEVER in my entire life sat next to a young white guy.

I've never shaken hands, or hugged a white guy, and now, I'm supposed to express how I feel, talk about my experiences? Because also I have had a terrible experience of living with someone with HIV and AIDS, so, I was like eish. Firstly, I was like, 'Eh, no, no. I'm not sure what these people get up to.' But I saw that they were all FREE, so I ended up being free and we did many exercises from painting, to writing, and feeling things together.

It was so upsetting to me that each and every time when I am watching television and there is an advert, or a programme that is about HIV and AIDS, there's only one face that appears of which is a black face. And I said to myself, maybe HIV and AIDS is for black people, and a discussion arose there. People were like, 'No, there are white people that are HIV positive.' I said to them, I mean, I'd been involved with the TAC back then it was two or three years, and I said I've been working a lot with the TAC people and I think I only saw one white guy who said, 'Yes, I am HIV positive'. I started to say, maybe he was lying [laughing], you see.

In 2004, we made this documentary called *Facing the Truth* whereby we went to different schools. We went to black schools, coloured schools and white schools and questioned them around the issue of HIV. They were like 'Yah, yah, yah, HIV, yah, yah. We know, we've seen from TV'. We questioned them about it, 'Do you know anyone in your community who is HIV positive?' They said, 'No.'

I remember one young guy said, because of medical aid and stuff, they don't feel that [white people] have got HIV and AIDS, because they can afford to buy the treatment, and no one can know that they've got the virus. We saw the difference in perceptions when we were doing these interviews in different locations. And it came to me that 'real AIDS' is not just black people. There were white people that had HIV because of the statements that I got. There were coloured people with HIV, and they were out, they were speaking about it.

What I was most grateful about the Soft Cover project was that it was us young people saying, 'This is how I think, or this is how I understand when we talk of HIV and AIDS prevention.' And that's when we had people coming in, we had writers, we had poets, of which we had everything that we as young people by then, even today, we enjoy, we feel comfortable, in terms of listening, that someone was going to stand there and say, 'Beware of HIV, it kills. You must wear condoms. If you don't, you could die.'

Of which, most young people say 'Ugh, we know that, yeah ok. Just give us something of which it's exciting'. And then we did the *In My Life* book, which made a huge impact on us. What happened was we had people who were saying for the first time that 'I'm HIV positive. I've been having this virus for some time now, but now that I've met these guys in the Soft Cover project, I feel like I should just talk about it now.' Even in schools when we went to distribute the book, people were like 'OK, yeah, yeah, yeah, now we are listening, because someone who is my age is writing about it, writing in a way that I do understand.' So, for me it was working in that particular way.

Audience Member: 'Two of you mentioned that you had opportunities of mixing with people of other cultures, and by cultures, you meant race. And I wonder [if you could] say something about it. What did you get out of it? Why was that important? Why was that useful? And also, if you could say something about 10 years later? Have you changed your views about other races? Did it change your relationships with them, and the kind of relationships perhaps you established 10 years ago, have they continued?'

> I got excited because each and every time that we learned something, I want to share it.

Not that I have a problem with coloureds, or whites, but I'm from Khayelitsha. So, when we talk of someone who is coloured in Khayelitsha, you talk of someone which you do not know. Of which you've got these superstitions that they live 'this way'. White people, they eat in Hout Bay, you see? They're all the same mind. That's what you know where I come from.

When I met with all the guys, I was like, ok, even these guys, they've got problems. They are like us. You see? So, I got to know them better. I got to know their cultures and traditions. I got excited because each and every time that we learned something, I want to share it. Each and every time when I learn something, I want to share it.

I had people in my school who used to come to me and say, 'Hey,

hey kid,' saying they think they've got a growth or something, and asking me, 'So do you know how I can get help?' [laughs] Because normally in my school, even my teachers, they used to tease me too much. But now for me it was a shock for me to see some people who normally tease me now asking for advice.

They come to me and say, 'Hey, I've got this problem down here,' also, 'Do you know where I can get help? Please don't tell anyone!' And I would say, all smiling, 'This is where you could go, I think you can get help there.' So, for me, that's what it did for me. Because it did not only help me, but it also helped the others surrounding me.

# 2011

KK at 25
Individual interview
Khayelitsha

*By 25, KK had started performing and directing plays, and exploring activism in new ways.*

There was a show I performed in the city of Cape Town. I was required to write a play about HIV and AIDS and TB. I did that, and we were touring around schools around Khayelitsha. A mobile clinic accompanied us, of which we were encouraging the school learners to go to for testing. In each and every town when we'd perform, after we finished, a number of students would go and queue up for testing. It was one of those things where I said, 'Ok, this is working', and I shall keep on doing it. Regardless if it's HIV/AIDS or anything else, as long as I want to tackle it, as long as it's something that is a problem, I want to solve it.

When I was part of the Soft Cover project, I learned many ways of writing you see, and so for me, it helped me a lot in terms of what I'm doing now because I write plays now and it's part of what happened before. Basically, that's one of the things I can say I've kept with me and also one thing that I love most of all was the fact of doing it, of the freedom and that made me love it. To love using the camera in terms of documenting and using audio visuals in terms of trying to get the word out there, not only about HIV and AIDS.

I'm using what we learned writing in poetry, and in writing productions to document stories that I want to tell.

When it's good it's good, but when it's bad, it's very bad. That's life and you've got to [keep going] otherwise, that's what life does. That's what I've learnt. For me, whatever happens, personally, in my life with my family, nothing will stop me from wanting to achieve what I want to achieve. Regardless of what the situation is, you see. That's why I keep on striving for the best.

I never paid much attention to my Xhosa traditions, even though my father is basically a traditionalist person. At home we are taught that 'this is how things are done here', but at a certain age, I was like 'No, I want to do my thing my own way'. Suddenly, it was like now everyone was going to the bush [for a circumcision ceremony] at that age. It becomes a HUGE problem if you don't go away and then your peers go, and when they come back, you can't call them by name. You get bitter. Some of them do something horrible to you or to your family. They will go and they'll be fine. So, I said to myself 'Ok, no, let me just go there and see what's happening there'. I went up [to the bush], and learned a lot. So, then that's how I think I came into myself as a Xhosa person, into my life, and to pay attention to my traditions and my culture and customs. Though some of the things, even though I don't want to agree with them, I can't do otherwise. Something that has already been THERE for quite some time I cannot say this is wrong, especially at my age. I'll just have to say, ok, if you say it, ok. I bow down and that's it.

What I miss most about those days it was when we used to meet at the Centre for the Book with all of us. Those for me are the memories that I think I will always have with me. If it was going to be the weekend then I know that, ok, we're going to the Centre for the Book, and I know I'm going to meet white people, I'm going to be around different races, and it's going to be fun. You don't be like ugh, eh, there's white people, eish, there's black people, there's coloured people, there's Muslims. For me it was like, this is more the South Africa that was envisaged by the freedom fighters. It was like now we are all in one room, and we're not fighting, we were all smiling, having a good time together. For me those were the times we used to be at the Centre for the Book. I won't lie.

I've learned so much and I'm always keen to learn from other people. When we were there, we had different things that we were able to do and we are always sharing them.

> I think it did make an impact back then. When you talked of HIV and AIDS back then, it was still something that was taboo in a way in our societies.

I mean I went to Johannesburg for the first time in my life. It's one of those memories of which I can never forget. For the first time, I was on a plane. I was the first one in my family to go on a plane. They were like, 'Really, you were on a plane?' I remember I phoned my mother when I was in Johannesburg. I think it was the day the cricket captain got in a plane crash and I was supposed to come back. My mother phoned and said, you must take a bus. 'No, no,' I told her, 'Everything's going to be fine.' She said, 'Okay, we'll just wait outside and we'll just look up [at the sky] and see you.' I was just like, 'How you going to see the plane that I'm in because the plane is just passing by.' It was quite an experience for me and also for my family.

Even before, I was into art. I met these wonderful, wonderful people. I remember meeting [the artist] Wonder at the Centre for the Book, and he was doing these things with paper, and I was like, wow, someone drawing and creating something like a sculpture with paper. For me I was like watching how they're doing this and thinking I must try and do something MORE. I must try and find something which they're not DOING. For me it was like growth in a way.

Even in my school that I attended they were like, 'Are you still busy with the books? We've got some young people here and we would love for them to do what you did.' And I said 'No'. I'm not sure that can ever happen again, or that there might be another opportunity such as what I got right there. The teachers said to me, 'You must share, share, share. We want people like you. Other writers at such a young age', and I was like 'Well, I'll see if I can...'

I think it did make an impact back then. When you talked of HIV and AIDS back then, it was still something that was taboo in a way in our societies. And then, when you're young and you're talking about HIV and AIDS, people look at you like, 'are you crazy?' or worse, 'do you have it?'

I remember when I was about to go to Joburg, my teacher said to me, 'Hey, small boy, why are you busy with this HIV nonsense? What do you know about HIV? Are you even sexually active?' 'No, no, I mean people need to know about this HIV and AIDS thing.' And he said, 'Oh you are talking shit, you know nothing. You know nothing', so for me, I was like [shaking his head, sighs].

But eventually, when I brought the *In My Life* books to the school, I gave him a copy, and reading different stories personal to HIV he said, 'Oh, ok...'. Even if I was also involved with the Treatment Action Campaign by then, I was leaning somethings about HIV and AIDS at the Centre for the Book from a different angle than from what TAC HIV and AIDS information distribution is about.

Then I had to go back to my community and share what I had learned. And one thing that was real when we did the documentary presentation, going around and checking people's minds about HIV and AIDS since in most cases back then it was more like black people being the face of HIV and AIDS. And a few whites and a few coloureds actually, fewer coloureds and no whites at all then. And then we did the documentary *Fire & Hope*. It was quite an experience for me.

I even remember when I was in Holland, I was talking about HIV and AIDS and young people in South Africa. Even then, they were like, 'So, this is really happening to Africans. It's a huge problem for you in South Africa now.' Yeah, so. No, you must keep doing this and that, this and that, this and that, and even in my community now. Even today, I've got people who are coming to me. And say, 'I don't know how not to kill my partners...? I'm HIV positive.' So, I'm experiencing such things now. People are coming to me to talk about it. Some people they come to me when they've got problems in their genitals, they come to me and say, 'Eh, man, I've got this thing...' So, for me it's been like this. It did have an impact on people.

It shows me clearly by the fact that now they're coming to me, and I sometimes advise them in terms of this HIV and AIDS thing and related issues or infections. So, you see, I think it did something to me. And something in my family and something for the community where I live and abroad.

# 2018

*KK at 33*
Group discussion
Centre for the Book

I'm a theatre-maker. Firstly, I'm from Khayelitsha, and back then, Khayelitsha was mostly populated by black people. And in that time, whenever you spoke of HIV and AIDS, one thing comes to mind, the black face. And for me, it was like 'Ok, really, this is our thing', but when we came [to the Centre for the Book], and we met with other guys from Atlantis and having to share experiences around matters of HIV and AIDS, and then it brought to light that, basically, this is not only a racial thing, and this is a human thing, of which all of us had been affected by it. One of the things I still remember as part of the writing, I'm not sure who was giving it, I think it was you [gestures to Abigail], we were doing this exercise of just write without stopping. Don't think, write whatever comes to mind, just go, and write. Fortunately enough, I still have all of those writings. I kept it. One of the things that I loved the most was when we had to make our own books. How big a thing were those books and dispersing them? That's what I think I can still remember. I loved that memory. I'm just trying to structure it now. I want to make sequels of everything that we went through, you know?

In my line of work, because I also act and other things ... we have our own theatre in Khayelitsha, it's a shack theatre. Sometimes we have these workshops for young writers and I apply the same techniques that I learned here. It's like, come on think on your feet, just write non-stop. You find that people come out with stories of which they never knew were there. You know. It's up to this day I am still applying many things I've learned from the project.

I think you guys know the kind of work that I do. It's been one great chain for me, up until now. I'm no longer young, but in some spaces, where we practice our work, we are always painted as 'young theatre makers' or 'young artists' or 'up and coming' or 'emerging' you know? But through all that, I've managed to do my work in a way that I'm known in many spaces, in many institutions, in terms of what I do. Especially when it comes to directing. That's where most people they know me, and also in acting. There's only one problem that I've had with acting. It's my height. It's been a problem for many years. Because my height is not corresponding with the age in my face.

> this is not only a racial thing, and this is a human thing

Sometimes I go to auditions, you know, and whereas they have my picture of me in front of them, they would ask 'so ... is this you?' and, I'm like, 'yeah, that's me'. And ... and they would say, 'Awe man, if you were a little bit taller', you know. That's the only problem that I have encountered in my acting career but I've managed. Even so, I've managed to get roles. Even so that I am this height. Also, me and also in some of my friends we have started and built a theatre. It's a shack but it's a theatre and it's based in Khayelitsha. Since Khayelitsha is the second biggest township in South Africa, unfortunately, it has no theatre. It has no arts centre, of which we managed to build our shack theatre. Later on, after building that theatre we were fortunate enough to get people from Switzerland, and we are now in the process of fund raising for the space to be more permanent.

In Khayelitsha, the money is not there for people like me. This is why whenever I see these programmes on TV or somewhere like *Cape Town's Got Talent*, or *Idols*, or *Strictly Come Dancing* or whatever, and our work, especially for someone like me from Khayelitsha, we are only being recognised when one has been nominated for a certain award. Or maybe one award and that's when you have your premier or your mayor coming into your space acknowledging you, that you are someone who is existing. That you are an artist that exists in Khayelitsha. But there are many artists of which are not being recognised up until you get your Fleur de Cap Award, you get a Naledi Award. You get yourself whatever award, and then they come to you as though they know you, you know? And for me, that's one thing I've been saying to many artists, it's like, if Hellen Zille comes to me and says, we've heard that Khayaletu Mofu has won a Tony Award and now she wants to come and shake my hands in front of camera, she could do that in hell. I would tell her exactly where to go. Personally, I would do that. I would acknowledge her, thanks for coming, but ok, the Tony Award. I don't need you! Or the Fleur de Cap Award or whatever award I won, was not for you to acknowledge me, it was for the work that I've done. So, if you want to do something about the arts in Khayelitsha or in Gugulethu or wherever, go to the artists there, find out their problems, if they have an arts centre, is it working, is it functional. Don't come to me because now I've won something and you want to shine on my own spotlight, you know. So that's what I've been saying. Even around the institutions, they know me. You go to the theatre, they know me. I don't hide anything when I feel like it's not on. For me, it's not on.

You have to fund Xhosa-written plays. They come as second-hand commendations only. It's only English and Afrikaans, but you've got many Xhosa-speaking people working in this institution. Then how come you guys are not acknowledging that you ought to have Xhosa-speaking theatre-makers. Even Zulus or Sothos, but mainly because Western Cape is mainly Xhosa- and Afrikaans- and English-speaking people, you know, so how, why is that we are not accommodating all these Western Cape official languages, you know?

It is where my activism has gone. It's been a great journey.

# 2018

*KK at 33*
Individual interview
Makukhanye Arts Room, Khayelitsha

I am 33 years of age. I met Shannon Walsh almost like 15 or 16 years ago, I think? And back then I was still in high school. Being a passionate and ambitious person, and being a person who was involved you know, because I was in the SRC, I was also part of the school government body, and also part of an organisation Treatment Action Campaign, of which in my thinking, it was influenced by Treatment Action, a group from America.

I was an artist, because I was an artist even before I met Shannon Walsh. After high school, I went to school, and I did theatre and performance. And I came back, and I did a lot of shows. The only problem was one, for me, up to this day, is still the same problem. When there are no provisions. When I'm having a gig and then like getting this huge amount of money, and everyone in your family is like loving you. You are hearing of uncles of which you've never met.

> You have to fund Xhosa-written plays.

⁓

The way how I grew up, I never knew my grandfather. My father's father, I never knew him. Even his mother. The only person that I knew was my mother's mother. And she was a political activist. Around about '94 came the first democratic elections. When they came I wanted to go and vote. My grandma was in exile, my grandma was a cadre, and there used to be times when we were there in Philippi when she heard gun shots, she would tuck us under the bed. 'The attackers are coming.' You know? And she went on to teach in Tanzania. She was in exile.

When my aunt had shingles, that was 2001. I was clueless of what shingles were. Even though I did know that the infection was a yeast infection. My aunt had only one son. Up to this day her son is still living. Before she died, I remember, she gave me her gold watch. Of which, I don't know what happened to her watch.

⁓

In my years of being an artist, as an actor now, as a theatre-maker, and as an activist, we now have this space: Makukhanye. It's called Makukhanye Arts Room. We have so many graduates and many qualified theatre-makers and theatre performers, and artists, you know. We came about to build such a space. And now because Khayelitsha is the second biggest township in South Africa, we have Makukhanye Arts Room. I do theatre, I'm in it myself. I do act, and when I do act, I do. It's a pity you've never seen me, when I do, I do deliver. And when I direct, I do direct and I love my work. And I love how things turn out to be.

Because when I grew up, the only thing that I wanted to be was to become an MK member, part of uMkhonto we Sizwe, the political arm of the ANC. That is what I used to see my grandma doing. I was like, I want to kill the Boer, you know. And I remember meeting Shannon Walsh, you, with Mandla. And I said, 'I really must talk with white people.'

Around about 1992, a white man once pointed a gun at me. They were termed Caspers back then, they were yellow. We used to call them Yellow Men. And this guy points at me [uses fingers to make a gun]. I was around about like, Standard 2. Very young. Very young. This was after Mandela's release. And the guy just pointed at me, and I just stood. It's still here [points to his left temple], and I stood. And then they just laughed, and they drove off. That was the first time a white man pointed a gun at me.

I know how my father was beaten by white people. Taken off our land. Of which now, it's my land, but [my father is] still alive. I know how, when he went hunting, he was beaten for hunting in his own land [injoli]. That's our forest. That's where we hunt. You know? All of that came back. I was a gangster. I was shot at. I even lost my tooth. A bullet came to here [gestures with finger into his mouth]. I was shot even here [gestures to thigh]. I was arrested, I got away with it, because connections with the police, you know?

One thing stood out. Who are you? Do you still know your mom? Do you still know your dad? What are they expecting from you? Didn't they name you Khayeletu? Khayeletu means in Xhosa 'our home'. So, must I keep on doing this and keep on stressing my mom, my dad and my sisters? I'm the older one, unmarried, you know. Must I keep on doing this? But it was hard work we did. I've done so many things.

But with *In My Life*, up to this day, I have a right to say I'm an author. I'm an author. I've met people who read the book *In My Life*. I've met so many people who read the book. And they were like, 'Is this you?' 'Yeah man.' 'Ah, you're lying.' 'No this is really my aunt who I wrote about. I used to cut her hair to go to the clinic.' Back then I was clueless of what HIV was.

☞

I'm not married. I was supposed to be married, but I am not. And reason being... When I love, I do love. And I still love the very same person that I'll talk about, but ... after disappointments and mistakes that happened in between. I think you met her once. Even today, it's ... Shannon, this is difficult for me, because I never express such things. You do know her, but not in detail.

I am 33 years old now. And I am the first born. I had a kid that died.

And the very same mum, of the kid, we stood together, like we, stood, you know. And so, we ended up getting a separation, like. At first it was like, we were open. Like in an open relationship, you know, you can date, you can do this and that. And then after a year she became pregnant. I was with the guys, and she came to tell me. And I'm like, yeah ... because our kid died, 'and now you're pregnant and you'll give birth. I'm good for you. You do know that I still love you?' And I know that she still loves me, you know, so ... There was the fear; the fear of having a kid again. That fear is a fear that you'll have a kid that won't last, of which you had a kid before of which didn't last. So, what happens next? You know. And I said to her, 'Can we just like, have sex and use protection?' We had a promise ring. Me and her. This should have been our eleventh year of marriage, you know. That's young love, of which it never ends.

☞

The only reality we are having now is for work to survive. We're not living in the ancient times, where I have cows, or let me go and grab that impala or… Now you just need to go and buy something.

I'm a thinker, I regard myself as a thinker. And I do know that I am a thinker, and I always try and make meanings.

Maybe one day you'll see Khayeletu Mofu winning a Tony Award. Maybe one day you will call Khayeletu Mofu to come and perform in Canada.

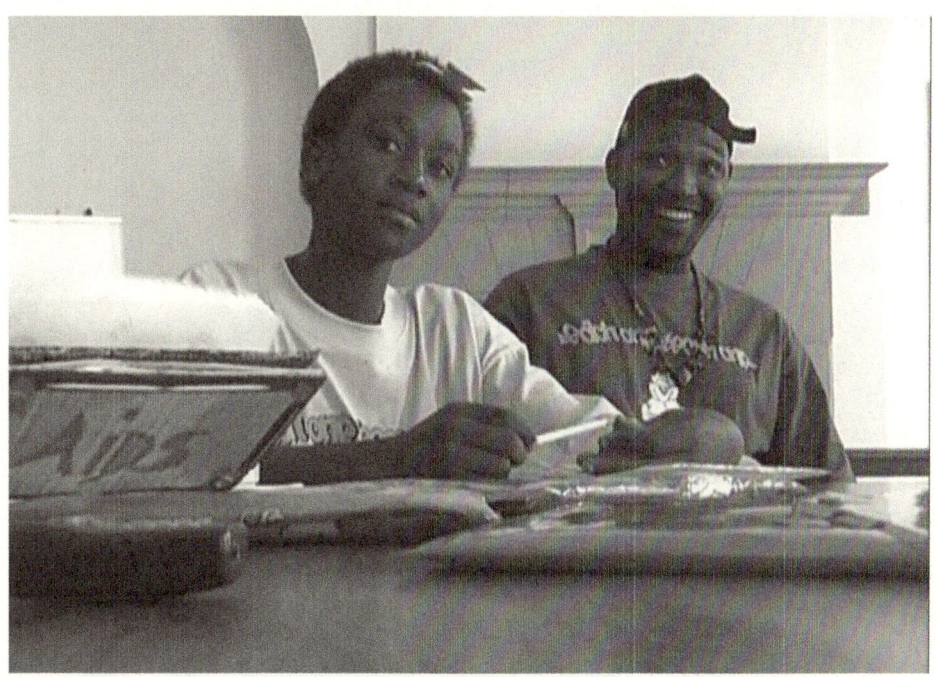

KK and Mandla at 'Soft Cover' workshops, wearing 'Each One Teach One' T-Shirts, 2002

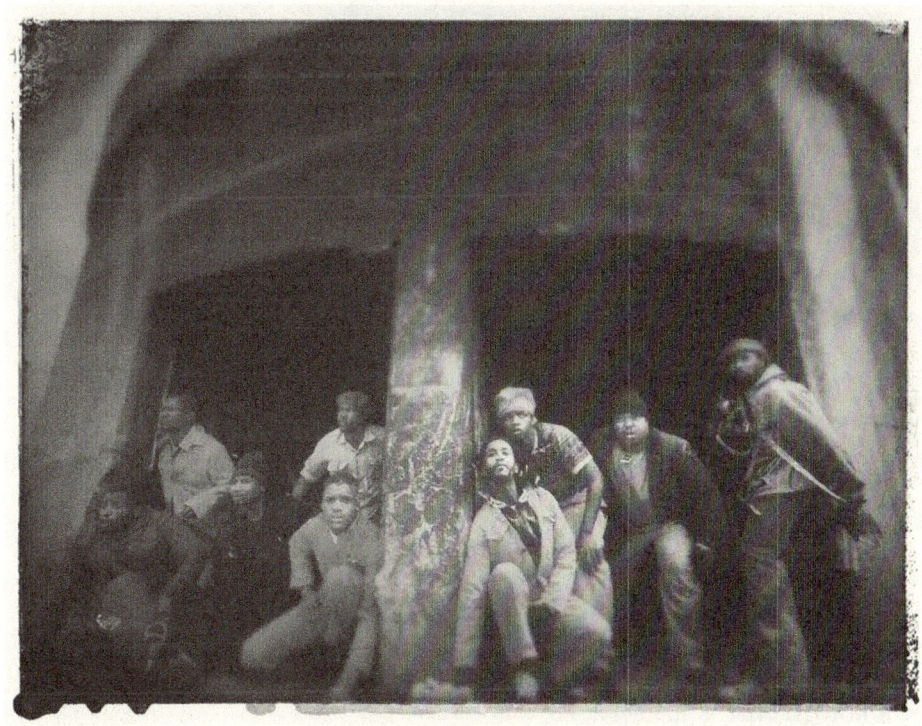

KK, still from play 'They Did Sing' by Toto Tsodo, 2014

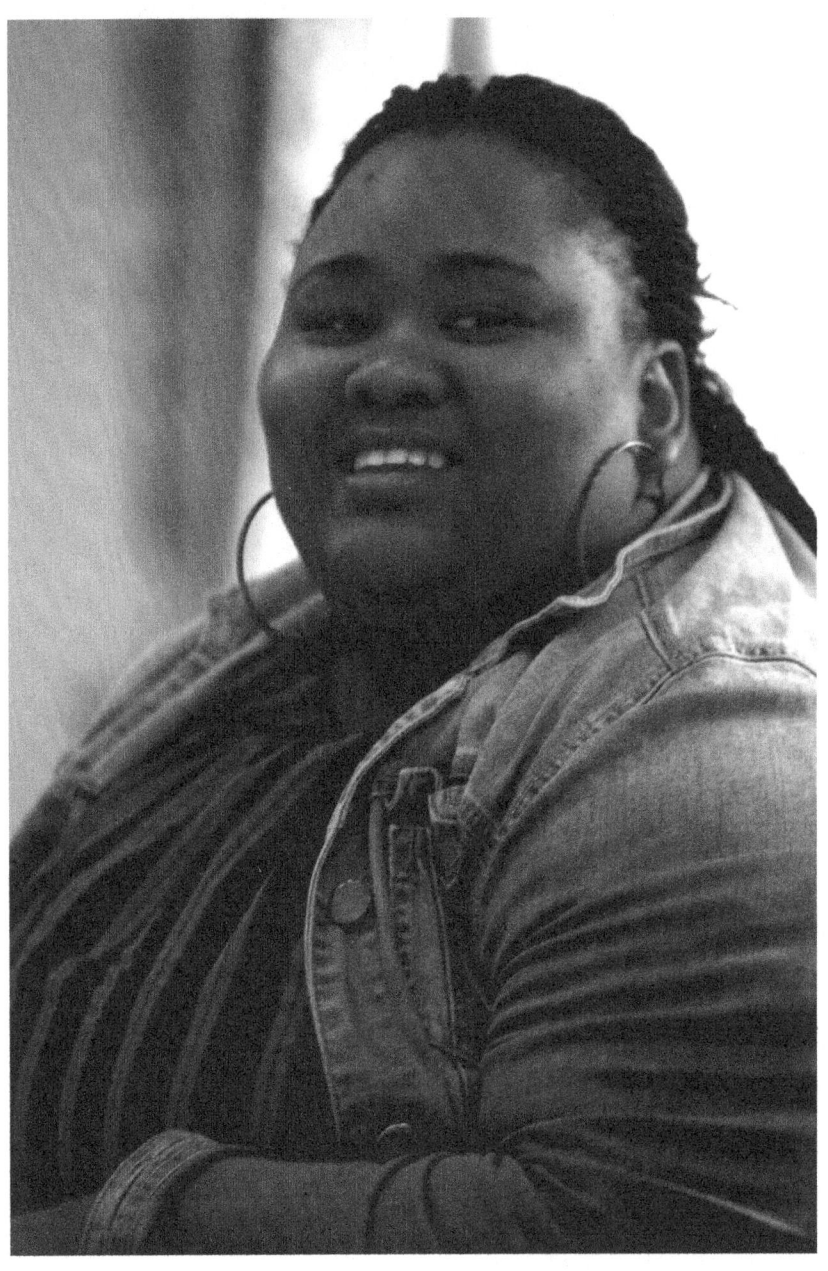

Photographer: Eugene Arries

# 7

# Lindeka Cynthia Rwida Joka

As a teenager, Linkeka was grounded and caring with deep empathy for those around her. Lindeka missed the first series of workshops that were held at the Centre for the Book and the Getting the Word Out symposium. Yet, she was already active in the Treatment Action Campaign in Khayelitsha then and was well connected to some of the other group members like Mandla, KK, Mphumzi, Bridgette and Thozzi. It was through those connections that she joined the In My Life writing workshop at the Centre for the Book in 2003. From then on, Lindeka was an active and committed member of the group.

Lindeka's writing struck us from the beginning as expressive and honest, as did her commitment to activism. She has continued to keep a writing practice over the years and talks about the importance of writing in her life. She was also active in the participatory video-making workshops over the years, both for the *Facing the Truth* and the *Street Fear* videos. Lindeka was technically skilled behind the camera, as well as being an excellent interviewer. She flourished in these projects and has said over the years how meaningful it was to her life's journey to get out of the township and to explore her creative side.

Now a mother of two children and a graduate with a degree in nursing from the University of the Western Cape, Lindeka has always been a leader and caregiver in the group. In many ways, she has been part of the glue that kept us all together. For her, the creative element of the research work we did together, combined with her passion for making a difference in the world, is a vital ingredient to instilling hope for the future and sparking young people towards real and significant social change.

Lindeka continues to do the work on HIV that she started as a young woman, now as a clinic manager at the City of Cape Town Health Department. She often says it was the creative experiences she had as a teenager that set her on her current path.

# 2003

*Lindeka at 17*
Excerpts from *In My Life*

I am Lindeka Cynthia Rwida. I am 17 years old and I live in Khayelitsha.

I am doing matric at Harold Cressy High School in Cape Town. I have many friends who adore me as much as I adore them. I love learning new things especially when it's fun and informative at the same time. I thrive on challenges.

I am an AIDS activist and I'm proud of it. I became an AIDS activist because I wanted to change a bad experience into something good.

Unlike some teenagers my age, I am too busy for drugs and night clubs. I can say that I am safe for many things because I don't do everything my friends do. If I know it is wrong, I will tell them and I won't do it. I do go to the occasional birthday party but if alcohol is available, I won't touch it. People say you must live life to the fullest and I couldn't agree with them more. If you do drugs, you are not living your life to the fullest – you will die before you get anywhere in life.

I would like to write the kind of books and poetry that everyone wants to read. I want to develop words or important sayings that will affect people in many ways. When I talk to people or say a speech, I often quote other people's words. I'd love to write something that the president would quote someday and say, 'I want to end my speech with these words from Cynthia Rwida, a famous writer.'

I don't want to limit my writing. I'd like to write about anything from my saddest moments to my happiest moments.

## AIDS

*I've always seen it from a distance*
*It's always been too far to affect me*
*It's always been someone else's problem*
*I've never even had to think of it*

*I don't even care about it*
*It never existed in my happy little world*
*My perfect world where everyone was happy*
*Where no one was sick*

*One day like thunder*
*It came knocking at my door*
*In the form of thin sick girl*
*It was death walking on two feet*

*It was someone I knew*
*She turned my world upside down*
*My wrongs into rights*
*My happiness into sadness*

*I wanted to keep her away*
*but I wanted to hug her too*
*I wanted to pretend it was a dream*
*But it was all too real*

*I wanted her to blend into my world*
*But she stuck out like a sore thumb*
*She was always sick and always crying*
*She was so fragile*

*She joked about it while we pretended to laugh*
*She called it Joburg's Curse*
*Every time she spoke*
*All I could think of was that she was going to die*

*Lindeka Cynthia Rwida Joka*

*I will never forgive AIDS*
*That's what I thought as I heard her crying*
*in the middle of the night*
*The pain ripped my heart apart*
*All because of AIDS*

*She was so innocent*
*She did not deserve it, no one does*
*It is so unfair*
*I hate it.*

### IN MY NEIGHBOURHOOD

I usually wake up late on weekends so I already hear children playing outside. Inside the house I always wake up with the sound of running water because my room is near the bathroom and my mother is usually doing the week's washing. If my brother is up before me he will turn on the music loud to remind me that it is late to be still sleeping. When my cousin used to stay with us, I was woken by the baby's crying.

On Sundays I wake up and do my washing. I see people going to church and my mother wearing her blue-and-white uniform going to her funeral or savings club with the other women. There are always traditional ceremonies on weekends and the smell of African beer and sheep dung is always in the air. There is one lady I always look out for. On Sundays she always wears one colour, like she will wear everything pink this Sunday and some other colour the next. We cook dinner early on Sundays, and we always have visitors over. My mother's friends from church come over for lunch or my cousins and their parents. I think it's tradition or some ritual that the house must be clean on Sunday, so we spend the whole day cooking and cleaning.

At night too when I switch off the light in my room to sleep, I hear the sound of dogs barking and gunshots from far away. I also hear the sounds of crickets and other noisy bugs. But what I hear before I sleep is the sound of my radio next to my bed. When I sleep early my brother is still sitting in the living room watching TV so I listen to that and try to make out what the people are saying. My parents like to have late-night conversations, talking about what happened that day.

The people in my neighbourhood are very friendly, they will always greet you if they haven't seen you that day. If they're going to church, they will invite you to their church if you're not doing anything. If they have children your age and they are going out, they will invite you to join them. If they're having a party or a traditional ceremony, they will personally go or send invitation cards to everybody to invite them. I love the women of the neighbourhood because of how they stick together during everything, and when there is a death in the neighbourhood everyone will go there to send their condolences.

## WHEN AIDS CAME KNOCKING AT MY DOOR

One day, when I came home from school, my mother told me that my cousin from the Eastern Cape was very sick, and she was going to come and stay with us at the end of the month. I knew that the reason was that there is better hospital care here in Cape Town than on the farms. I didn't put this to mind because I expected my cousin to have some odd sickness but the doctors would give her a cure for, and that we were going to have fun after that.

When the end of the month was close, I started thinking of the good times we have had in the past. I had not seen her in a while and I missed her very much. I remembered her as a little plump and very light in skin colour. I remembered how I used to style her hair for her and that it was very long and beautiful.

Finally, the day came. I was the first, wanting to hear the sound of the bus outside. She was not alone; she was with her sister and her baby. I was shocked when I saw her. She was thin, dark and her hair was shaved off. She looked like a man and her lips were very pink and her skin was strangely dry. She could not even walk, but had to be carried from the bus to the bedroom. That morning was very confusing. I had not even known she had a four-month-old baby, which she now could not even hold because she was sick.

Everyone was hugging and kissing each other and when I came to her, I was scared to kiss her because her lips looked like they hurt. Later that day my mother served mielie pap, my cousin called me to the bedroom and begged me to eat her pap because she had no appetite. I refused, and I told my mother, who made her eat it.

That night I could not sleep. I kept thinking about her and how she got sick. I was told that she went to Joburg the year before, to look for a job. She had come back with the baby and she was already sick.

Her sister left the next week to go back home with the baby and left my cousin with us. She was due at the hospital the following Monday and I was curious about what the doctor would say.

I could not concentrate that day at school because I was worried about her. When I came home from school they were already back from the hospital and she was sleeping. I saw no change in her, and she was coughing non-stop. My mother told me she had TB but I could not understand because I knew that TB was an illness of the lungs and I thought it only affected people who smoked. No one explained this to me because they were also clueless.

She was given a lot of pills and she said to me that it hurt to swallow them. Her next appointment was the following Monday at the same hospital in Khayelitsha and of course my mother would take her there. The trips to the hospital are very difficult because she could not walk on her own. My mother had to pay taxis to take her from the house to the hospital which was very near. On days when she could not get transport, she had to walk a few steps and rest along the way.

The next Monday, I got through school fine because I thought if nothing went wrong the first time she went to the hospital, nothing would go wrong this time too. When I got home my mother was sleeping and my cousin was not there. I was too afraid to ask where she was so I said nothing and went out. When I came back, I was told that she had pneumonia and had been transferred to Tygerberg Hospital and would be kept there under observation.

She stayed there for two weeks and when she came back, she had gained her appetite and she was eating healthily. Everything seemed better from then, and she wasn't so thin anymore. We shared a bedroom and since she could not walk to the bathroom, we kept a small bucket under her bed for her to use. One night I got up from my bed and went to the bathroom, when I came back, she asked me why I didn't use her bucket instead of walking to the toilet and I said I would remember next time.

The following week she was due at the hospital to get results for a test she took the week before. The day when I came from school my mother was not home and my cousin was alone at home. I asked her how things went at the hospital and she just cried. I asked nothing else, and just left her alone. Later that day my mother told me that I should not use the bucket under her bed because she had AIDS and it might infect me. That night I could not get a wink of sleep and I could hear her crying and I could not blame her because I was also shocked. I felt that something was wrong with the way my mother told me this and that it was not her place to tell me.

My feelings and actions changed totally after I heard the news. For a while I could not look her in the face. The fact that I did not have any information about AIDS did not help the situation. Then I started reading everything I saw that had the AIDS ribbon on it and I started listening to AIDS programmes on television.

When my cousin was fit enough to walk on her own, she started attending support groups and became more informed and confident about her status. I wanted to go with my cousin to her support groups. She told me that she was not ready for that yet. She had joined the Treatment Action Campaign in 2001 and she took me with her on June 16 to a rally they had. I enjoyed myself and learned so much. Every bit of information I received, I brought it back home with me to educate everyone.

**This is a true story and I am the narrator of this story.**

When my mother started separating and marking my cousin's dishes and telling us that we should not use them because they were for my cousin only, I told my mother that she was wrong to isolate her like that and that I had read that AIDS does not spread that way, and she actually listened to me.

I am glad my cousin came to our house. Because of her I gained so much knowledge and I became so much wiser. Ever since then I knew that I should not discriminate against people who are HIV positive. This was a real eye-opener and I can now make sure that I don't get

*Lindeka Cynthia Rwida Joka*

infected by this virus, and I know how to protect and care for those around me.

This is a true story and I am the narrator of this story.

# 2004

### *Lindeka at 18*
*Street Fear* video project
Cape Town

When I started in this project, I thought I might do some interviews or help with the ideas, but I can't believe how much I enjoyed being behind the camera. I never thought I could do something like that.

# 2006

### *Lindeka at 20*
Individual interview
Khayelitsha

My name is Lindeka Rwida, I'm 20 years old right now. I live in Khayelitsha, Little Bank. When I was with you the last time during *In My Life*, I was in matric. After that I worked for a couple months then I went to school last year. I did a diploma in marketing, which I'm going to finish next year. This year I'm doing an internship with Shoprite. I am working as a cashier.

At home here, first there were four of us. My mother, my father and my younger brother. But now my brother lives in Waterfront. Now it's just me, my mom and my dad.

There were impacts left from being part of the projects we did together, definitely. The information we were giving each other. I'm wiser now and I've grown up. I can make wise decisions now about my life and I'm still interested in the topic of HIV and AIDS. I also like to write about it as well.

I've stopped now, but I was trying to write a mini novel or something. Not particularly my life, but everything that goes on around me. I've stopped now. I got writer's block or something.

It was a story about a girl. She comes from this Khayelitsha family who become poor just like that. She has to adjust to being poor, and having new friends, not going to the same school she used to. In the surroundings is a little bit of HIV, like her new friends, the issues they're struggling with. It's about how she adjusts.

Actually, I wanted to write poetry but it turned longer and longer so I decided to turn it into a story. Right now, I just don't have the time now and I'm running out of ideas. But I'm going to continue.

I think I'll always be an AIDS activist, even though I don't have time to go to events or workshops or whatever. I'll always be an activist. It'll never change.

There are challenges now because, you used to be inspired when you were in school by the groups. Now that I am working and there's no groups at the workplace, like HIV/AIDS groups. We used to be together as friends, the activists. Now we're separate. Everybody's doing their own thing, now you are left alone. So, it's not the same.

All of the activists in the community who were with me have now moved away.

My friend Barbara she went to live with her other family in Site B. Bridgette she stays in Harare but most of the time she's in Constantia where her mother works.

Being involved in those groups influenced my sexual behaviour. Like I said earlier, I'm making wiser choices now. I have a lot of information and anything wrong that I do, would be an informed decision. Like, I recently went for an HIV test, which I was scared to do but actually I'm negative. I'm proud, and I'm going to keep it that way.

We talk about getting tested all the time with my friends, but some of them are scared. I try to encourage them the whole time but it has to be you, and you need to be ready.

There are a lot of challenges, but you have to know why you want to practice safe sex and not just say I want to use a condom. You have to know why you want to use it, and try to convince your partner as well.

It's very hard to convince the partner at times, but as I said you have to know what you're talking about. That's what helped. The activism helped me. To know the myths from the facts, and to know how to convince someone else.

More people are coming out with their status; that I see has changed. There is a lot of information now. Everybody is doing their own thing and making informed choices. At first it was because of lack of information, but now I think there is a lot of information and people know how to come out status free. It's just a shame that more people are getting infected every day. I don't know how you can prevent that though. Everybody knows about it now.

People are also admitting to being positive now.

I think the difficulties we had, and I think we still have now, is the age gap, actually the information gap, between the parents and teenagers. I think if there was some way to convince the parents to talk about it, to talk to their children, that would have been a great help. I don't know how we can bridge that gap. I don't have any ideas about that.

Otherwise, nothing negative I can think of about the projects we did together. It was really nice projects, and I think we made a major impact with those videos and books.

My goals haven't changed. They haven't at all. Actually, if you were to tell me right now that there was this new project, I would jump in. I've been missing the guys and all the work we did.

Everybody is doing their own thing right now, I'm not sure what the other guys are doing but everybody is busy with their own lives. When you come, you like, bring us all together. So, I think we need your help, some way, somehow.

# 2018

*Lindeka at 32*
Group discussion
Centre for the Book

Relationships. So, I've been through a lot. I've been through a lot and a lot has changed. I've come far to be where I am today. Let me draw you a picture from where I was back then. Seventeen years old. I was in high school. And didn't really know much. From then on, I didn't go straight to varsity. I worked a little bit. I worked in retail, worked everywhere, organisations. But I had demons that I was fighting that I would escape.

Like most of us, I'm sure, I was under the influence of one of the top demons, alcohol. It kind of flows into, fits into, relationships. You start as experimenting with a little bit of alcohol, and then you find that you have an unhealthy relationship with it where, instead of using it for what it's made for (because wine is a celebratory drink) you end up using it to hide. You're hiding from people, hiding from yourself, hiding from your environment.

It was such a relationship that I had, where I wasn't happy with the way I was, or who I was, and then I used alcohol as an escape for a couple of years. I really didn't start at a young age with alcohol. I think I was about 19 or 20 years old. I think it stemmed from having a father that abused alcohol. That's one of the things you tell yourself.

I remember this one day, I think I was walking with Bridgette in my area. We were walking home from my house. We saw this old man who was so drunk. He was staggering and leaning onto stuff. It was just starting to be dark and he almost fell over. But luckily there was this shack or something that he held onto. Then as you came closer, we were looking, actually we were laughing at him, from a distance. And then when we came closer, we were like, 'Oh my god. This is my father.' Yeah. So, that was one of the things I said. I will never, ever put alcohol into my mouth. I detested, I hated him. Come varsity, there I am with the bottle.

It brings out such a character in you that you didn't even know. Especially when you're this inexperienced teen that's going in there to this world of freedom. Because once you stay on campus, you don't have parents any more, all inhibition is lost and you're just free.

That's the way relationships came in. We were laughing about ... what were you saying ... [to Bridgette] something about past boyfriends or something, and you said you had one guy and I was at like twelve guys! Yeah, so, I shut up then.

I found that with that alcohol came a lot more things where there was no inhibition. Sex was in the mix there. Reckless living. That's where I think my background in HIV helped, because comparing myself to other people my age, or people that have my background, I think being here definitely helped because I went through that stage of multiple partners. I went through that stage of reckless alcohol abusing, but safety was always first.

> Being that wild daughter that I was to my mother, now, it's like karma, I now have a daughter.

Even being in the HIV field, like we were, the thing that pushed me into it was having an HIV-positive cousin come and stay with us. I think that's where my story in the book *In My Life* came from. Because HIV, we knew about it, but it was always there, far away, until someone in your family tested positive and it affects you in that way. That's where my curiosity around it came from, and where I wanted to find out more.

At the back of my mind, whatever I was doing, drunk or sober, I kept thinking, I don't want to, I'm not going to, be infected. I don't want to expose myself in that way. Relationships for me were very much unhealthy.

I was also facing body shame issues. I remember at one stage I tried to commit suicide because of just one thing my mother said. Actually, I still believe that suicide is quite selfish, because you are going to kill yourself because of someone else. You're going to write that note and leave it there. You die. Whatever happens to you after death. But what about the people that you leave behind? That person's name that you mention in that note, that 'I killed myself because Mathew said this…' How are they going to live with themselves?

I think it was a Sunday morning. My mother said something to the likes of, 'I wish you were like your cousin, like, not so big. I wish you were …' something like that … 'tinier'. Yeah, so, she didn't know the impact of what she said. She left to go to a church meeting. I went straight to her bag, took every pill that she had in there. I drank down all of them, and then I went to go sleep. She came back hours later. I remember hearing her coming in. I'm like, 'Why am I still alive? Why can I still hear her coming in?' I tried to stand up and immediately when I stood up, I started vomiting. Everything came out. Everything came out.

I didn't even need to go to the hospital. She asked me why was I vomiting and I told her 'I drank every tablet you had in there.' Later on, I found out that that would have killed her more than me. Because she was blaming herself, she was regretting everything she ever did, she ever said.

Yeah. So relationships. But our relationship improved from there.

And then, another scary part in relationships is having a daughter myself. Being that wild daughter that I was to my mother, now, it's like karma, I now have a daughter. I have a five-year-old. She's turning six next week. What do I teach her? What do I say to her? What do I want her to know? How do I mould her into this powerful woman? What do I wish my mother said to me or taught me? Yeah. I think that's one of my big responsibilities now. I'm trying to nurture that relationship and mould a powerful, bold woman out of her. I think that's my blank canvas. Where I can either break or make her, I think. Relationships!

And then I got married. I married a nice man. Being that wild child that I was, and seeing the pattern of boyfriends that I was having. Very destructive. I married the opposite. He's a down-to-earth, serious man. He's four years older than me. He grounds me so much. I can say, a side effect of my past, that I wanted to change so much.

I got that change.

They say the pattern that you have, you attract the person in your spirit. Like I would have someone that I attract. It's not just meeting, like falling in love, at first sight. Some of who you attract, and your friends, are a reflection of who you are. Yeah, so I think it's just what I needed in my life at the time and then I got it.

# 2018

*Lindeka at 32*
Individual interview
Khayelitsha

I'm Cynthia Lindeka Joka, previously Rwida. I am now 32 years old. I was part of *In My Life*, the book, and I was also part of *Fire & Hope*, the short film, and the part of making the video *Street Fear* with other girls, that video I shot back then. And I was also part of making the *Facing the Truth* video.

As a teen I was involved with TAC, the Treatment Action Campaign. I was an AIDS activist and also peer educator along the line. I was also part of LoveLife where they helped us to start an AIDS activist group at my school.

The things that I can look back to in the project was how I started with the HIV field. I had a cousin of mine come stay with us, like I wrote in the book, *In My Life*. I was 16 at that time.

Back then I basically knew nothing about HIV, or just heard about it on TV, but it was always something so far away. And then here comes a cousin of mine to come stay with us. She was sick obviously. She had the virus, and then I was so curious about it. She would attend social support groups.

That's the way I got to accompany her to TAC. That's where I first learned about HIV.

They were giving workshops and informing us about HIV, so that I became really interested in that. From the group there, the TAC teens group, we were taken to go participate in the Fire & Hope project with you, Shannon.

That's when I remember us having to explore our inside stories, and to put them down on paper. Something that really stood out for me, because if you were to ask some of the things that we wrote, we wouldn't be able to tell anyone. You couldn't voice them out. But once they gave a pen and paper, blank canvas for you to put your thoughts and feelings out. It was really interesting how we were able to. The pen never stopped writing. We were able to pool all our thoughts onto that paper, and how HIV affected us and our lives back then. I think the impact of that project, like I said before, was immense in my life, because I can see that I wouldn't be where I am if not for that. Because all of that information that I got there, I carried with me and I was able to make smart choices because I was educated. I felt empowered to go through my youth and to be where I am today. Yeah.

Now, my life 15 years later: I was in high school at the time so I went to go work a little bit after that. I worked in retail. I worked in the Treatment Action Campaign for a little bit, and then I went back to school to go and study. I studied full-time. I did a nursing degree. I'm now a professional nurse and I went on to do a postgraduate diploma in HIV management.

Right now, I'm acting manager in a small clinic in Crossroads, and I'm also doing the initiation of ARVs to clients and I'm managing their HIV programme right now.

From that point on, that field of HIV just became so interesting that I carried on with it.

I'd like to do more because I see a gap that is there with the youth. As much as HIV was new to us back then, it's still new to some people now. Even with the loads of information that is available out there, there're still a high rate of new infections. And it's still amongst the youth that is more at risk. I think there's still a lot that needs to be done and I want to do more with the youth, so I am involved in the HIV field. I'm a professional now, wanting to do more.

I feel like in my growing up, I was privileged to be part of this project we did together, and it did so much in my life that I want that to carry on. I see its need and I know what it did for me. I see that the youth out there, they use information like I'm saying, but they are still uninformed, they're making stupid unplanned decisions. Spur of the moment. They need to be kept busy with something like this. They've got all this pent-up energy that they don't know where to direct it to. You see them experimenting with alcohol, experimenting with sex, with drugs, gangsterism. That is all the youth, with bright minds that need to be put some way. They need to be directed along a more positive route.

> She was sick obviously. She had the virus, and then I was so curious about it.

What I wish that I could do is to give the skills that I was taught. To pay it forward. To also start a project like what we did. We were talking with the group from *Fire & Hope*, the group that we worked there with *In My Life* as well – Mathew, KK and the others – that we would like to start such a project as well, to be able to pay it forward to the youth that is up and coming. To help them shift their minds to put them to something more creative. Yeah, that is a passion of mine. Something that I'd like to do.

For me, personally, being able to be put in a room together with youth from different backgrounds, different communities and different races was really important. To be put in a room together to find out how much similarities that we have towards each other. Some of us are battling our own demons from our own past, some drug abuse, abusive families, domestic home abuse, depression, mental illness, body self-harm issues, and all these issues. We come from different backgrounds and to be put in this room together, and to actually find the similarities within each other; that is something that stood out for me.

You make life-long friends. We are still friends more than 15 years later. We don't see each other as much as we would like, but we are still friends from that time, because we shared experiences together that will last us a lifetime. So that stood out for me.

Also, the creative writing part of it was really important. We also learned skills. We were dabbling in filmmaking. We were dabbling in filmmaking, where we shot some videos. We had a concept that we carried through, like with the *Street Fear* video, which actually came to life. It's so inspiring to see an idea come to life. And you see it being able to help others. Those are some of the things that stood out for me.

Since you've last seen me, I'm married now. I met a wonderful man. We actually met at university. We got married a year after we met. We've got two children. We've got a daughter together, and his other daughter that came to stay with us. So, we are this happy family. I still have both my parents. My brother was staying overseas for a while and he's back now with this big happy family.

I have had lots of challenges. Self-confidence issues. I struggled a lot with that. I struggled a lot with that.

Now having a daughter, I think that is one of the most wonderful things and also a big challenge. It is sort of a scary thing because having been a wild teenager, you know they say a daughter and a mother will clash at some point. I have such a sweet mother, but when you are teenagers, you hate all parents and you want things to go your way, and then you want to experiment with things. I think I now have a chance with my daughter too. To show her things that I wished I had been shown by my parents, and to teach her things that I wish I had been taught. Because growing up especially in a black family or township, some topics are taboo. You don't even touch, you don't even go near, some topics. I think that's where you have an opportunity now when you are a mother yourself, to be different, to try out many other ways.

You'll find that when you grow up, I wish that my mother had told me this. I wish that my parents taught me this and this. Now you have an opportunity yourself to actually do that for your child. You have an opportunity to shape her, to mould her, to be a powerful woman. To guide her away from the mistakes that you made growing up. Because you have insight and you have experience.

Sex is the one big issue I'd like to teach her about, because otherwise you find out from friends like I did. It would be nice if you could first be introduced to it at all from your mother. And then when you go out there, you're already making informed choices. You know what you want. You know what you don't want.

And also, self-confidence. Being told that you are beautiful, no matter what. That it's not a guy that comes around to tell you that you are beautiful. That you believe immediately that person when they say that. If maybe you grow up hearing it, maybe you believe it. Maybe you're more confident when you go out to the world. Stuff like that.

⁂

We are the ones that were given those opportunities. We are the ones that were given that chance, that information. Now we need to give it to the youth, because it mustn't stop with us. What was the point if you are given something and it makes you successful, it works for you, and then you don't give it to the next person? It stops with you. Which means, what was the point?

The rich guys in Khayelitsha and everywhere else; no one wants to share their method, no one wants to share their success. How did I get it? How can I help someone else to get it? If it made me rich, I keep it to myself. I don't need to help another person. But that's what is needed because we are the generation that was, I couldn't say, was saved from HIV infection. So, what worked for us? How come we now can go confidently to have an HIV test and have it become negative? What was different with us?

I think that's what we need to relay to the youth, to share with them. Because it really can't stop with us. And it has stopped with us if we don't do anything. That means it has stopped with us now because we are already seeing it with younger brothers and sisters. What's happening with them, they are falling into that same trap that we were saved from. I think we need to let it continue.

I can say the government isn't really into prevention strategies anymore. At that time, treatment was still new. In 2001–2000 treatment was still new, so they were focusing on prevention methods. Now it has all been about treatment. All the Global Funds and other funding, they all want to fund treatment.

Who's doing the prevention now? At Stellenbosch University where I was, my professor, Jan DeToit, retired with our graduating year. He was saying that they lost their funding around teaching prevention.

No one is focusing on prevention anymore. There still is a need for prevention because not everyone is HIV positive. Not everyone is positive, and we don't need everyone to be positive. I think even government's focus has shifted now into treatment and funders are exhausted now because they've been on treatment, and no one is doing prevention.

I think that the pharmaceutical companies are the ones benefiting now. You see. They are making money now. It isn't just about condoms. Condoms are everywhere. There are lots of condoms. I can't say there's a shortage of those. Maybe in some remote areas we still need to get them to reach there, but condoms are more than available now. It is not the only prevention strategy.

I think we need to focus more on prevention, especially with an understanding of consent.

I don't even think there are still HIV test teams in schools anymore.

I think that we just assume that the information is out there for everyone. But why is the infection rate still so high? And why is it still amongst the youth?

I think government did a great service in getting rid of mother-to-child transmission. In that sense, it has done a great job. But now there still are new infections. What are we doing towards that?

I don't think the issues are very different now than they were when we were young.

Some issues have always been there, like drugs. It has always been there. But now I think it's worse because the unemployment is also so, so much. I think now, because of the high unemployment, good guys are actually not doing so well, and then the bad guys – the drug dealers, the gangsters – they are the ones driving the flashy cars. They are the ones owning the big houses, and they are looking more attractive to the youth. Even if the youth do know that it is wrong, this guy looks more attractive than the other one. More attractive than that guy who carries a bag to work every day. He works all his life. He works hard but he doesn't have anything to show for it. The good guy who sits at home, he doesn't want to do crime but is unemployed. And what does that get him. But the one who is given a bag of drugs to go sell at school, they are driving flashy cars. They're wearing expensive clothes. I think that was existing even in our time, but now I think it's even worse. It's on steroids.

> I think we need to focus more on prevention, especially with an understanding of consent.

I think it's still the same issues, but social media has poured fuel on that fire. On social media, everything is easy now. Everything is painted colourful and bright and attractive. So even the bad things, they look attractive.

Still, I think that the future is looking bright. I think it is looking bright.

I don't know if it's feminists or women empowerment that gives me the most hope. I think we are rising towards that. A lot of women are in business. A lot of women are feeling empowered and positive about the girl child. I think there's lots of opportunities for girls now. Everybody,

*Lindeka Cynthia Rwida Joka* 133

like the women in business, they are giving back to girl children. Look at that Oprah Winfrey School for Girls. I think they are doing great strides. I think more schools need to be like that where they're not only teaching the curriculum, but also grooming strong and positive young women.

I think children of today they have such bright minds. They need to be put to good use. That is one of the positives.

We need a youth camp where we can have this group, like we had, where we can fill them with all this positivity. Take them away from everything. Fill them with ideas. Give them hope for a bright future so that they go back to their homes. They spread it to others, that they could share that drive to be something better in life.

I think that's how we can change South Africa, through the youth.

# 2022

*Lindeka at 36*
Personal writing

## DEEPEST, INNERMOST THOUGHTS ON PAPER

I keep my feelings inside so much over the last 25–30 years that I don't know how to communicate anymore. If I have to talk about anything re feelings, I choke on the lump in my throat, tears fill my eyes, and I end up saying 'I'm fine'. Angry, sad, disappointed? I cannot express these feelings. I've become so good at being silent that people have stopped asking if I'm fine or not. The few times that I have tried to express myself did not go very well; the other person listening but not hearing me, they come to their own conclusions and give a solution that does not work for me, but I just smile and say ok, and let my life move on. When I was 16 years old, I argued with my mom and felt attacked so I overdosed on her pain and hypertension tablets. It didn't work because I changed my mind.

I'm not sure why but I carry around a lot of guilt, like I'm not good enough as a wife, that I'm not a good enough mother or that I haven't done enough for my parents. I feel like in my life and work, I am just on autopilot. Like my life will happen the way it does whether

I participate or not, that the decisions I make, or made are for others not for me. I may understand their benefits in the future but right now I gain nothing. I'm not happy and I'm uninvolved. I can't remember a time where I made a choice/decision for me or about me that I didn't have to defend or explain or justify to anyone. I sometimes feel judged for my choices before I even make them so I don't, I just let things be or I just agree to the 'politically' correct one or go with the flow.

I feel like crying all the time. I feel like I'm hanging off a cliff and if I let go, everything will fall apart. I feel like I'm wearing a tight rubber band around my head and some days I can't feel it and other days it's so tight I can't breathe. I want to be alone in a quiet place all the time, then I feel guilty when I think of those around me. I've become so good at pretending I'm fine that I don't know when I'm really happy. Nothing is making me unhappy, I just am. I feel like I know what to do to be happy but there are too many things stopping me. I just lose interest and energy just in thinking about it. I walk around with a lump in my throat hundred per cent of the time that I need food, water, cool drink, and basically, I use everything to push it down. I love my family, friends and everyone around me but sometimes I just want to be alone.

I feel like my mind is always occupied, it's never quiet. I feel like I don't sleep enough although sometimes it may seem like I sleep a lot. I don't remember a time when I woke up because I was done sleeping or that I slept enough. I'm always woken up by someone or something, it's not always external. Sometimes my own mind wakes me up with obligations that await me. I feel like my days are too short, not enough hours, I get overwhelmed by a lot of responsibilities, home and work. Not that I have more work than anyone else, just that I lose time while at home or at work. I would sit and think then realise that an hour went by or two hours, and I know I have things to do but it's like I'm stuck or paralysed by my overactive mind or the number of responsibilities I have that I end up not doing any of them or not finishing them.

I feel sometimes like I'm a bystander, watching my life go by like a movie.

I will sometimes be on the way somewhere and the last thing I remember would be starting the car then I find that I have reached my destination. I drove safely but I was checked-out. I thank god for His Mercy to make me drive safely. I sometimes come into work, get into my office and shut the door. I will realise the time is 11:00. Three hours later and I have done nothing but sit on my chair and open the PC. I will go through emails and answer calls but on autopilot. Then it would be home time, and I would leave so tired, in fact exhausted, from my mind to my body. I cannot talk to anyone about my feelings, mainly because I'm scared of the response and also, I may not like the solutions I get and that also becomes another burden I have to deal with.

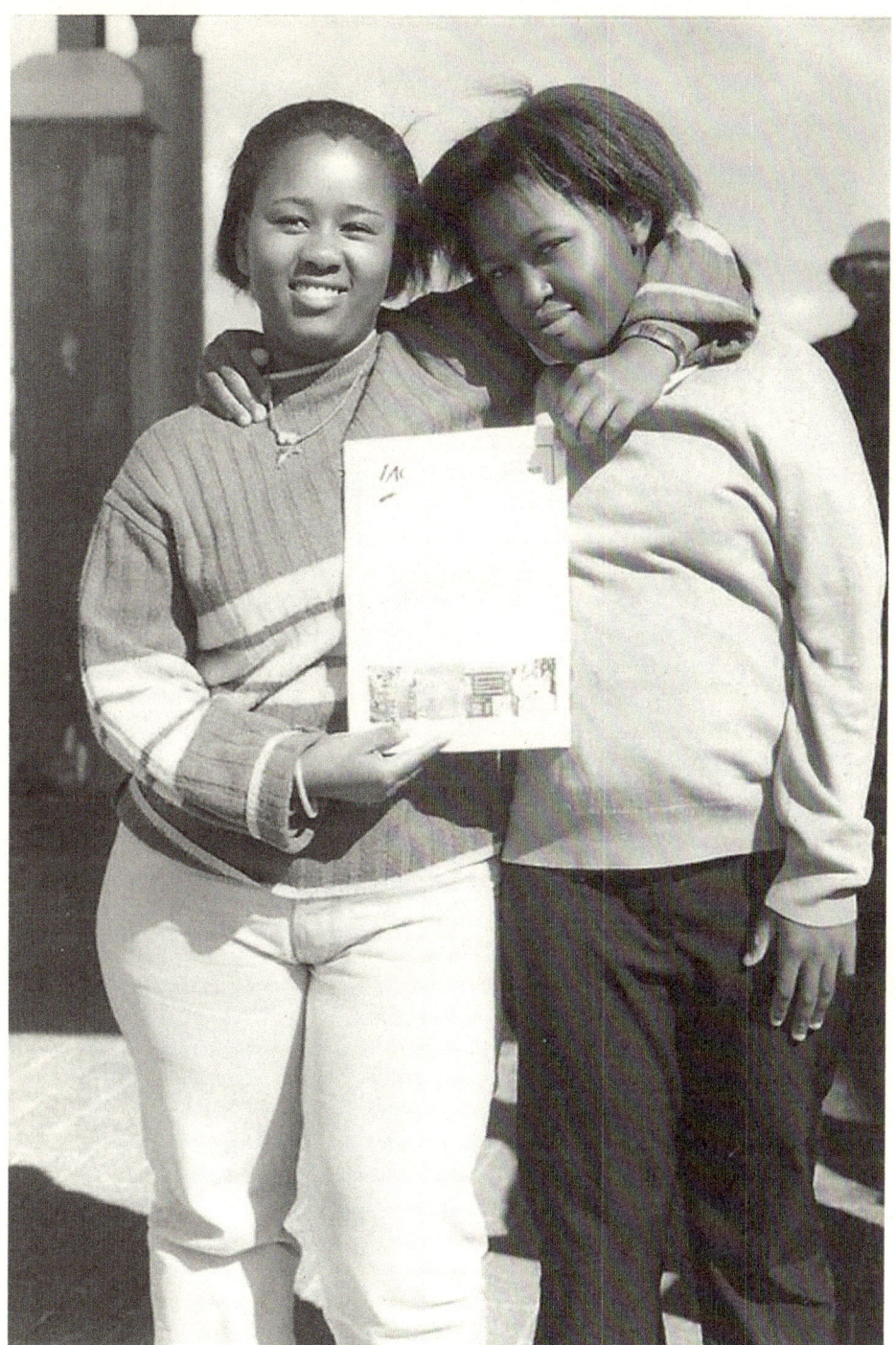

*Lindeka and Bridgette pose with a TAC flyer, 2000*

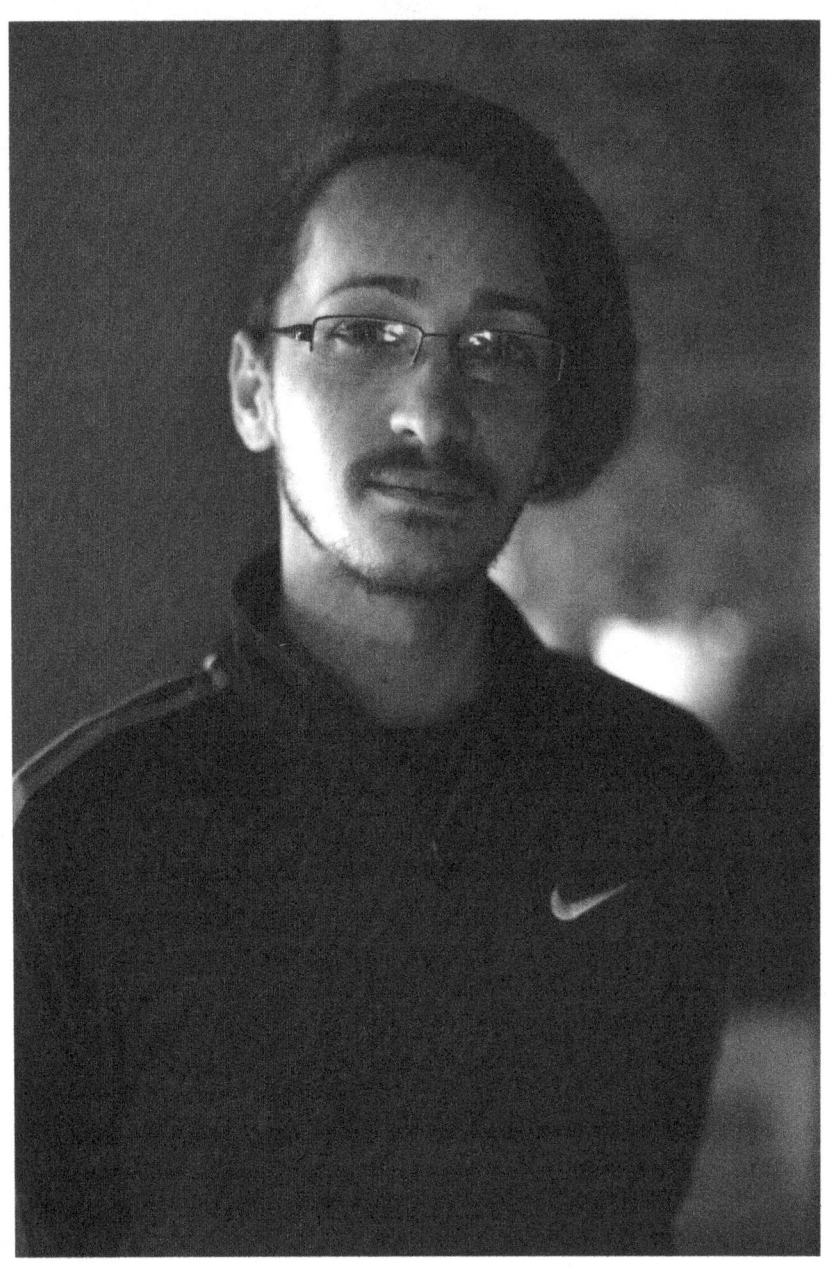

Photographer: Eugene Arries

# 8

# Mathew Johannes

FROM THE BEGINNING, MATHEW was open and curious about other young people and cultures in the divide of South African society. He has been involved with every phase of the project from day one, including participating in the short documentary *Fire & Hope*.

As a high school student in Atlantis, Mathew was already active in his school and community. The son of a car mechanic, he had grown up in a masculine, and often violent, gang environment in Atlantis. In the workshops we did together, he was persistent in exploring questions about gender identity and sexuality, and was performative in his approach towards creative work. Coming out as gay in the environment in which he lived was not easy, but he felt that it was essential to live in his own truth. Mathew managed to go to university at Stellenbosch, but the environment made him all too aware of his identity as a coloured South African in a sea of white Afrikaans speakers. He studied biological sciences and began actively pursuing ballroom dancing as a hobby. He was competitive and excelled as a dancer and was soon winning awards. Tragedy struck when Mathew lost two siblings to violence; one was stabbed and the other was killed in a car accident involving the police. Things could have gone awry, but Mathew persevered, and has always been ready to learn, adapt and grow. As a young adult, he became involved in the drag community in Cape Town and created his drag persona, Eva Torez. In 2011, Eva/Mathew starred in the feature documentary by Lauren Beukes, *Glitterboys & Ganglands*, where he competed for the title of Miss Gay Western Cape.

Mathew sees this phase of his life as a continuation of his activism in following the trailblazers from his own community who pushed against stereotypes and norms. For the moment, he no longer competes in drag, and identifies as non-binary. Mathew has applied his creative skills to becoming a dance instructor, training others from his community in self-expression. His life has been through many ups and downs, but through it all, Mathew remains committed to being the voice for change even as the focus of his activism has shifted over his life journey.

# 2003

*Mathew at 17*
Excerpts from *In My life*

I am Mathew, 17 years old, and I live in a small town called Atlantis. I am a Grade 12 learner at Atlantis Secondary. I am a fun-loving, 'forever late' guy who is in love with being a student. I love to participate in anything the school has to offer me – except sport! I simply love drama, acting, reading, going on workshops and socialising with friends. I love listening to all kinds of music, especially rock, all the time. I also enjoy being alone, and am always trying to improve every aspect of myself. I remember how it was to be lonely. I remember how it was to feel rejected, an outcast. I remember fun days in the sun, and the bliss that innocence brings. I hate seeing other people suffering. I dream of a world without AIDS, a world without prejudice. I wish that South Africans would be proud of who they are and work together so that we may overcome all obstacles, including HIV and AIDS.

Once late at night I woke up to the sound of sirens in my street. There had been an accident. A car came around the bend too fast and crashed into a wall. As it hit the curb it shot up in to the air and landed on its roof. The whole neighbourhood was outside in an instant dressed in their pyjamas. We found out that the driver of the car was drunk. He did not get any serious damage. Besides this, my street is pretty boring. Only a few children play outside during the day. Our street has never really seen any real violence such as gunshots or robbery.

When I feel afraid, I get cold shivers. My heart feels like it's beating in my throat. I feel agitated and annoyed by my inability to overcome this phobia. After a while my whole body seems to want to shrivel up and die. I get lame. I can't speak properly and I just feel like going to bed and sleeping, sleeping to get away from this thing.

To feel brave is exhilarating and wonderful. It's a mixture of feelings like happy, proud, strong and yet also afraid. My whole body seems to want to do the impossible. I stand tall. I feel like I rise above my earthly body, undisturbed by the phobias of this earthly realm. I feel like I am on a natural high. It feels so good that I would not exchange it for anything.

The music is thumping. I'm sitting alone in my room. With nothing to do and no one to help. Totally oblivious to all disruptions outside. My time to be with me, myself and I. Bored to the bone. Alone just like I was for nearly all my life, even when I am with my so-called friends and family. Distant, undisturbed, I laze around, waiting for the next day to come and take away the empty feeling.

But something happened to change that. I heard that there was a drama club at our school. I decide to join. In the school hall, the laughter of fellow students eases me into the atmosphere. The drama Miss invites us to come and sit. Hesitantly everyone calms down and pays attention to the teacher. I am the only new pupil to join that day, and feel very nervous, I introduce myself to the group. Then she says that we have to do a play on HIV and AIDS. Most of us do not know much about HIV and AIDS. So, we set out on a mission to find out all we can about this disease.

I am horrified by what I find out. Horrified to see what HIV and AIDS does to people and how many people are affected. Horrified by the idea of what the after-shock will do to my beloved country. When I think of all the AIDS orphans it makes me sad and depressed, and yet also motivated to do my bit in the struggle against HIV and AIDS.

# 2003

*Mathew at 17*
Interview for *Fire & Hope*
Atlantis

I think one of the biggest challenges youth are facing is this whole thing about sexuality; who you are and your sexuality. Should I do it, shouldn't I? The whole subject of sex, they've kind of thrown it in our face, and so now we have to deal with it. And in between that, we still have to find out who we are, too. So, it's like kind of complicated. It complicates life!

'I think we should use a condom', but then, somehow or another he just gets her not to, or says he doesn't have one, or says this one has a hole in it, or says, 'No I'm not going to use this, it's cheap, it's going to break so rather go without…'

You have to be true to yourself because if you are not true to yourself, who can you be true to?

Young people can speak to each other and there are no pretenses. It's not, 'Look, I'm the doctor and I'm telling you everything about AIDS now.' You can speak about it. I think it can be less formal too, as long as each one just has a little information and they can come together and speak about it.

Don't worry too much about the stereotypes. If it's in you, it will come out. Just try and be yourself in everything that you do. Speak about everything. Have an open relationship. Talk, because if you don't talk, no one is going to know what you are feeling.

It's like working with HIV/AIDS in the workshops – everything I have done this far in my life – it has changed and improved me as a person. People at school asked us if we could speak to the standard 6 class and teach them all that we know. So that they can teach it to the next group of students, because we won't be there.

# 2006

*Mathew at 20*
Individual interview
Atlantis

I'm a student at the University of Stellenbosch. I'm currently in 3rd year Bio Genetics. I'm 20 years old soon to be 21.

Right now, I've got this hectic social life. I can't remember the last weekend I could honestly sit down and say I did nothing. Which is, yeah, it's quite taxing. And my studies. But it's been holidays so it's been fabulous. I've just been enjoying the time, but yeah, soon it's going to be back to normal.

I always try to do a lot of community work, but I don't get much time. Since our work together, I did run more workshops at my former high school in Atlantis. We did another one on World AIDS Day last year, as well as clinics and talks in a few primary schools. At the high school we talked the learners through what to expect around sexuality. We've been through the whole thing ourselves, so, just to guide them through and point them to the right direction at least. You have this information, so use it or don't use it.

It takes some work to get to people. Actually, it means doing it again and again because having a workshop with them once is ok, but it's only once. We even had a three-day workshop with them and we were hoping that they would take initiative and continue, but yeah, we couldn't be there all the time because of our studies. We couldn't be there to help them. I didn't hear anything about if they continued.

At university, I started off with just plain molecular biology and then I went down to a bit more into plant bio-technology and finally ended up in genetics. I totally love plants. I prefer working with plants, and you can do much more with plants, it's more hands on and you can see what happens, when like, in one of the practicums we did, we cut pieces of a plant and grew a whole new plant from that.

It's fabulous, the shift from high school to university. There's a total mind shift in lots of ways. I sometimes thought, 'Why do my parents always treat people that have degrees and such differently', or [why do] the people who have degrees, they seem to be different in some way? I've come to realise and appreciate that being in university is not only about academics, it develops your brain. Your whole thought pattern changes, you learn to become more open, at least a little more open, and you perceive stuff quite differently, you're always searching for the bigger picture. Where does this fit in? You don't just take anything and everything for granted; they tell you the sky's blue, you ask 'why is the sky blue?' That is something I love.

I've changed, since the time we spent together. I can't really point to it but there was a shift. I think just becoming more mature in a way.

I started ballroom dancing in my first year. I just started; I didn't dance any time before that. The society I'm at is the social societies. We just earned up to three-bronze level, that is like entry-level competition. At the moment, before you get that, the three-bronze competitive, if you do it socially there's like three other levels… Social 1, 2, 3, 4. So, this year I'm doing bronze now.

I'm doing social competitions. I'm not doing the competitive. One of the most major social competitions we have is Intervarsity, each year in August. I'm looking forward to that. Universities all over South Africa – seven or eight other universities – they come together and each one has their own dance school so we all compete with each other. Stellenbosch has been quite good. We were either first or second in both of the categories. You get one that we call formation. We've got a group of at least five couples on the floor and they have to do whole choreographies and different sequences all incorporated. Each university has to put forward a couple to represent them in a certain dance, like the Jive, Cha Cha, Rumba, Waltz, Foxtrot and so on. I've been on the team since first year, so it's quite nice. Mostly Jive, which I love.

The projects we did together definitely made an impact in my life. I don't think I'll ever forget it, all the experiences. Growing up in Atlantis, you're totally sheltered in this cocoon, this mini world. You don't get exposed to much of the issues.

The youth here, they don't get exposed much to the issues and they're not, how can I say, facilitated. No discussion is promoted between them on issues of life, just like normal everyday life. They don't actually talk about issues, like South Africa and the whole apartheid thing. We're 11 years away now of being free South Africans, but South Africa still has a long way to go and I believe that we should speak about it and get discussions going and find out more and just learn from each other's cultures. It's not promoted here. I've learned to do that.

The workshops that we did, it has given me a few skills. If I'm in company it's much easier for me to bring up those topics and wanting them to discuss, 'what do you think about this?' Even now, just a couple of weeks ago, we had a part in Habitat for Humanity. We organised for underprivileged people, people that can't afford to buy their own houses around here, so Habitat for Humanity gave them a loan and we build the houses for them. They just buy the materials and then pay it off as they can. But at the build, as it was the international build, we got students from Ireland and from Botswana and all of South Africa as well. I appreciated it, because we sat down and we spoke about apartheid and why there are the Irish coming down to the South and between the churches. It was nice talking and seeing their views, how they perceive themselves and which issues are raised and what are you going through, what they're passionate about. It was nice to know.

The project definitely affected my personal development, gave a real boost. As you can notice I'm not a public speaker or somebody who can make connections. I'm not very articulate in that manner. It helped me a lot! In primary school I started to realise this at first and my teacher said that I was an introverted-extrovert. I'm somebody that likes my little close world. As soon as I come into a new environment, I stay in my world and then gradually I'll come out, I let down the walls, and when I let down the walls, I can be quite talkative. That whole experience with the workshops … it allowed me to speak more freely about myself. Speak more freely period.

I feel a definite improvement in my communication skills. I know it feels to me like something I'm still lacking and that's something I can work on. But the workshops came in into a part of my life I really needed. I was seeking self-improvement and to see how I can improve myself. Because being in high school, you come to grade, what was it, ten (or standard eight as we used to call it back in the day) ... When you get to the end of high school you realise, ok, I'm 18. So, I'm not actually good. I was not one for sports, if you can call ballroom a sport, I think it's a sport, but yeah ... I'm not one for sports. I was just looking around and I thought, what makes me different from all these other people? If I was a big boss of a corporation, why would they hire me? Why? What skills do I have, who am I? The workshop just came at the right time and it helped me develop in that way. I think that if I didn't go through that at the workshops, I would have definitely been in a totally different place right now.

Something that I love, when we get off time and all of us are at home, maybe in the weekend me and Danlia, we still sometimes just come here to this little spot, then we just sit in the garden and speak about what is going on in our lives. Besides the social aspect, we talk about issues that we are facing as well, which is so nice. Sometimes I'm in Stellenbosch, the friends that I've created, we don't have that same connection. They all grew up there. It's always nice to come back here and actually discuss something.

The activism and workshops we did made an impact on my sexual behaviour. It made me much more cautious. Now that I think about this, ok, I've been naughty. I know, I've been naughty sometimes. You know, yeah, quite a bit, but, um, yeah. I've learnt... I knocked my head once and said, 'Ok!'. Then all of that knowledge kicks in and I think, 'You were telling people not to do this and this, and now you do it?' It's a hard lesson.

It's like the whole big discussions we had around when is the right time to talk about using condoms. What I've found, it's the state of the moment. Like, you see something is going somewhere, and you just put down and say, this is what I want. I think that I learned from the workshops we did together, and I became more open.

There's a show on the radio called 'Talking Sex', which I really love. Lots of my friends have been known for asking for advice from Doctor Eve. I think she's totally fabulous because it made me much more open to my sexuality, and being ok with the fact that I'm a sexual being. I want to have sex. I'm young and there are always a lot of issues and stuff like that but, yeah, it's normal. You have to have your boundaries and stuff like that.

It's nice because the thing is I realise that some things that I've heard of now and again is that we are told to love, but we are not told how to love. I think going through teenage years, and being a teenager, and trying to find your own concept of what is love, and how to love. It's just like growing up now, like being older, out of school and stuff like that, you get to a point where you more or less have an idea about what you think love is. And now it's more about how do I make it last.

How do you show, like, trust and honesty? All the key elements in relationships. Lots of people perceive stuff differently. If there's honesty, a little fib is ok now and then.

I'm in a relationship now. It's been almost three months. The honeymoon period is definitely drawing to a close there [laughing], but I'm still battling for this one. We'll see. It feels worth it. Just have to see where it can go.

I simply love being single. I just love the freedom. Freedom is ok, but you know these little thoughts like, I want to have romantic outings and I want to have someone to just give a hug. Sometimes, you know, it's exactly at the moment that you're not actually looking for a life partner, but for a friend and companion. I think they're just cool people actually. I think that's all I expect, a friend, companion, somebody you can speak to, confide in; just they should understand you. I know I can be a horrible person to understand. I've got all these little walls and stuff that I put up, yeah.

I'm very open, but you know I'm a Sagittarius. We only allow you to see what we want you to see. It's like we give you a searchlight into who we are. You can only see a certain spot at a certain time. All the rest is dark, and I like it that way.

At one of the workshops they said, you're an expert of being yourself. I was an expert in being a teenager going through high school then. I don't think I would do anything differently because times change. It doesn't matter if it was three, four years ago. Still there is a definite shift and I don't think I would have said anything differently.

I'm still passionate about this whole apartheid thing. What do they think as young adults, us adults should do? Because I'm considering that South Africa is still developing and is still, I think, in its infant stages. South Africa has a lot to grow still and what do they think to get apartheid out of the way. Because apartheid is still here and it irritates me. It irritates me that people are just like, apartheid ended in 1991. It did not! The laws were changed but apartheid is still here. I want to find out what did they think should change?

> South Africa is such a melting pot of culture, we just need to turn up the heat

One thing that I was so surprised about was something that we had a discussion about at some point. I believe that we need to integrate people's living spaces to get people to live together. There are a lot of issues that go with that as well, because we don't want some homogenous country, you know. We still want to keep our diversity, yet we don't want to separate people and stuff. We still have to get the middle ground.

I was so surprised when I saw this coloured girl coming around here with a little black girl. They were running in the back and they were speaking in Zulu or Xhosa together. She was speaking the language like [...] it was her mother tongue. I was so surprised. It was so nice seeing the coloured girl next door ... just sing little Xhosa songs all the time. It was so nice for me. It totally struck me, District 6 or Sophia Town where people were forced to live together, brought the diversity we speak about, and our heritage. It comes from little places like that where people were forced together. Just look at South African music, how it changed. Sophia Town had a huge impact on that.

South Africa is such a melting pot of culture, we just need to turn up the heat, I think.

What is working is that this process is such a slow one, that people take it for granted that this is a slow process. They think that they can just speak to the children now and again about this. But it's a mindset that has to be changed. If you just speak to the people and give them advice [it's not enough]. They need to feel that 'OK, it is my country.' I see a lot of young people, they don't take ownership, saying, 'This is my country'. They're not proud of being South African. I'm proud of being South African. I don't want to be anywhere else. This is my South Africa. I was born here. I love this place. OK I don't know much other places, but I still love it. I have this feeling. I've got this connection with here.

Stellenbosch was the first time I got to know whites. I really didn't have experience with white people, being brought up away from whites. For the first time I actually saw there was even infighting between the whites because there's the English whites and the Afrikaans whites. Ooohh! There was some lovely ... what we would call it ... action, you know. Lovely. Ooohh... Then I just thought, what about the auntie on the street, who stands at the gate to see what is happening down there, because I would be one of those people. Just watching.

The coloureds are a minority at Stellenbosch because the university is an Afrikaans university. Now they're trying to integrate, to become more acceptable, you know, according to the laws and stuff like that, but I don't think they have. Afrikaans is a language and it has its people, both white and coloured, who are predominant Afrikaans speakers. Stellenbosch is trying to get more coloureds into the system, which I think is great, but now the difference is that, they're going to lose. They need more black people as well.

We've got major language policy issues now because there's these lectures that are strictly Afrikaans, only your textbook is English. My first-year chemistry lecturer – I'm not going to mention his name – but he's from the Netherlands. He speaks Afrikaans with that accent and sometime the accents are so thick. I used to go sit right in front in class and I still didn't know what he said. You laugh for the first two months and after you get used to his accent. But for people who didn't grow up with the language it's even more difficult.

I've got a university bursary and that covers most of my costs. Two thirds of it was paid for by the university. It was affirmative action. They come around in high schools and they ask for the top 20 students and then you had access tests. You write two tests, one to see if you can access the university and the next for your ability to study. They are grading you on whether they think you will have good grades in university or not, and they give you a bursary according to that. I don't think I would have gone to university otherwise.

# 2010

### Mathew/Eva at 23
Interview for *Glitterboys & Ganglands*

*In 2010, Mathew/Eva had been in the Lauren Beukes feature documentary* Glitterboys & Ganglands, *which followed a number of contestants who were part of Miss Gay Western Cape, including Mathew. Mathew was a lead character in the documentary.* [See photographs in picture section]

I'm a motor technician. My father is a mechanic and his father did it before him.

When I first started working here, I needed to prove myself, and when they found out I was gay, I had to prove myself even more.

I lost two of my younger siblings very violently. The one got stabbed outside of his house, and a few months after that my little brother was driving on his bicycle on the road, him and his friend, and a police car knocked both of them off their bikes and cracked open his skull. [See photograph in picture section]

# 2011

### Mathew/Eva at 24
Conference panel
Salt Rock

*In 2011 Mathew had transformed into Eva, his drag persona, for our conference. He dressed in drag frequently at that time, including for the panel we held with a public audience. Ahead of his comments on the panel, he showed a clip from the* Glitterboys & Ganglands *documentary.*

Two years ago, I started actually working on this art of drag. It's a form of expression, and I think why I chose to show you guys this.

I'm not always good with public speaking. So why this clip? Just to show that this is a form of art, and a form of expression for me. It is a platform that I would use. I think there are various issues that can be dealt with debate that can be initiated by the drag queen. A well-known drag queen once said, 'As soon as you step outside your door with a pair of heels and a wig you are an activist. Knowingly, or not.'

The thing is, I think after all these years and after these experiences, I could realise and cross with this concept, that this is a platform that I can work from.

In terms of the initial workshops and project, I think it was more about the process.

Everything we were given: we were given a task to make books, a writing schedule and speeches to make, and it wasn't about the speeches or the books or the writing. It was more the process thereof. Sitting down and somebody actually coming to you as a youth and asking, 'How do YOU feel about this?' Giving YOU a platform and opportunity to focus on YOU, and how you are dealing with this. Making that important.

I think that is the greatest thing. Like this, working with the arts. I think that's the greatest benefit. It's not in the result of the product, it's about the process. Because you are sitting there thinking 'How does this really affect me? How do I want to portray this?'

The avenues of thought that projects like these open up are very important. Crime happened in our community, and we were very sheltered. We were isolated. We weren't exposed to the others, to society and other cultures and other thought patterns. It was just what we grew up with and told this is right, and this is everything.

I think doing projects like this, and especially interacting with others from different communities, that interaction around the project helped majorly in opening up other avenues of thought for me as I developed.

*Audience Member: 'I was very interested by what you said when you said, that you feel you are not transgendered, that you use this as a platform to exhibit talent and to express yourself. I wanted to ask you if you feel that because, as you say that this is a platform to express myself, that it allows people to enter into discussions about sexuality or HIV and AIDS or race more easily?'*

I think this is me. Just being here and being in drag. I think that is enough to spark a conversation and interacting with me on a personal level. That is where I feel comfortable, sitting and chatting with you. I mean, me already sitting here in full drag, and just showing that I'm comfortable with who I am. I'm comfortable in expressing myself in this way. And sometimes I find that it does make it easier for people to relate to you.

# 2011

*Mathew/Eva at 24*
Individual interview
Salt Rock

Some of my memories of our project: Not wanting to wait a week until we could all be back together. Kaylene and everyone. Getting back together.

What stays with me the most is the growth that we went through. It was like a little family that we created, growing, and just being there for each other. In a way, the things we did, the thought processes, the discussions we had, that is what stuck. The idea that we are experts at being ourselves.

I think it had a huge impact, because it came in a time of my life where I was really just grasping at straws. I needed something to focus on, and the idea that HIV/AIDS was a major thing, and it still is, and I'm doing my bit and in doing my bit, growing as well. I think that was something exciting.

I am in drag now because I have been doing it for almost two years now. It's been going on for almost two years.

It started as a dare to enter a pageant. Initially to just go to a party, I took up this idea. And then after the party, my friend dared me to do the pageant. Me, thinking it was a one-night thing, agreed, and it turned out to be three months of drag, being in drag every weekend. And it opened up another world for me and I realised how important the drag image, and drag is, in my community.

You are the ones that stick out and people notice you. If there is a message you want to get across you have a better platform because you incite discussion with people. When I walked into where we are now [at the conference in Salt Rock], those guys, they all came and grouped together, and they were looking at me. So, if I was not in drag, I don't think I would have got that response.

I think, coming out in drag, and being out in drag, is really a tool for expressing myself. In that way, I'm also showing that it's ok to be yourself and to express yourself in a way that might not be a social norm.

The thing is, where the Soft Cover project fits in with that, is that I came to understand that process now led to this. I can see it as a platform, because of the way that we took things, like the writing about everyday life experience. The Soft Cover project showed that we can share our experience. It actually means something to some other people.

The stories we wrote, other people could relate to them. That's something that we didn't know. I didn't know that people would actually need to feel that it's ok, and that they needed to relate to somebody else that is going through something similar. Or it is drawn to their attention that, 'Hey, something is happening over here'.

I think that is the biggest things that I take from the Soft Cover project, knowing and coming to feel comfortable with working with different mediums, and not just thinking, standing on a pedestal and saying a speech is the sum total of activism or doing your bit. There is a whole creative process. I am not a painter or poet, but drag is my creative outlet. So, using your individual strengths to do your bit.

I think one of the weaknesses of the project was that I think we could have done more for the ones that fell to the wayside to keep contact with them.

I think that was what made the Soft Cover project such a success in my eyes, and that it was such a great experience because it was not just one snapshot we worked at. It was something that developed over time. We grew as we grew. We grew together, and ... we grew together but apart in the same time.

I think more people could have had the opportunities that we had, and the experiences. I'm just thinking, just that, more attention could have been made to those who fell to the wayside. More attempts. It was sad to lose people.

What I'm doing right now: my life was supposed to become a little quieter now, after what I call drag season. As you move to the effective end of the year and all of the pageants start lining up, and culminating to the goal of Miss Gay Western Cape.

Eva's been keeping me very, very busy. But I'm enjoying it. There's charity gigs we do, doing cabaret, so lip synching as well. So, yeah, the money we raise at events we give to various charities, and even get to get a word in or two about some issues that we face. So that comes in with 'creative emceeing', as I like to call it.

And then, I'm studying part time again. I'm dead set on finishing my degree, even if it takes forever! I am studying part-time by correspondence trying to finish my biochemistry degree from UNISA.

I'm also working with my father. We fix cars. Yeah, it does face you with challenges. It's not always the best, because I think we are so alike that it doesn't work out. We argue constantly. But it's good.

I'm still living in Atlantis. I moved back. I've been living in Atlantis for a year now. Things are OK. It's... It could be better, but I'm not complaining. It was tough; really it was hard, for a few years, definitely. It has been.

# 2018

*Mathew at 32*
Individual interview
Dance Studio, Bellville

I live in Parow now to be close to work in the studio which is based in Bellville. I have been living in and around this area for the last eight years.

What's happening at this moment? Right now, I am just easing my way into the thirties. Focusing on my work and family.

I've noticed that over the years, I have got so caught up in my own little world that family time hasn't been a high priority. So, that is something that is shifted. I spend a lot more time with the family, instead of friends. And it's basically work, which I love, and home. Just keeping busy and trying to make sense of what life is.

I'm in a stage of my life where everything is sort of on a roll and going. It's also because I've been used to a lot of turmoil and things and now it seems like I have to catch up emotionally on the backlog. So, I'm seeing a psychologist weekly. So, at least getting there. Getting to somewhere and making sense of what is happening. What I have to deal with. It's so good, so good.

We are currently in dance class studio. It's a studio that is very close to my heart. I've been working here for five years. I teach Ballroom and Latin predominantly. And then I do some cross training, me being the student, with some capoeira and belly dancing. I tried Hip Hop, but it's way too free. There's freedom in boundaries and hip hop just doesn't give me that.

Studio Good Life is a real social studio, so a lot of our patrons are people who need some distraction. Some people that, like me, don't really tune into the gym vibe. Whenever I think gym, I think about putting something down, pick it back up, put it down, pick it back up, put it down, take it back up. And that's it. Whereas with dance, you get to be a little more in touch with the music and you get to enjoy music, and you get to chat with people. You interact with people. And it's a break away from everyday mundane life, or hectic life, or whatever. It's a little oasis at times.

As a good dance instructor, you're constantly trying to improve yourself. Dance is a journey you have with yourself. As you get older, you notice that certain things don't come as easily, so you need to have a work around. Like the splits! I've somehow lost the splits due to a torn muscle, and it's a mission trying to get it back. I have to be more creative with choreography that does not lean on the splits as it used to. So, things like that, but it helps me and the team that work here.

Each dance teacher is qualified in their own section. We do various things. We've got ballet. We've got a special needs programme, so that is kids with autism and learning disabilities and physical disabilities. We have ballet-barre which is also like fitness. We've got Hip Hop fitness. We have Contemporary and Modern. It's a lot of stuff.

I love my job because a lot of the time I find that I get to put people back in touch with their body. I've realised that people totally get caught up in their heads. My biggest challenge as a dance instructor is to get people to trust their body. A lot of the times, the movements that I want them to do, that they would really like to do, would come naturally if they stop thinking, and just do it.

Being a person who has struggled with anxiety issues, and things like that, it does help just to let things go through, and flow through. Instead of just overthinking. Your body literally freezes up once you overthink something.

I started dancing because I needed a hobby. To get away from books and just overall stress relief. And for me, not being a gym person, I thought, 'Ok. Music and dancing sounds good.' Then I got an opportunity to dance with another student and she was a few levels higher than me and she very much wanted to compete. She basically forced me to speed up my training, which was good. That got me into the competitive scene faster than most, because I was forced into a higher level. I didn't start right from the bottom. That meant hours and hours a week. At least in a normal Monday to Friday, nine hours a week. And that was besides whatever you were doing. Evenings, it was basically, get to the studio, music on, repeat, repeat, repeat. Yeah. So, it was good. We competed. Then she graduated and I got another partner, and then we moved away from varsity. And then I got another partner, and we started to work in different areas. It was always a mission to find a partner.

During that time, in my section, I was South African champion, both Ballroom and Latin. It was something that I enjoyed and loved. When you get to the higher levels, it requires more commitment. When you dance at a competitive level, at like national Championship level, you really need to be focused and really put in the work. A lot of the times, dance partners will compete up to the level where they can wear the fancy dresses and get into the VIP section, and once they've reached that level, they just fade out. That made things slightly difficult for getting a partner and maintaining a partner.

Then I started work at the studio, which meant working Monday to Friday, one to ten. That means when I have my mornings free, my dance partner is at work. When she has her evenings free, I'm at work. And then weekends and dancing all week. I still find myself dancing most weekends. You see, once the bug has bitten, it really becomes a way of life. Even December holidays, the summer break, you'll find that after the second week and I'll be like, 'This was fun, but I want to go back to work.' My body starts to feel stiff because it's not dancing every day. Your body starts to crave dancing and moving. You feel withdrawal.

I probably would still compete but finding a partner is not easy. Even when you do, it is a lot like a relationship. You see that person more than you see anybody else. And you have to manage it like a good relationship. I mean having clear rules that partners have their own friends – we do not have mutual friends. 'I see you enough!'

I'm also having long-term relationships, but you get people that aren't so comfortable with having their partner spending more time with somebody else than with them.

I am single at the moment. There is someone, but it's not anything official or anything, but there is something that might be in the pipeline. For me, it is the stage of my life where we'll see where this goes but … I am not willing to settle. Or just jump into a relationship. I'm too old for that. I got a few lovers, but it's like, been there done that. If it's not something real then nah. What's the use? I've got other things to focus on.

I'm perfectly at peace with myself. I am totally fine being single. You have to compliment my lifestyle. And I have to compliment yours and somewhere compromise. I don't need somebody else to do, or to be, my other half. We can be a good team together but that doesn't mean that you're my half. Nothing messy.

The phase where I was doing drag as Eva was quite a major change in my life, where I actually got into drag. It was eye opening for me because it was a part of me that I didn't know existed and it opened up so many avenues and questions. Since then, I've developed and I found that I don't subscribe to the two genders being binary. It's fluid. I accept that, and I'm comfortable with that and I wish more people would at least just be cognizant of that idea and acknowledge that gender is not binary. It's not. You don't have to say you're a female or male or whatever. And then besides that, sexuality is totally separate from gender. The whole spectrum and just exploring that spectrum and the way that I feel comfortable in that.

When you first come out as gay there is a lot of soul searching that happens, and a lot of trial and error, and 'Is this for me?' So, there's definitely a path to walk in that regard. Just being and expressing that side of me as Eva has been very empowering. I've also seen that a lot of people don't get that chance, or don't have the freedom to do that.

Going through the phase of being in drag gave me a great respect for transgender people and empathy for their struggle. A space in my heart goes out to the transgendered individuals. I can choose to wear drag and I'm also comfortable dressed in men's clothing. But there are individuals for whom the mere fact that they have to shave feels alien to them because it's not who they feel they are, and who they know they are. It's not easy and a lot of the time they are the target for homophobia and transphobia. How do you hide something like that? They are thrust into the spotlight, when they just want to be themselves. Everything becomes activism for them, where a lot of them don't want that. They just want to go be the girl next door, the boy next door, find a partner, have two children and a dog and a house with a picket fence. They end up on the front line. The last people that would want to be thrust in the spotlight, and yet they are, constantly.

It also empowered me just to be myself more, because I can do this. Even if people notice, ok. No, he's slightly androgynous or he/she or whatever.

Just being and creating new norms and challenging heteronormativity as a major thing. I don't feel that I need to be shouting off the rooftops. It's everyday life, the way we handle things. I'll be doing capoeira and belly dancing. And it's like ok, it's like, one minute I'm kicking somebody and the next minute I'm shaking my rump and vibrating my nonexistent fat. So yeah!

I'm just expressing myself and being empowered enough to do it and not shying away from it because of heteronormativity. That is a big thing for me. That is like my Gandhi – 'Be the change you want to see in the world,' You don't need to accept or believe in somebody else's way of life. It's just, that is their truth. Does it affect you? Does it harm you? If it harms you, if there is harm being done, ok, this we need to speak about to find some middle ground. But a lot of times it's just senseless.

I haven't gone out in full drag in a while. I don't feel that that is something that is needed for me to identify my gender fluidity. I don't need to go out in public all dressed up. To prove to who … for what? Sometimes I would go shopping and I would decide that I want to wear heels while I do my shopping, or I want to put on some makeup and then I do that. I've gone out with full-on makeup and a beard. It's not for seeking attention. It's just, I felt like that, and that's what I wanted to do.

> Going through the phase of being in drag gave me a great respect for transgender people and empathy for their struggle.

Standing in queues, especially with my hair being different colours or slightly longer, a lot of times with little kids in the shopping centres, I would hear 'Mommy, Daddy is that a boy or a girl?' and then I just think ok maybe they should have that discussion now, because just getting it out, that is something.

This is my form of activism right now. Actively being in organizations and things like that is not exactly where I am at this moment. I've got other things that I am managing. I have to keep my cup full before I can fill others.

The one talk we had back during the programme was around 'when is the right moment to talk about condom use and HIV'. That is always something I think of in a new relationship. It's like, when is the right moment to speak about that. I've found just making it a normal, saying, 'now we get tested every three months or six months.' 'Ok, but why?' 'No. Just because I do.' And then, just like 'Ok, we're going to the clinic is anybody coming with?' Making that more of a norm. So that it doesn't become a major thing. And I found that this is very daunting for some people to even talk about. Talk about, much less go sit in the waiting room and wait for the nurse to come out, or the counsellor to come out. When they hear there's a counsellor first, then, 'What do I have to speak about? Just get the thing done! Just prick me and tell me!'

That is a big thing. Going with a friend, just holding their hand.

Just last night I was chatting to another friend of mine and she said, there was a gap where she didn't get tested for a long while. She went to the doctor and said I'm too nervous to have actual test done, is there any other test you can do that might infer that I need further testing? So, she had a CD4 count done and all the other tests instead of just a rapid test because she says she's not willing to put herself through that at that moment. The doctors assured her that everything was fine, and then she got into the habit of regular testing again.

It's just being open about HIV and realising that through the workshop and all that it was just to get talking about it. As soon as you stuff it under the rug, that's how shit happens. Ignorance is not bliss.

The transition into adulthood as an activist was hard... It was easier in the teenage years to focus on what was put in front of you. HIV and AIDS were huge things. Racism was a big thing. As you got older you get to realize that there were more things, and more and more issues. And you kind of have to choose your battles.

I've always said, why didn't anybody tell me that in my twenties I was going to have another 'finding myself' moment. I sat on my bed and I was like, I want to talk to somebody older, because they didn't tell me I'm going to go through this again! Nobody warned me about this! I thought, you get through your teenage years and then everything is fine. You'll be very equipped to handle things. And now I'm in my 20s, I don't know what the issues going on with life and having to find yourself again in your 20s, and then like, it's apparently a 7- or 12-year cycle, so... Yeah, so, back to the drawing board. And

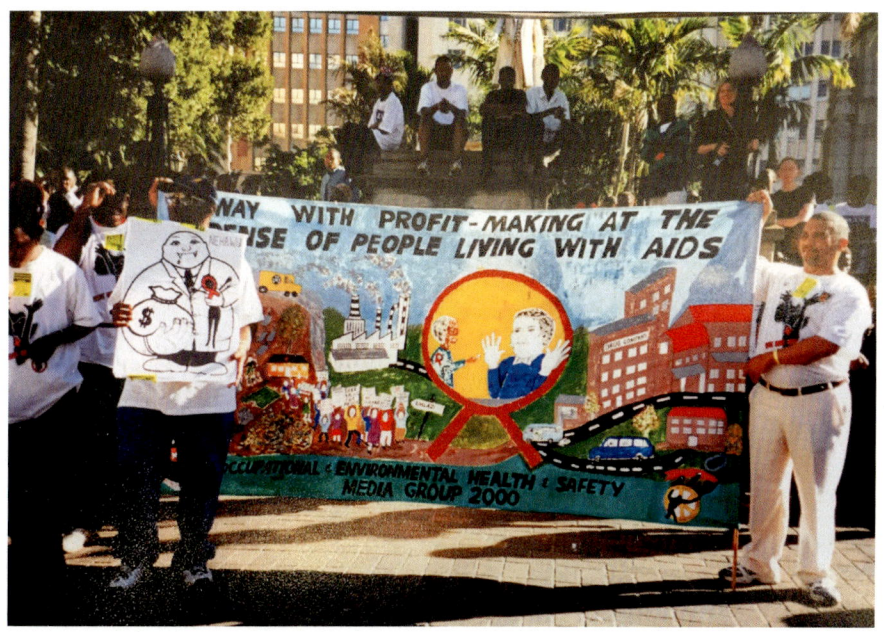

*13th International AIDS Conference, Durban 2000*

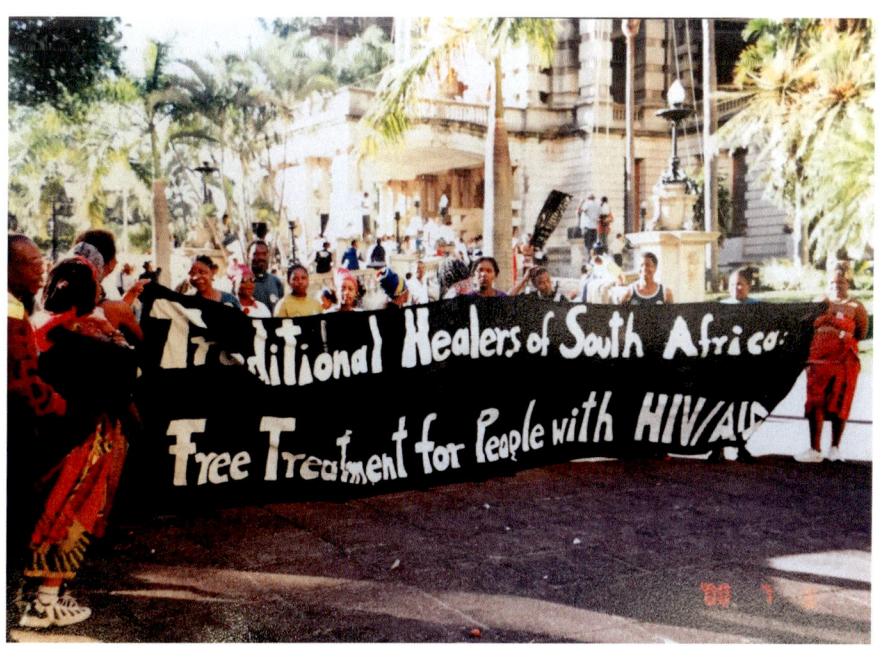

*Traditional Healers of South Africa, 13th International AIDS Conference, Durban 2000*

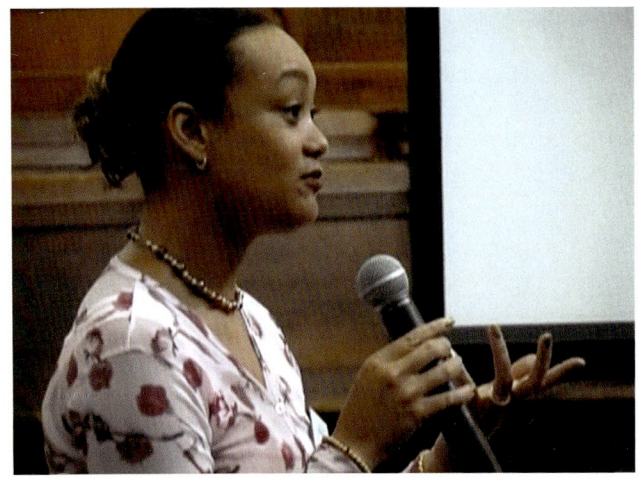

*Abigail Dreyer, 'Getting the Word Out' symposium, 2002*

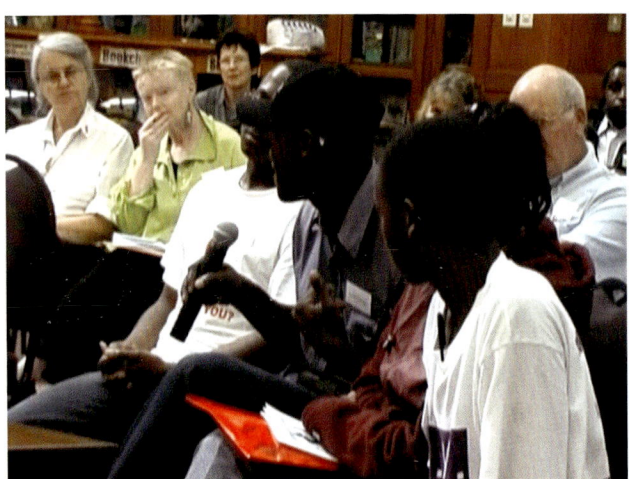

*Mphumzi on the mic, sitting with KK, Danlia and Thozzi. Claudia Mitchell, Ann Smith, Sue Williamson and Robin Malan look on. 'Getting the Word Out' symposium, 2002*

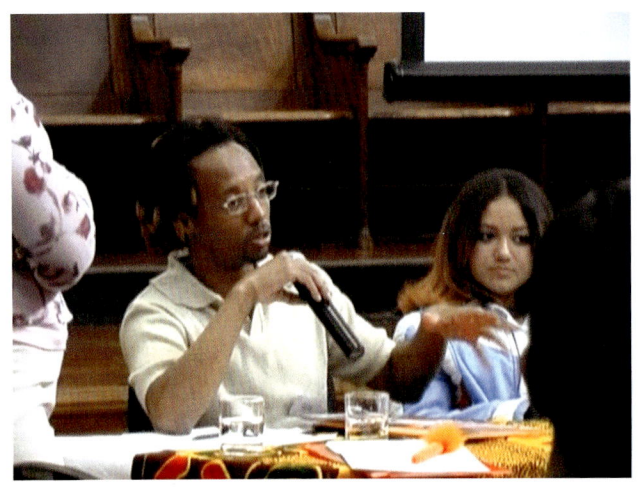

*K. Sello Duiker presents on panel with Kaylene, 'Getting the Word Out' symposium, 2002*

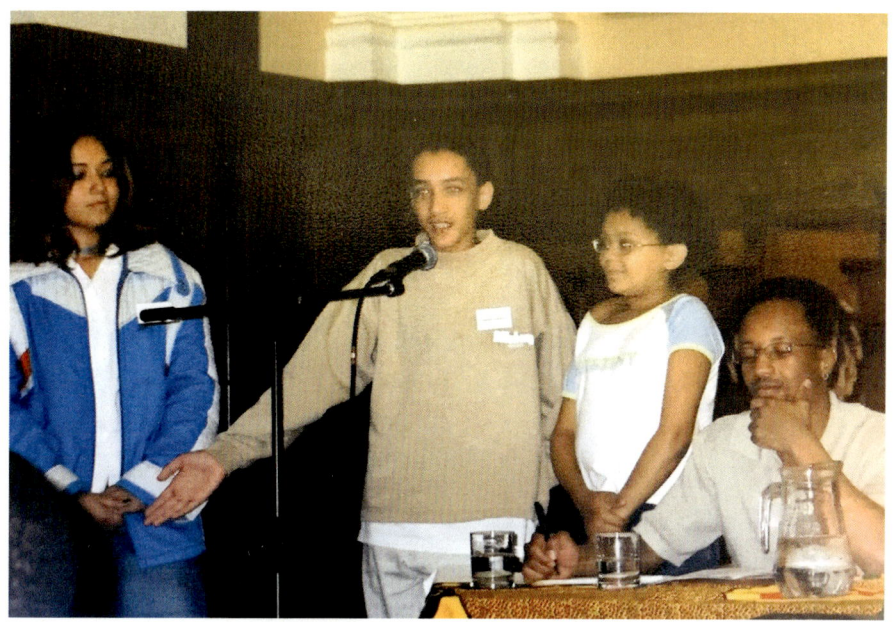

*Kaylene, Mathew, Ruth (L to R) speak on panel, K. Sello Duiker sits to right 'Getting the World Out' symposium, 2002*

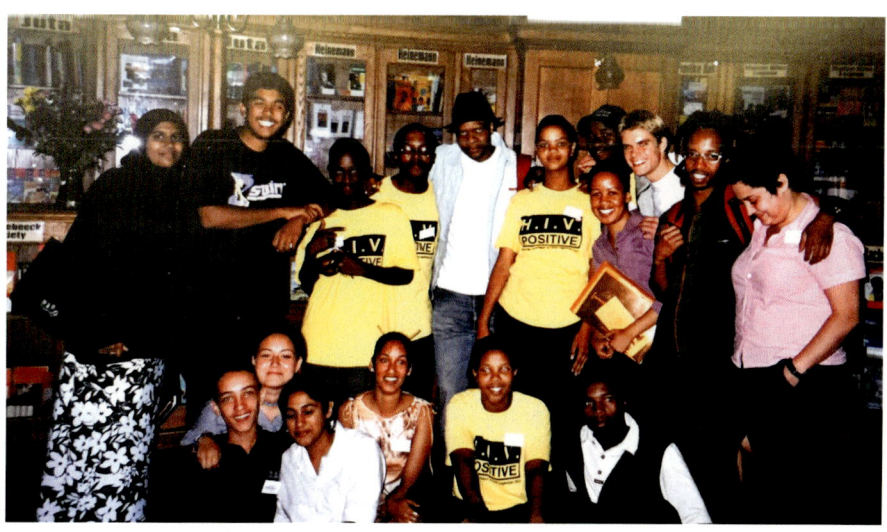

*'Getting the Word Out' symposium group photo, with all workshops participants and film director Teboho Mahlatsi, novelist K. Sello Duiker, and artist Mara Verna, 2002*

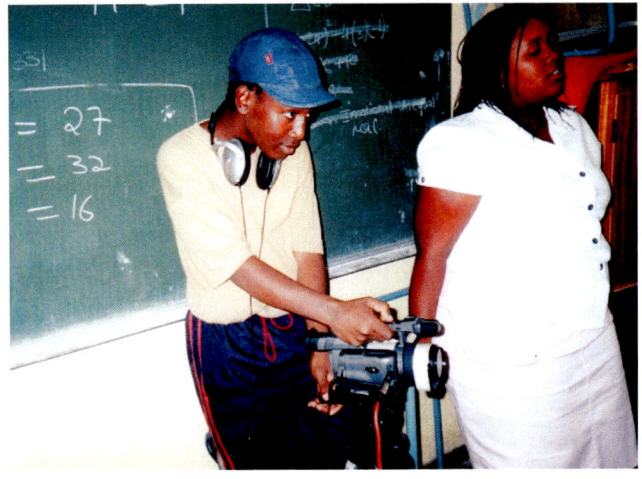

*KK behind camera and Lindeka interviews learners for the FAcing The Truth (FATT) project, 2004*

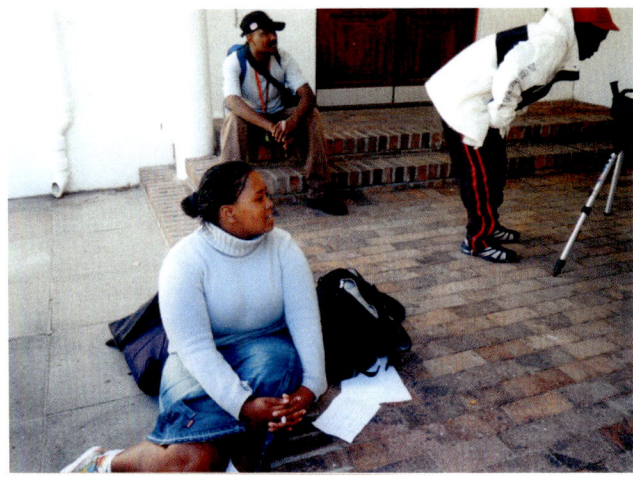

*Lindeka, Mandla and KK at Rustenberg Girls School, filming for the FAcing The Truth (FATT) project, 2004*

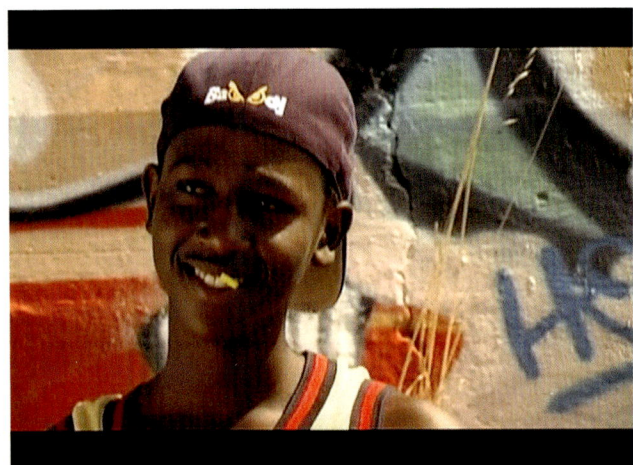

*KK, film still from documentary 'Fire & Hope' 2004*

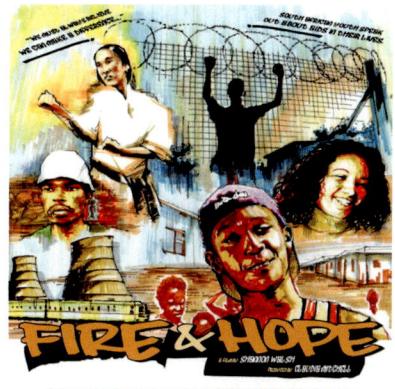

Poster for 'Fire & Hope' 2004

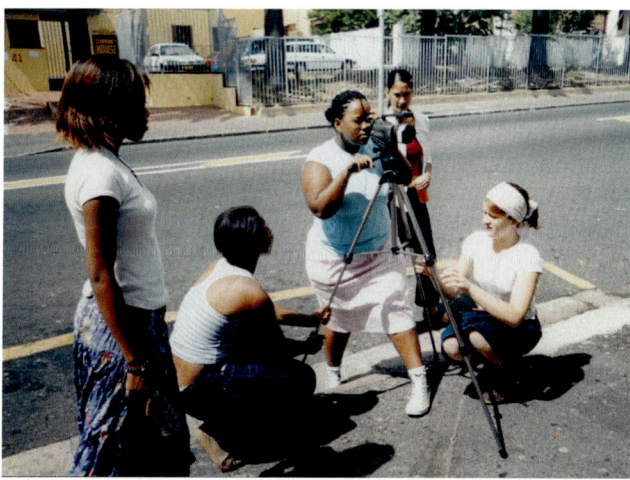

Filming 'Street Fear' 2004 (L-R: Nosy, Wendy Tapleni, Lindeka, Chinomy, Nadia Brown)

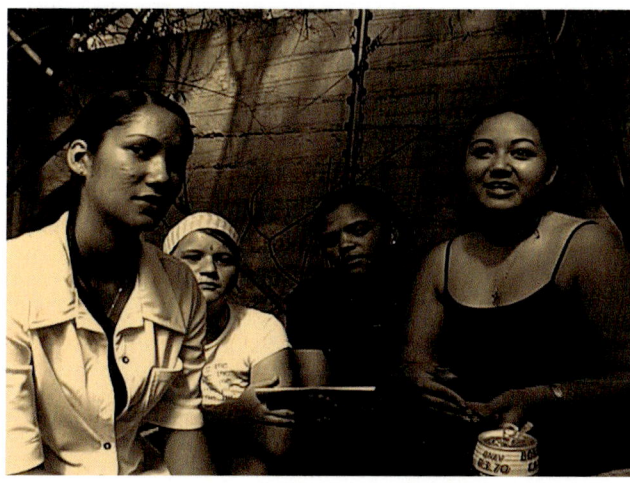

Film still, 'Street Fear' 2004 (L-R: Chinomy, Nadia Brown, Ann, Kaylene)

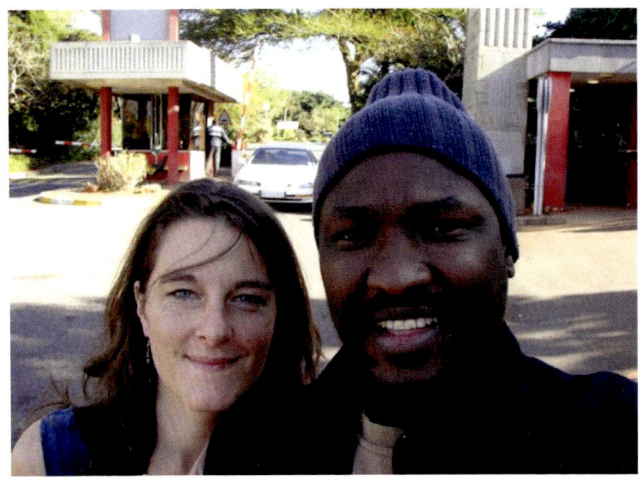

*Shannon and Mandla, Durban, 2009*

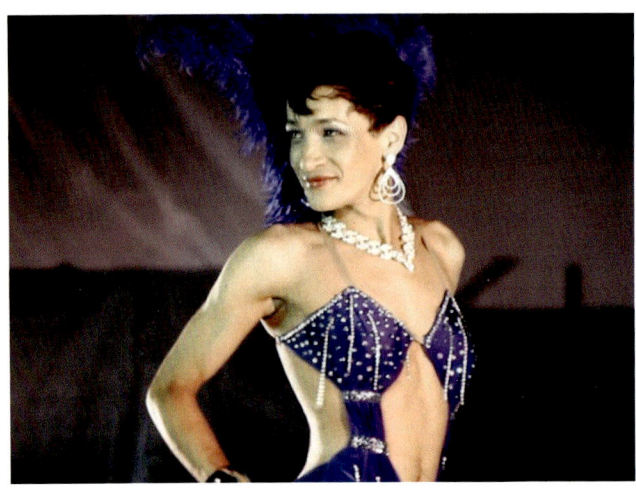

*Mathew as Eva during Miss Gay Western Cape, film still 'Glitterboys & Ganglands' by Lauren Beukes, 2011*

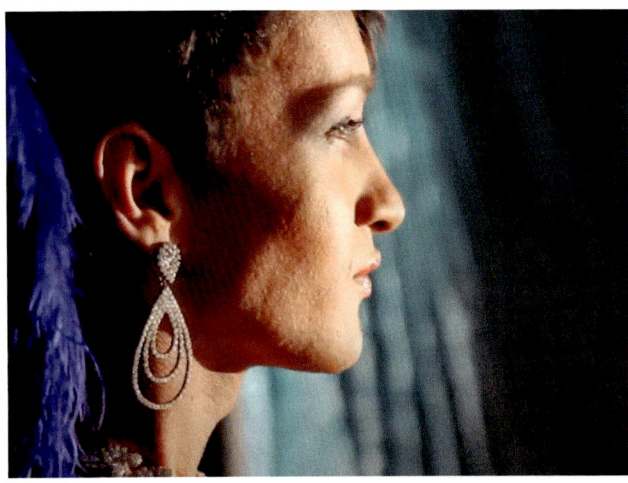

*Mathew as Eva during Miss Gay Western Cape, film still 'Glitterboys & Ganglands' by Lauren Beukes, 2011*

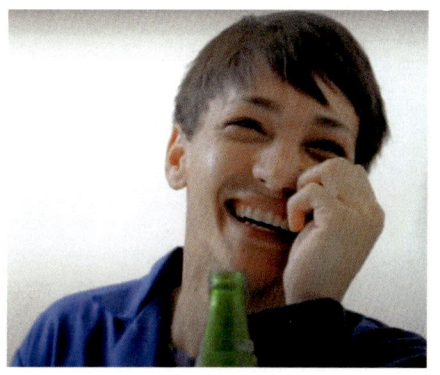
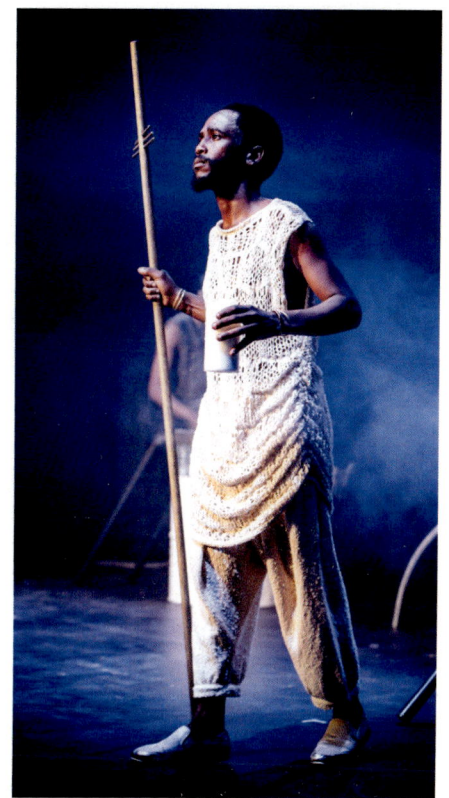

TOP LEFT *Mathew at work as a mechanic, film still 'Glitterboys & Ganglands' by Lauren Beukes, 2011*
RIGHT *KK, still from play 'Holy Contract' 2016, photo by Neels Kleynhans neels@nkphotography.co.za | nkphotography.co.za*

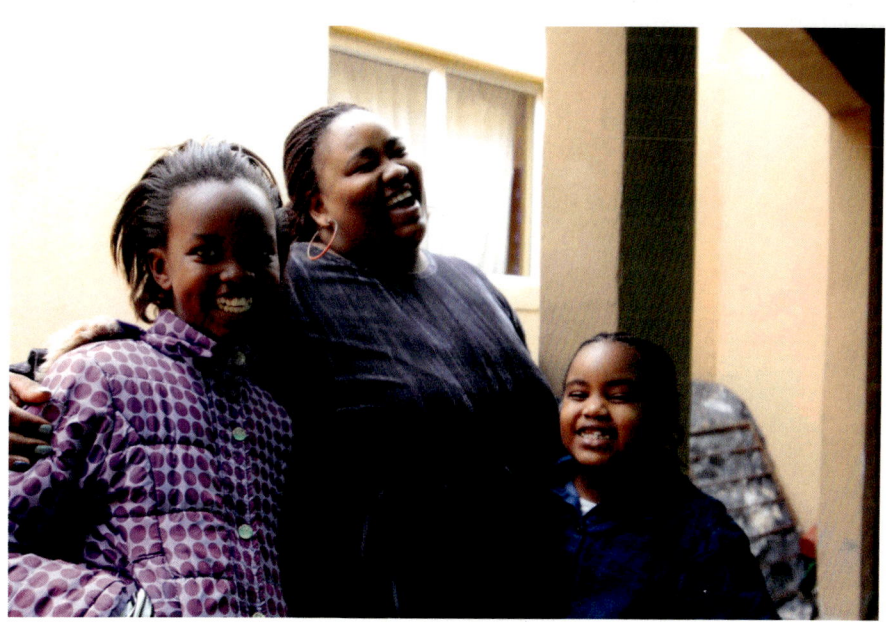

*Lindeka with her children, 2018, photo by Eugene Arries*

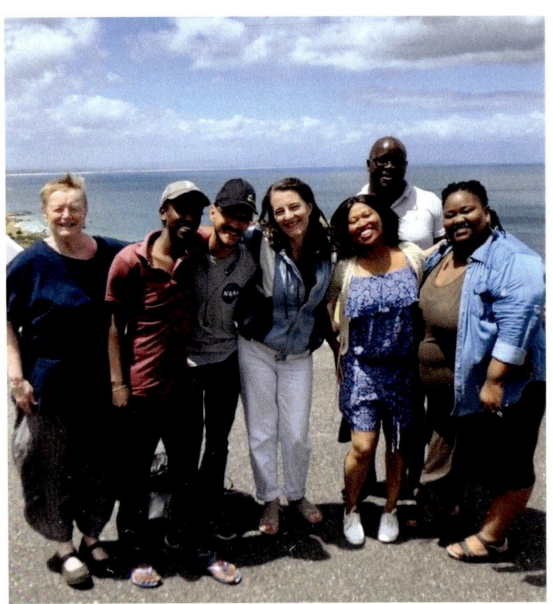
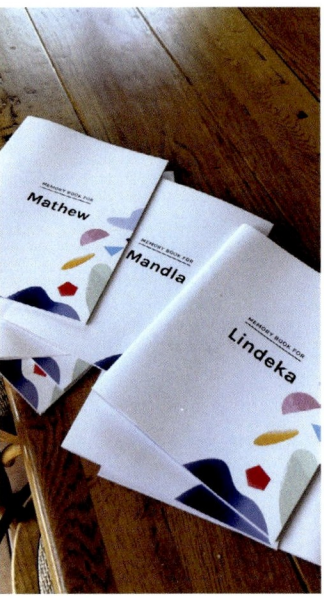

LEFT *Simon's Town retreat and workshop, 2019 (L-R: Claudia, KK, Mathew, Shannon, Nosibusiso, Mphumzi, Lindeka)*
RIGHT *Memory Books for Simon's Town retreat, 2019*

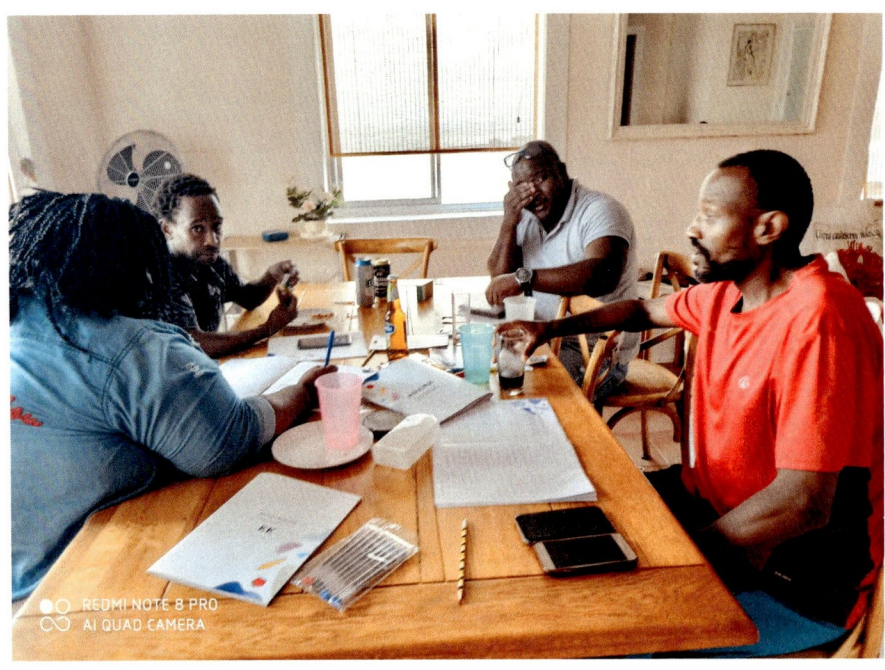

*Simon's Town retreat & workshop, working with Memory books (L-R: Lindeka, KK, Mphumzi, Mandla)*

you're going through that all over again.

There were a lot of opportunities when we were young. You were more or less thrust in the spotlight. In the teenage years you were given more opportunities, whereas in your 20s you actually had to make that happen for yourself. You needed to be the driving force. You needed to decide what are your battles? What can you give and where you are going? Like, you could go vegan because cows are totally fucking up the ozone layer with all their shit. Or, do you really want that piece of steak? Are you going to go all organic or are these GMO foods really that bad? Things like that. For me, evaluating and seeing, that was just a transition from being given the opportunities to do things, to making it happen in your own right, and finding what you can do.

You can't save the world on your own. You have to see where and what you can do. Finding that balance was for me what it meant going from a teenager to 'adulthood'.

I think knowing that there really is change that you can effect was good to know, because I find a lot of people complain. It's like ok. Now do something about it! Do something. Do Anything.

⁂

Where I am today, like as in TODAY, today? Oooof. I had a breakthrough with my psychologist today, so that was good. I was crying like a little baby. I am at a point where I can actually start to face things that I was not willing to do before.

It means that in a sense, I am at a low point and a strong point at the same time. I'm down in the gutters and yet, not defeated, not in the slightest.

That is where I am presently. I am finding everything else in my life is more or less settling. I'm in a job that I like. I don't have to worry about huge debt, bills, or keeping a roof over my head and things. You find at this stage of your life it actually brings a lot of skeletons out of the closet.

Now I am busy cleaning out the closet. For me it's spring cleaning at the moment. Being able to do that is very empowering. It feels good getting to a point where you can do that. That I'm there in the first place.

In the last while, it's been quite hectic. I can't use public transport anymore because I was attacked on my way to work in a taxi. I'd gotten into a taxi on my way to work and then they decided to have it out with me and emptied my bank account. Three different ATMs. While I'm lying in the taxi with a knife at my neck. Then I get out of the taxi, they kick me out of the taxi, and there's a police van just across the road. I ran to the police van and they tell me I have to report it to the police station. They can't help me.

I flagged down a law enforcement officer that was city police, and they said the same thing. I walk into a random shop, a mattress shop, to call work to tell them that there's no way I am going to get to work today, and then I walk back a few blocks to my aunt's house.

Yeah, so that was a thing.

That was only a month after I had gone to that same aunt's house to pack lunch. But I didn't make it. I was on a scooter and I went to go get some take out. And then a young bloke decided that he didn't want to stop at that intersection while I was crossing. He crossed. I was in the hospital for about three days.

So, I was still recovering from that. That was just so... I was so glad that I could immerse myself in work after that.

Dealing with all of that, and then the whole idea of grief, and how to deal with it.

With all the family members that I've lost, I've realised I haven't really quite completely dealt with that. And it's difficult to deal with. As somebody that is not very religious and trying to make sense of it. The biggest problem is once you see how cruel and unpredictable the world can be, you can't really unsee it. And somehow you have to get to a point where you... Rationalise it...? Or something?

Having two brothers taken away in three months. One stabbed, one being knocked off his bicycle by a police van. My brother-in-law being shot. My cousin being caught in a vehicle accident. He always said he never wanted to drive because he was always scared of dying in an accident, and then he drove under the influence of alcohol and he died. His friend survived. The friend didn't tell the family that they were in an accident, so my cousin laid in the morgue for a weekend, unidentified.

To start that all off, it was my aunt, she was going from one of her lectures, she was a lifelong student. She was on her way home from varsity evening courses. And they thought that her new car was not hers anymore. So, they hijacked her. And raped her. And emptied her bank account and left her naked on a sports field in Mitchells Plain.

So, in a span of two years having to deal with all of that was like ... it was like, it was just ... at the time after I was feeling raw.

That's a lot to try and process and I understand that, very clearly. Like, yeah. It's not going to happen overnight, but, yeah. Those are the things that have happened. I guess you have to make sense of it somehow.

But life is good. I still try to live like I might die tomorrow, and plan like I will live forever.

But life is good. I enjoy what I do. I do try to live my best life.

Do I have hope? Yes. I have hope because I see a lot of the youth and people in general still fighting and wanting to fight for what they want on social media. Yes, it is a whole new level of bullying and it also opens up a lot more of the dark spaces. The dark spaces may be shifting.

Light is being shed where it wasn't shed before. People are seeing other people doing more and saying more. It's like, I'm not the only one going through this. It's not the feeling of isolation. It's a bit better. Not 'no longer', but it's a little better. It's much easier.

When I was thinking, and trying to get to terms with my desires, 'Ok now... Girls? Boys? BOYS! Girls? Boys GIRLS, BOYS, girl-boy?' Back then all I knew was, ok, that's something that that person said, that auntie said, and this auntie... But now young people have it in their faces. There are very strong gender non-binary people in the media and they can see they're out there doing things. Just showing who they are, what they are. All these strong women ... they can see that a female can be president. We've got a black president. Yeah. Things like that, they are exposed to more.

Yes, it comes with its own bad things but it gives me hope that they are still fighting.

If you see the recent thing about the university students that are fighting for fees to be lowered or taken down. They are fighting for something. They are not just lying down. The culture of fighting for what we want is still there and it's still strong in South Africa. Fighting for what they want is good.

I can't believe it's 15 years since we did our first workshops together. That flew past. But honestly the experience is always great. The friendships that we've had over the years and the exposure to things and the ability to speak freely. I'm always thinking about that, and even talking about it to a friend last night as well.

Besides that, I consider myself as a safer sexual being as well, because it opened me to that. There are so many more ways to interact with people. We are not in the jungle anymore.

We don't breed just to procreate, or hump for stress relief, like some of our fellow dolphins and chimpanzees. There is more to human interaction than reproduction and things, and that's good. People should embrace that. I'm glad to have been exposed to a little more than I would have.

---

I think it was having all of that exposure to the arts and to yourself [Shannon] in a way as well. I was speaking to my psychologist earlier and just the idea of how I could actually sit and speak to her about things. That was something that was gradually coaxed out of us, because we would just sit there and do exercises like, 'Tell me something about your life' and it would be one-liners and things.

The reoccurring thing I think about it is about, 'being expert on who I am'.

If you ask me, I'm expert at being me, and this is my situation. That was very empowering. And then being given the opportunity to see how different people choose to express that idea, because not everyone is a linguist, not everyone is a painter, not everyone is a singer, not everyone is a dancer, and it brought about a great love for the arts. Really... [gestures to the studio they are in]. Great love for the arts. Just to be exposed to that, and being exposed to people that weren't necessarily in your community. Meeting KK and the others. The black people I've made friends with, and they're great, I love it, Cynthia, Nosi… I smile when I think of them.

> The culture of fighting for what we want is still there and it's still strong in South Africa.

It's great memories that we made. It was eye opening for coming out of a community that is segregated. Whenever you thought about another race it was 'Ok the whites are doing something, or the Boers', but you got to see different ways of how people live and experience things and think about things. That made you think a little more about, and sometimes reaffirming, the way you're doing things. Or opening up some thought patterns or ideas or avenues you could possibly go down.

I think that's what stood out. That self-exploration. And that you are empowered. That was good to share, because you got there and after a workshop you would feel – now I can go share. It's like, you have your hands full of things and now you can't wait to get to school because you can just hand it out. And then yes, it's like 'You didn't know?' 'Ok let me show you how to put on a condom'. Yeah… I was always the one showing how to put on a condom!

I also really saw myself as a peer educator. I could relate in my own language and I always found that very effective when we did the workshop at school because kids could relate, and I could speak their own language. Or mention things that are relevant to them. It was nice. Those interactions and being able to share what I'd learned was, as I said, empowering and it opened up so many avenues.

I wish I could find that again, being 32 now. In my life I've seen a lot of people who have not been exposed to any of that. And I sometimes feel sorry for them that they didn't get that, they didn't get the opportunities to explore things in that way.

# 2019

*Mathew at 34*
Individual interview
Simon's Town

I am 34, living in Brackenfell now. It's a bit closer to work.

Work has changed. I have opened a new studio with a business partner. It's early days, exciting, stressful. Yeah, just cribbing in the owner seat instead of actually being an employee, so it's interesting to say the least. It has its own challenges but it's good. Besides that, I'm also helping my business partner with the restaurant that she has to manage now, after her business partner passed on. So yeah, it's a very, very busy year ahead getting the studio up and running.

The first couple of months of any new businesses you're not really raking it in. So yeah, just getting through that and marketing and setting up the systems and everything. It's a welcome change compared to last time we spoke because I was in a space where I was complacent or just comfortable. Too comfortable, but also too scared to take the leap and go for it. It was just monotonous. Same-same. No challenges. I was hungry for more challenges, but also too scared to actually take the leap and do something, and I didn't know what I wanted to do.

Then this opportunity came up to start my own studio. I took it, and grabbed it with both hands. It was as if you were standing at the edge of a ledge, and jumping for a rope. Yeah, so I am holding onto that rope very dearly.

It's good so far. I've been getting into the swing of things. I am very optimistic and hopeful for the future.

In that sense, it's not been easy. I had to maintain my regular visits with my psychiatrist and psychologist. The dentist seems to love me as well. It's a mission impossible! It's each time I go in, they say I have come back for another appointment, another appointment.

I feel that I'm settling in nicely to this new kind of routine. I feel that I've actually invested in the support systems I needed.

Even now, when I was going through the Memory Book, and

some of the things just reminded me of how important it is that I manage my anxiety. It's not something that I can just forget about, unfortunately. It is some chemical imbalance, and past trauma. It's an amalgamation of a lot of things. And yeah, it wants to work. It needs to work. It has to work.

I got so scared because of this whole transition. Leaving a job and starting something new. It's like, 'What the hell are you doing?' For the first time in my life, I had suicidal ideation. I was like, busy painting the new studio. I would imagine, oh, okay, so if I kill myself what do I have to use, what am I going to do? If I'm going to cut my wrist, I don't want any blood on the dance floor, but I want to be at the studio, so what colour should I paint the walls? [laughs] As I'm painting, getting everything ready. That was a struggle.

I've always been too conceited to think about suicide. For the first time, I needed to actually put into practice the tools that I've learned. I was so grateful that I had actually reached out, beforehand, and made sure that I had support systems in place. It could have gone south very quickly otherwise. I had great support from family and friends as well. Yeah.

It was so weird to me. I just didn't know that. It just made me realise that it could be about mindset or headspace, you don't just think about suicide out of the blue. It affirms for me the need to stay on my antidepressants, and manage, and choose my battles. Busy work is not always good. Taking good rest is as important as work.

I am happy now. I am in a good space.

Last time we spoke I had alluded to a relationship. It was nice and good, but I have become too independent. Sharing everything was too much work. The partner that I had was just a bit too clingy. He loved me dearly, poor guy, but I think he loved me too much. There's a song that I used to listen to that totally sums up our relationship, something like, 'You know I love you, but I can't miss you if you are always around.' I needed space, and he couldn't give that to me. He didn't get the picture. After a couple of months of repeatedly trying to reinforce some boundaries, it didn't quite work.

I'm proud of myself for having gone through these things this year, and being at a high point now, comparatively.

Life takes work. Taking time out just to enjoy life is important too. With anxiety and things, it's more about keeping busy so that you don't just end up in your own headspace. Being in your own head without parental supervision isn't a good idea! Yeah, it's not a good idea. You can go there for day visits, but don't live there!

Last time I saw you, it was dramatic. I was getting out of survival mode. It was a major challenge. Of course, I'm still getting things started and it's not really perfect, but I'm actually reaching for the things that I want. Things are happening. Even if things don't happen or whatever, I'm okay with the process. It's no use just pissing into the wind.

When I was down, I told my mom, 'I know I'll get through this and I'll make it to the other side and everything will be okay.'

I think life is so sadistic. It knows that I can bounce back, but that doesn't mean I'm a ping pong ball. I'll bounce back, but I don't want to be a ping pong ball. It's just given me some space to really roll for a while. I think therapy, especially talk therapy and CBT, has helped. There's a lot of black and white thinking that I've had to adjust, because I'm uncomfortable with any grey. When it comes to relationships, that is something that I'm working on.

Where do you find the balance of, okay, this is good compromise, instead of compromising too much? Am I just being way out there, or not? I think everyone is dealing with that. There are no easy answers.

Going through all this interior stuff, and going through the Memory Books again today, I think in the end, it's like same shit different day, different flavour.

We are constantly learning and relearning who we are and how to love. That's life. We can't run away from that. You could, technically, but I wouldn't advise it! [laughs]

*Shannon: 'What was it like seeing yourself in* Fire & Hope? *Yeah, what did you think about the boy that you were back then?'*

Mathew: That boy... Whoa, so I still could feel the same need to just be. I'm getting to a point now in my mid-thirties that I see it's a journey we had to go through. I'm still the same person, but different. I feel that I am growing more into myself.

I was constantly censoring everything back then. That is something that I've grown out of. Now I'm more like, this is me, deal with it. That was always what I wanted, and what I did in small sections or little controlled environments. That made me happy and is what is keeping me happy at the moment. Just being me, whatever that is. Sometimes I don't know what that is. It's okay. It's life. Who really knows themselves perfectly? The Dalai Lama doesn't know, maybe the Buddha had a good idea. But there's a few billion other people that are just stumbling around in the dark, just like me.

At least we've got some stars in the sky.

My coming out. I had a 'a-ha' moment when I was in Grade 8. I just had a 'a-ha' moment one Monday morning. I woke up, and it just made sense. All the puzzle pieces just fell into place, like oh! And then I went to school. We used to have a register period first thing in the morning with your class teacher where we caught up on whatever work we wanted to do. I went to my circle of friends, and I'm like, 'Guys, I'm gay!' Kaylene was in that group. And they said, 'Okay, let's see what happens, let's see how this goes. You don't need to go tell anybody, just figure it out for yourself. We know that ... and okay, what kind of guys you like? When did you think of this?' And so, that was good.

I always have been blessed with great friendships. There are many people who have not been as blessed as I have with the calibre of relationships, and friendships, that I've had, and still have. How many people can count on one hand friends that they have for more than 10 years? I can't even count on two hands how many friends I have had for 18 years! The time and space apart doesn't really affect that connection that we have. Sometimes just touching base now and then even, and it's like, was that last week or was it two years back? [laughs]

Friendship is the thing that keeps coming up, and it is what really remains from our work together.

So does the way I approach life and issues and ask questions. I want to know why. I don't just accept things. I think when I went to varsity it was like lighting of a fire, or more like rekindling something for me, because I felt working on the Soft Cover project, and being exposed to that really shifted me and took me out of my comfort zone. It had me talking, opening up, and thinking and questioning.

Why is the status quo exactly that? Does it apply to me? I think that stood out.

Also, just the habit of giving back, and trying to do something for others. Even now with the studio, I have set aside time on Tuesdays so when I am not working, I'm at the children's home and I'm volunteering. So that time is a no-go. I'm not making any compromises or whatever. If need be, we can work it into the studio's social responsibility or something. That is something important to me.

Previously, I only had my Saturday morning to spare, and I like my weekends. I like to have time to myself and I was a bit too selfish to offer that up.

The Durbanville Children's Home is a government-funded children's home, so when children get removed from their family they go to a children's home. Most of the children are longtime residents, and a lot of them don't go into the foster care system. A lot of them are kids that the courts removed from their families. Just being there and spending time, it's just nice. Watching them develop and seeing how they are. I always ask them about good habits and how they are doing. I insist on asking them to tell me what made them laugh today. It's tiny, but it's good. That is something that I enjoy. Giving back.

We're also working on a dance school competition. We got Grand-West on board, so they are assisting with everything, adding them onboard is a huge help. There's a lot of nitty-gritty to work out. Maybe mid-next year we'll be announcing the dance competition.

I haven't really felt the need or want to go out in drag. I haven't felt it was something missing, going out on the scene or being part of Miss Gay Western Cape now. Still, I clean my house in heels, I can attest to that. If I feel like cross-dressing, if you want to call it that, that day, I'm going to put on makeup and wear my heels to the shop.

When I think of myself as that young boy to now, I really wish that young boy knew that gender is non-binary. There is so much grey when you look at gender and sexuality; they are two different things.

That brings back something that KK brought up, how over the years the focus has changed. HIV is treated more like a chronic disease now instead of a pandemic, of which it still is. Our mindsets and the causes that we are interested in also changes. Sometimes it changes, but it stays the same too.

When I look at the things that I wrote in 2004 about drugs, violence and gangsterism; it's still there. It's still there. It might have a slightly different face, but it's still there. I'm learning to get a balance – there is only so much you can do. I did what I can.

On the scene, yes, I could do more but at what cost? And me, just being the friendly 'it' next door: they, him, she, whatever. Whatever you want to call me, it's your label, not mine.

Unless it is for business purposes, dressing appropriately would be dressing appropriately. What I think is appropriate. If I feel comfortable, because people look at the way you present yourself. You're not going to be all dishevelled if you want to be respected. But if I want to wear a short skirt that is shorter than most people's g-strings, then that is my prerogative. If you're offended by it, am I in your place of worship? Am I physically breaching your boundaries? If you have a problem with me, call me. If you don't have my number then you don't know me well enough to have a problem with me. Call me, call me, and we can sort it out. Sure, yes!

I have adopted not to say I have had a difficult or challenging year. I'll just call it interesting. I'll leave it grey purposefully. I need to remind myself that as much as there were bad times, there were good times, there was progress. You think you're going forward sometimes, and you walk back.

It's always up and down.

This dynamic over the years – I know that, especially today, KK was really talking about what is being given back. I think this is a relationship we have developed and maintained over the years. And also, if you look at it in the academic sense, it's like, how many people or how many cases have been followed this far? Where there is this paper trail, so to speak, to just see how things affected us? It really does change you, as I have said, and certain things get kindled. Just the way you look at things.

It definitely changes you, being empowered at such a young age. When I'm at the children's home, I'm always reminding them every day that the power is in their hands. Just because they are at a children's home, that does not need to define them. What happened in the past does not need to define them. Life is still happening. Life is not guaranteed. Forcing them to sit down and think about it.

As I said before, I had kind of a panic attack when I got the invite to come to this gathering. I was just keeping busy and not allowing myself in my head. Then I was like, 'Oh shit, they are going to ask me about my life! What has been happening in my life? Who am I? What am I? What did I do? Am I a failure? Do I exist?' I was totally shaken. My therapist was very pleased, though, that I was shaken up. According to her, we made some progress, and that meant I could also start further unpacking things as well.

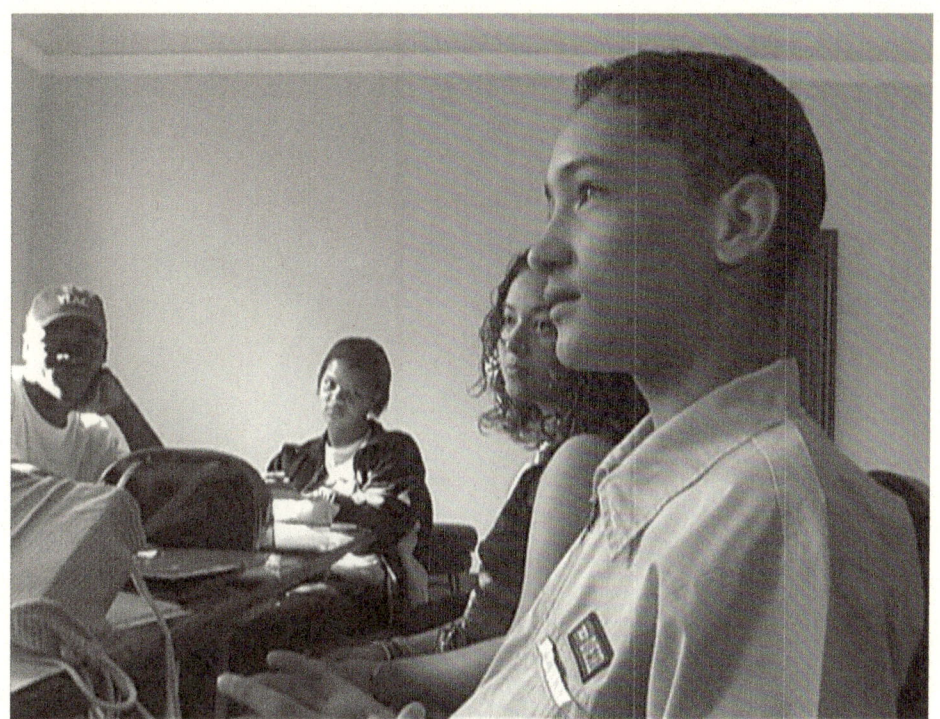

*Mathew, Kaylene, Ann & Mphumzi at 'Soft Cover' workshops, 2002*

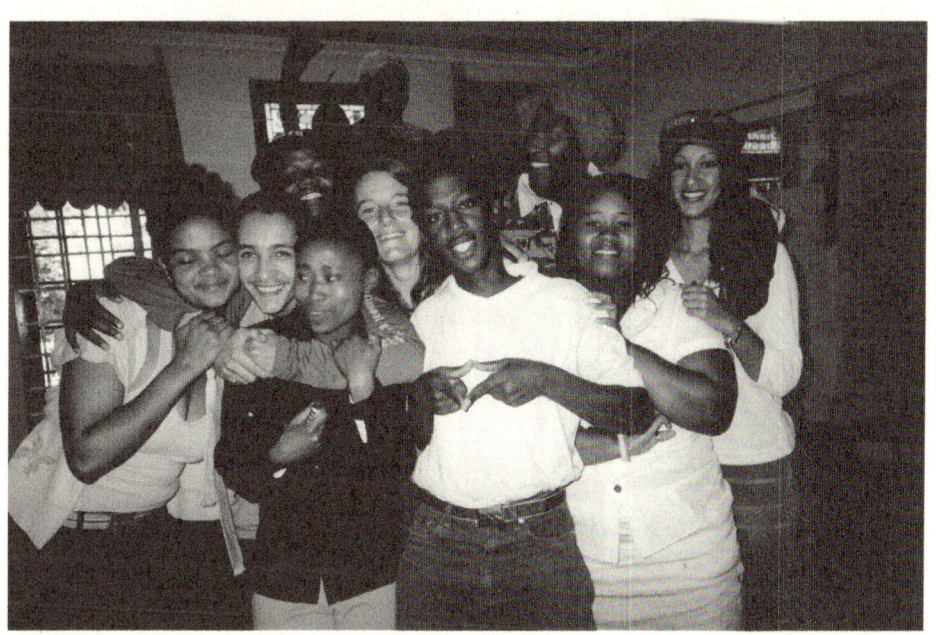

*Evaluation review session, 2005 (L-R: Ann, Mathew, Nosibosiso, Shannon, KK, Mandla, Lindeka, Chinomy. Mphumzi in far back)*

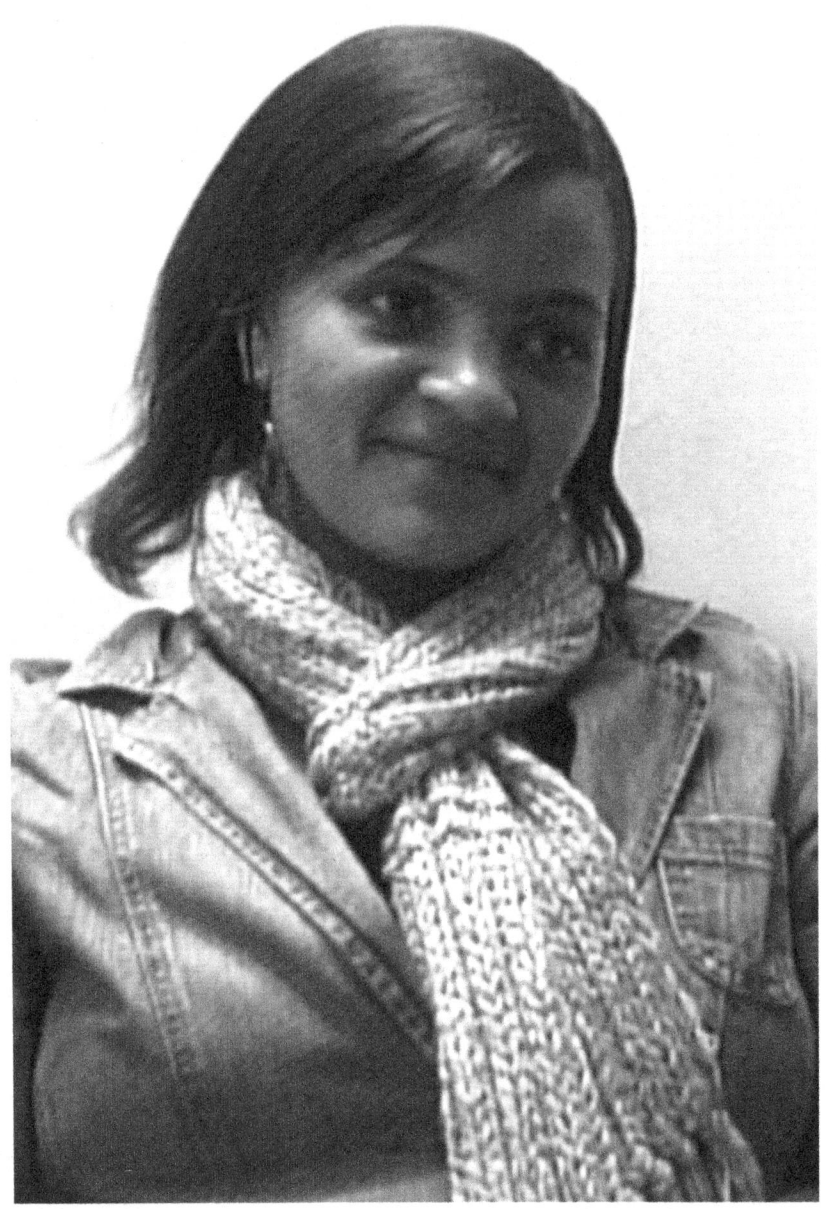
*Video interview still, 2006*

# 9

# Ann Thembeka Dipa

ANN WAS QUIET WHEN WE FIRST *met her at the Centre for the Book, but this hid the forthright, vibrant and strong woman we came to know over the years. During those first workshops and interviews, Ann kept to herself, but once she started writing and sharing her story in Xhosa, her confidence grew. She became able to read her poems aloud in front of a packed audience of learners. Ann has had a challenging life and committed herself to building something different from an early age. Growing up in Khayelitsha, she faced struggles in relation to violence and poverty, and had direct experience of HIV and AIDS with her family and friends. These experiences made her a staunch ally and activist, a role she has continued to play. Alongside her writing and poetry, Ann was an active part of creating the* Facing the Truth *and* Street Fear *video projects. She studied at the Cape Peninsula University of Technology and now lives in Cape Town and works as a bus driver with Golden Arrow.*

# 2003

### *Ann at 18*
Excerpts from *In My* life

My name is Ann Thembeka Dipa. My grandma used to call me Pinky. I'm 18 years old. I'm a student in Manyano High School in Khayelitsha. I'm doing Grade 11. I live in Site B, Khayelitsha, Cape Town. I live with my mom, dad and three brothers and one cousin.

I love educating people about HIV and AIDS so that they can know the difference between HIV and AIDS. I would like to be like Zackie Achmat one day, be a struggle hero, be a role model for everyone in the country.

I remember the time of Nkosi Johnson's death. I was hurt at the time, and angry at the president for letting people die and not doing anything about it. I wish that the president would see HIV and AIDS the way I see it, and do something about it, and that he would stop saying antiretrovirals are toxic, because it makes people distrust them.

I also wish that everybody would know their status and do something for their lives. The thing that I would like to highlight for you is that HIV and AIDS is real, and it is there to stay. A person with HIV and AIDS is still a person, your friend, your family. Take HIV seriously every day. Play safe, because… I care – Do you?

## IN MY NEIGHBOURHOOD

I hear a train sound in the morning at 4am and dogs chasing cars. I go out and smell the sea breeze, the flowers in my neighbour's garden, and hear the sound of police chasing a robbing gang, gun shots. I wash. Mommy's cooking breakfast. On Sundays, I go to church, people singing, especially gospel, joyful of god. Some people don't go to church, they just go to drink, and chase one another, making noise. Visitors on Sundays, telephone, ring after ring, cooking lunch.

In my neighbourhood, young people are smoking dagga and drinking alcohol, doing drugs and robbing the people. Young people carrying guns all the time. They kill people, they get arrested every day, but they don't change. Instead of changing they do more killing, sometimes even innocent children. People get infected with HIV every day. There are people who are dying every day, people who are arrested every day, people who are killed every day, people who are robbed every day, people who are raped every day.

All the time there are people shouting and laughing loudly. People drink every day especially on weekends. Gangs shot one another, they rob the houses and hijack cars and kill people. They also kill one another. But we had a meeting in my neighbourhood where all the people in the street got taught by young teenagers about the disease,

HIV and AIDS, and that was good.

On 24 December 2002 this guy was carrying a gun. He was going around the area alone because his friends had been arrested and he was not found yet. Later he found out that there are people who are looking for him and they were going to kill him. He went looking for them. But in the meantime, this gang went to his house and found his mother. They asked her where her son was, and she said she didn't know. So, these guys shot and killed his mother, then they went looking for him. When he got back, he found his mother dead in cold blood and the neighbours told him who did it. He went after them, but they shot him in the head. He fell and the police came. The gang had run away. The police called the ambulance. He was crying and he was sad. He said he was going to be ok, and go after them and kill them all. But he didn't have enough time – he passed away. And that was the end of him.

## MY STORY

First, I didn't know anything about HIV and AIDS. I didn't know the difference between HIV and AIDS. Although I was curious about everything happening around the country I live in, and had heard about HIV, I wasn't very interested. I thought that if the person had AIDS, they were going to be locked in their room, not to be seen by anybody. I thought that HIV was not in my country. I even thought that if a person had AIDS, everyone would be able to see it, that they would have a special colour or something.

Then one night, I was with my friends in my house. We had a girls' night that day, and we were talking about issues. We talked about HIV, and then my friend disclosed her status to me. I didn't know what to say. After that I didn't know what to do. She was healthy and beautiful. We always did everything together at that time. It was then that I realised that HIV is something real. I became interested in HIV and AIDS.

We went to the workshops together and got more information and we have ended up being informed. After that I realised that I have to know my status. I thought about it first and then the next week I went for an HIV test. I tested HIV negative.

I am proud of my friend because she has accepted it. She told herself that she is going to fight it, no matter what. I joined her and we became very close. She is happy that I accept her and I do all I can to make sure that she is happy.

I think that HIV changed my life. First, I was scared, but now I know that HIV is there to stay and if it gets into your body, it is going to stay for the rest of your life. I realised that you have to love it and take care of it. It's time to stand up and fight it. Now I feel the pain of people who are being discriminated against, as if it is happening to me. I take HIV seriously. I take it personally. People in my heart are all those people living with HIV, and those who died because of HIV and AIDS, like Nkosi Johnson.

## NOMONDE GCAZA

It was Monday and Nomonde Gcaza came to visit our school. She was educating us about HIV and AIDS. She came with her daughter and she disclosed to us that she was HIV positive. Everyone was shocked because she was beautiful and she was healthy, and there were many questions from the students. I found one student outside and she was crying. I asked her what was wrong, and she disclosed her status to me. Everyone else was inside and listening to Nomonde, so I tried to comfort her, and from that time she became my friend.

Nomonde stays in Khayelitsha. She's a mother, a counsellor, a nurse and also an educator in the community, in schools and shebeens. After Nomonde saw me talking to my friend, she asked me if I would help her when she's educating, and I said ok, it's my pleasure. Many of the teachers and students have problems, and I can't help them all because I am also a learner. So, I asked Nomonde if she could help me build a support group at school and she did.

Nomonde is like a mother to me because I can go to her anytime and ask for help. She never turns me away. She always helps me, and we discuss things together. When I get sad, she always sees me and talks to me. Nomonde changed my life. She calls me Pinky, my grandmother's name for me.

### When I am afraid

*I have a stomach pain and my legs*
*are not standing properly*
*I feel sad and then my emotion changes*
*and I become angry at everyone*
*I can't concentrate*
*I do everything very fast and*
*end up messing everything up*
*I don't want to be outside*
*I always stay inside the house*
*and when someone knocks on the door*
*I jump and go to the bedroom.*

*when I feel brave*
*my stomach feels free*
*and I feel like a queen*
*I feel like going out anytime,*
*not afraid,*
*not being scared of anybody*
*I feel like I am living in my own country,*
*and I do everything on time*
*I am nice to everybody*
*and to concentrate a lot*
*feeling at home and welcome.*

### Selfless spirit and champion in the struggle against AIDS

Found poem by Ann Thembeka Pinky Dipa from a newspaper article

*Every struggle gives birth to its own heroes*
*the apartheid struggle had Steve Biko and Chris*
*Hani*

*Tupac Shakur was shaped by the racial dynamics
of life in New Jersey's inner-city
and by the meaningless existence
of the black youth in capitalist society*

*The HIV and AIDS war has its own warrior
Zackie Achmat
who leads the country's battle against
the multi-national drug companies
and takes on the South African Government
over its confusing HIV and AIDS policies*

*Nkosi Johnson and Gugu Dlamini
gave AIDS its face
in their fight for treatment*

*Achmat, a founder member
of the Treatment Action Campaign (TAC)
mobilizes AIDS activists to take to the streets,
go to the courts and to parliament to prevent
pharmaceutical companies making profits out
of dying people's lives*

*TAC, assisted by unions and other lobby groups,
demands a roll-out of antiretroviral drugs
in the public health sector*

*HIV-positive Zackie Achmat,
refuses to take antiretrovirals
until they are given to all who need them.*

# 2002

**Ann at 17**
Group discussion
Centre for the Book

Like girls, when you say to the boys, let's just break up, he will say you can't do that to him, and will beat her. The girls are afraid because you don't have power to beat him. It's like that... Those guys they make their own ... their own kind of like ... go and steal this ... or force their girls, and say let's go ... they don't want to give their girls a choice to say ... when they decide it is time to have sex, the girls always say 'yes, yes, yes' because the girls are afraid of them – because they beat them all the time.

# 2006

**Ann at 20**
Individual interview
Cape Town café

My name is Anne Thembeka Dipa. I'm 20 years old. On 9 September I'm turning 21. I still live in Khayelitsha, Site B.

Now I'm studying at Ashiva. I'm doing computer programming. I'm still active but I don't have that much time in terms of going with the workshops and other stuff. I'm working on Friday to Sunday, going to school Monday to Thursday.

I'm helping my mom. I'm paying my fees for school. By doing the job I'm helping my mom to pay my school fees, yeah. I'm living with my mom and my dad, my sister and my young brother, and my late brother's son, he's five months old now.

It's been a long time since I saw you.

I was still in high school. After we launched our book, I set up a group at Manyana high school where I was attending. When I started, we were three at first. Some of the students they came, and as they felt comfortable, they came talk to me. After they felt comfortable to come to me and talk about their problems, some of them disclosed their status. We had to open a separate group so that we can chat. We did workshops, we educated students at school in our free time. Sometimes we'll ask the principal on break time or after school, or to give up just a period when their teachers are not busy and then we'd do workshops.

I did attend the TAC Information Campaign. Not full time right now because I'm doing so many things. It's been fun.

Last year I passed my matric. Before I passed, I had been saving for this dream of mine to go to the matric ball. Just before the ball, my older brother passed away. He was stabbed in my area. So, I couldn't go to the matric ball because of what happened.

My brother passed away on 13 August last year. It was a sudden. I left him there in my place, he was sleeping. Then later we found him. We heard the news and all the stuff and, yeah... The following week there was supposed to have been my matric ball and I couldn't go. I couldn't go. I had to be there for my mother, my brother, and my sisters, so I couldn't go. But I just told myself that I'll graduate, and next year in January I will try to just go. So, I just... I will graduate, I will, I will.

My friends called me that night. They were having fun and I was at home in the dark and all that stuff. Yeah, but I did cope. After that, my uncle passed away within a month that we buried my brother. I was writing my final exam then, and I told myself that I will do it, I will pass this matric, and I will go to school. I will go to college.

I did tell my teachers, but it's like, I'm having this pride. I told myself that, well, I'm having a problem, so it's my problem. It's nobody else's problem, it's my problem. I need to focus on school, focus on my books. Yeah, I'm having a problem at home and all this stuff. Sometimes I would feel emotional, but I just tell myself that well, I'm going to school and going to write, so I have to study. I have to go and write. I come back at home then I can start thinking about things. It was like that.

It is a big deal what happened. Honestly when I feel lonely, I always call my friends, 'Guys, I'm not sleeping now.' Sometimes late at night or around 2am, I have to talk to someone. I can't wake my mom or somebody else. I just call my friends, because I need someone to talk to. My friends always help me, because I'm always there for them! It's like that.

And I did finish my matric.

About writing, I always write. I even wake up in the middle of the night when there's something on my mind. I always take my book and write. Well, writing is like my life, yeah it is. Because, every little thing that is on my mind, I just don't want to think so much. I just take my book and write.

# 2006

*Ann at 20*
Individual interview
Workshop for *Facing the Truth*
Khayelitsha

Being part of the project made an impact on me. Very much. I was having this thing to do and I was very proud of writing a book, meeting other people, especially of other cultures. Working together, building a relationship with them.

It really opened my mind that we have to teach one another. It's like as we said, 'Each one, teach one.' I followed that slogan, 'Each one, teach one.'[54] I was told, I was taught, and I have to do the same to other people. They must know. Especially for black people, because we as black teenagers – I don't know whether to say we don't care about the future or we don't think about the future.

In terms of that what I've been told, I would tell somebody else. Maybe he or she will go somewhere with it. I did the same in school. I taught them and told them what I've been told. I showed them my book. When I first showed them the book, they were too excited, 'How did you get there?' I had to tell them everything.

I introduced the book to the other students, and they were very interested. There was so much interest in it. We decided that we would do something. It wouldn't be as perfect as our book, but how about we just buy some blank books just to write. We tried to speak to the principal to support us to buy those books. Then we wrote together.

Each one had a book, so maybe if you have something in your mind, just take a pen, your book and write something. Stories, poems. It's not easy to write a poem, but you just write what you feel inside.

I told them I really liked what they wrote, they were very interested and we wrote together so much. It was very interesting. Every time we would meet, we would come up and read what we've written. It's not like you have to read everything what you write, because some of the things are very confidential. Because we all have our problems. It doesn't matter how beautiful or how right you look or whatever, we all have our problems. All of us. Either it's personal or something from home, or anything like that. So, we did that and it worked very well.

> what you feel inside you could just write

Because at least what you feel inside you could just write and try to communicate with your book. Although the book won't answer back, but you could keep on asking questions with your book, writing what you felt inside. We did that and sometimes we'd find, like I'm reading my book and everybody is listening. And then we would ask questions like, how did you feel before, how did you feel now, and all that stuff, yeah. So, it did work very much for me.

I started first doing a workshop at school. It was about teenage pregnancy because the rate was piling up at school of teenage pregnancy. When they were in primary school, they didn't have access to information. Now they're in high school, and they're out of control. So, I did a workshop on teenage pregnancy to teach them about condoms, drugs and other stuff.

There was a lady that was very interested in what I was doing, Nomonde Gcaza. She's a community worker. I asked her to come and help me, because I'm a student and they know I'm from school, and they won't listen like they would to someone from outside. I asked her to come, and then we did the workshop together and I tried and explain everything to them.

The thing is that we as students don't want to rely on or disclose our matters to the teachers. We are scared that she will shout and tell the students my problems. So, we came together as three students, and opened up a group, where we can come together. Maybe I'm stressed, I have to meet the group. I'm having this and this problem. I don't know, whether I'm not like everybody or it's just me but I take other people's problems very personally. I always take them. I don't say, 'I don't see your problem.' Your problem is my problem. So, we have to sit down, we have to discuss, we have to talk.

Sometimes I don't have someone to speak to. Sometimes I'm just stressed. It's other people's problems, it's my problems and it's all in my head and my books. I have to focus. I have my own problems so I just say ok, when I'm having problems I need to speak to my friends. I just call them 'Guys, can we chat?'

After we did the support group at school, we found out that there were so many students that are having problems. Some, they're living alone. Some, they just come to school and they haven't eaten. What we did, every cent that I have I had to make sure that me and Lamande, we just collect the money. Let's say I have five rand and Lamande has seven rand, we have to take money and buy bread. When we are sitting in the support group, we have to at least eat, make sure that they eat and organise some transportation for them. Some of them live really far from school and they don't have money. Sometimes they don't come to school because they don't have money to come to school.

We did our best to help them. I was in matric and I had to focus on school, so to me it's like I'm leaving them behind. They had problems but I told them, 'Guys sometimes I wouldn't be there, you have to stand on your own. Don't rely on a support group, we have to stand on our own.'

They can practice to be alone and facing their problems the way we did. We did face our problems. At the end of the day, you have to face your problems, don't always rely on somebody else because that person won't always be there.

In this support group, we don't only talk about our problems and other stuff, we talk about what is HIV, what is teenage pregnancy and other stuff. We do everything, everything. They have to know everything. They have to know, because one day someone will say, 'I'm the member of this support group Rise and Shine', we called our group Rise and Shine. I'm a member of Rise and Shine support group and someone will come with a big problem, so we have to be aware, so when somebody else comes we must know how to help them.

My mom, she's doing very good work for me. Sometimes she would just say, 'Hey, we were taking a taxi or a bus and someone talked about a friend or sister in their family who was dying of AIDS', and my mom just said, 'Can you give me your number because my daughter knows about HIV and she can help you.'

She's always giving them my number. She'll come home and say, 'Ann, there's a person like this and this, who'll call you. Maybe she'll call you now, or tomorrow I don't know. But you must be aware that that person who will call you and that person needs help because of the person or the family or friend that is dying.'

I would have to wait for that call. I only stare at my phone, because that person is dying. I tell myself: 'Ok I'm told that this person is dying. When my phone rings I have to help them.' I always visit them. One thing that I tell myself is that, those people they don't just need to be counselled, they need to go to the clinic. They need to get antiretrovirals, they need to be in a support group where there's HIV-positive people. I always help them like that. It did work for me.

It's like to me, you showed me the world. You showed me how life, it is. Things are not always right, or always positive. You have to expect everything. You have to expect everything.

I'm seeing a lot of impacts of AIDS in my community. I don't know whether I would say that people really don't want to listen. Because, one of the things that makes me really, really angry, it's like my cousin who passed away in 2003. We weren't living together. I just heard that she's been sick and she's in the hospital. I went to the hospital when I got there and she was very, very sick. I asked again what is the problem? I was just told that she's sick, and nothing else. The family knew that she was sick. After, about a month later, she said, 'I need to talk to you, there's something I need to tell you.'

'What is it?'

'I'm HIV positive.'

I was like, 'Ok. I'm not shocked. When were you HIV positive why didn't you tell me then?'

I didn't ask so many questions, because she was already sick and she was lying in a bed. I couldn't ask so many questions because I would be stressing her, and so I just told myself, 'She needs someone to be there for her. I'll be there.'

We talked and she got better and better. I was angry, but I didn't show my anger to her. I was very angry! She was getting better. She couldn't eat, she had thrush. Her throat was sore she couldn't eat, she just drank some liquids. I supported her. In every way, I supported her.

I still remember it was the first of November 2003.

I got home late. I think it was around 12 at night. I got home late, because we were doing some symposium. There was a competition for schools, so we had to be there. It was about HIV and AIDS, pregnancy and drugs. Each school had something to say about it. It was a competition. So, when I got home, I just went straight to my room because I was tired, and the next morning I had to be back at the hall again.

My mom calls me, 'Ann, come here I have to tell you something.'

'What?'

'Lily passed away today.'

'Ok.'

I just went to my room. I didn't think about what she was telling me. The next morning, I went to the hospital because I made a promise to Lily, 'On Saturday morning I'll be here. I'll come and visit you.'

And she was fine, she was talking, she was eating then! That next morning, on Saturday, I went to the hospital and the bed was empty. I tried to speak. I went to the doctor that I always found when I got there, and she just said, 'Didn't you hear?'

And she told me again and I said, 'Ok.'

I started to remember that my mom told me this yesterday. I didn't listen.

I just said it to myself, 'Where do I go now? Do I go home?'

One thing I knew is I'd be stressed to go home because the family will call my place. They knew that we were very, very close. Especially when she was in the hospital. I would be stressed enough if I go home, well what must I do now? I must go to the hall, where I'm supposed to go. I went there and people kept on talking, talking, talking, and this thing came in my mind…

Someone came to me and said, 'Ann, you don't look fine.'

We went outside and I told him. He was the first person to know. He was the first person, whom I opened my mouth and told my cousin passed away. And I was very, very, very angry that she didn't tell me anything before, after she found out she was positive.

I was very angry. When my family got there, I called all my cousins and sisters into my room. I didn't want any secrets.

'Guys, if you are having a problem, with a boyfriend, or whatsoever, feel free to come to me.'

To them, it was like I'm joking, because I am the little sister of all the cousins. I was the youngest one, and they were old.

'Guys, guys, really. I'm serious.'

They knew that I was serious. I told them I was angry that Lily didn't disclose her status to me. I'm teaching other people, I'm helping other people, what about my family? My family keep on dying. But I spoke to them.

One of them didn't listen to me. In 2004, she said she was going to visit her mom after she gave birth. It was a week after. She said she was visiting her mom in Eastern Cape, and she was fine and everything. A month later we heard that she's in the hospital. And the problem? I thought that the baby was sick or something, but they said, it's her. She's not talking. The last thing she said, she said to her uncle that they must keep her child happy, make her child happy and all this stuff.

I asked them, 'What is the problem? Why is she sick?'

I was ready to visit her that weekend, and I found out that she's HIV positive. She disclosed it on Wednesday, and then on Thursday, she passed away.

I was like, yeah, you see someone outside, that person has a problem, but in your family, they will keep on hiding things from you. I was very angry.

I told them, 'Ok well maybe they don't want to be helped by me.'

I didn't notice anything. That cousin that I was helping, she would keep on asking things about mother-to-child transmission, antiretrovirals, what not to eat when you're pregnant and HIV positive. I didn't notice anything. I just answered the questions, telling her how it works. I'm just giving her the answers. Well, she knew what she was asking then.

I just told myself, ok, that just happened. Although I am angry, I mustn't focus on the negative stuff. I need to be positive now.

I had to be very close to them, so that they could tell me. We sat down, we talked. I even said to them, 'Guys, ok, we go to the movies. We go out. We go to the parties. I meet your boyfriends and other stuff, you meet my boyfriend and … one day, can we go like we go to the movies, and go to Voluntary Counselling and Testing (VCT) and go do a test?'

They were very shocked.

'I'm not going there. I'm not going there.'

So, then I asked them questions: 'How will you know you're sick then? When you're sick, you can't do anything, laying on the bed, and that is worse for you. If you want to live, we have to go and do a VCT.'

We did. We did go. My cousins, my sisters, even my brother, my late brother. We went together. It was unbelievable. We went to the clinic and they asked,

'Do you know each other?'

'Yes, we do.'

The lady said to us, 'We can't do a VCT for all of you in one day. You must know that you're doing the right thing, you're right, but you can't come with your friends or someone close to you, you must come alone yourself.'

I spoke to her privately, and told her: 'I struggled to be here today. It took me about three months to be here with these people. I begged them, so they can know their status. If you don't test them today, they will never come back. Now they are ready to hear whatever. They are ready to know their status. Can you please do your job? I'm just telling you to do your job. Not to focus on something else. Those people know what they came to do here. They're older than me, but they know what they're doing. Just do your job.'

And she was like, she didn't have a choice. I was telling her myself, 'If you don't do it, I'm going to the manager. I'm going to the manager and I'll phone the Minister of Health. I have the number of Manto

Tshabalala-Msimang. I have her number.'

I showed her my phone.

'Does this number ring a bell? Does this name ring a bell for you? Well, she's not the one who said to you, you're hired, now you have a job. But, this person can really, really, really, really make you do what you are hired to do, or otherwise you don't have a job anymore.'

On one hand, it was like I was threatening her or something, but I just wanted her to do her job.

Well, we did the VCT. There were seven of us, six of us were negative, but we found out that one of us was positive.

I found out because each one will go and come back, go and come back. Others came out happy. I noticed that my older sister wasn't happy. I didn't ask at that moment. We just went home. Everybody heard the good news, but she was ignoring us.

Before we went to bed, I went straight to her room and sat next to her. It was only two of us in the room. I locked the door and took out the key, so that nobody will expect that there are people inside. She started crying. I just knew. Well, there it was. I didn't have to ask.

I just told her, 'Well, now you know. Now you have to take care of your health. Now we have to fight this. You won't fight this alone. We have to fight this. Other cousins, parents, they don't have to know. You don't have to tell them now, but when you are ready.'

The family was shocked, they didn't believe it, but she told them. She's on ARVs at the moment. She's on ARVs and she's fine.

You know what happened? I still remember this, after my brother passed away, we went to the funeral in Eastern Cape and she was there. I buried him in Eastern Cape. Two or three months later, my uncle passed away, which was really sad, especially for my mom. She just lost her child and now her brother. Those two people they were very, very close. I'm telling you, she'll kill you for them. I just told myself, 'Ok this happened I have to be there for her, I have to.'

Then before the funeral of my uncle, one of my aunts, they were gathered with my mother, they were talking. I was very glad to see my mom smiling. I was like, the case is closed, my mom's smiling. She's becoming herself now. My aunt and her were talking about this HIV and AIDS thing. Some don't understand. Some they do, because they come from Eastern Cape. Some they don't know HIV. They know that if you have HIV, HIV is AIDS to them and you will die after. It's like they were talking, they keep on talking and talking. My mom brought up my name on the topic. And my aunt said, 'I'm not sure whether to say this or not, but I'm suspicious of your daughter in this HIV/AIDS thing. I think she has it. How come people come and talk to her when she's not positive?'

'I'm doing this for myself, I'm doing this for my tomorrow. I'm doing this to help other people.'

My mom, she was smiling because she knew that people will think otherwise about me knowing everything about HIV and AIDS. She just said, 'Ann has been involved in so many projects, she keeps herself busy.'

Other people will say I'm digging for nothing. Why am I wasting my time on this stuff? But I just tell myself, 'I'm doing this for myself, I'm doing this for my tomorrow. I'm doing this to help other people.'

My mom said, 'Well, it's her problem. It's no matter if she's positive. It's her problem, but one thing I know is that she won't let me down. She won't let herself down.'

I came with the certificate from our workshops, and she smiled. At first, she didn't understand, she was stressed because people were talking and I told her, 'I'm proud of doing what I'm doing. I don't care what other people think.'

People will think otherwise if you're active, especially in HIV and AIDS. They will think that you have AIDS. I would wake up in the morning and wear my HIV-positive T-shirt from TAC. Sometimes when I'll go to town, I'll wear this T-shirt and my mom will say, 'Don't you have clothes anymore?!'

'Mom, I feel like wearing this T-shirt. To me, this T-shirt says I support people. I can speak to them. Because HIV is not like a robot. When you have HIV, you just don't become red. It's a virus. It's inside. Wearing that T-shirt to me says, I support them in every way. I support them in every way.'

They must know that they have support, because if we all wear the T-shirt that says, I'm HIV positive, it's like disclosing yourself to other people.

It's either you're infected or affected. You wear those T-shirts to support those people.

We have to end this stigma and discrimination. We have to. Now people are educated and most people, they know about this HIV and AIDS. Yet, there are people who are stereotyped. There are people who are very stubborn. Who don't want to listen. Who do things to please other people. I can't please somebody else but myself. I'll never please somebody else. I can give you my money or something that I have, but not my body. I'll never do that. I don't have another body; this is what I have. I have to keep this. This is what god gave me. I have to take care of it. So, we have to end this stigma and discrimination. We have to end it.

> To me, it was like we are all positive, and we are all negative. There is no difference.

I talk mostly with women, it's not easy to talk to men, it's not. But, it's like the gentlemen... I always meet them, maybe someone like a sister or a cousin or a mother came to me, my son or my brother or my husband because I do meet all the people, my husband, my grandfather... I sit with them.

It was my experience with TAC and our group at the Centre for the Book that made me this kind of activist. The workshops taught me a lot, they taught me a lot. Before I didn't know about HIV. I didn't care about HIV and AIDS. To me it was like in Zimbabwe, not here. It was like HIV is for those people. I don't know how to say those people, what kind of a people, but other people, not us.

I had these best friends, we were triplets. We used to have girls' night; sometimes we'll sleep at my home or Narissa's or Nombulelo's. We'd always hang out on weekends maybe on Friday or Saturday, and the next week we go to my place, Nombulelo's or Narissa's. Our parents knew about it. One day we were in my house, we were just playing soft RnB. After the song Narissa said, 'Hey I have to tell you something.' I said, 'You know that you can tell me anything.' Narissa started to disclose her status. I was very shocked. I asked her again, 'What did you say?' 'I'm HIV positive. I found out about this in the previous year in June. So, yeah, I'm HIV positive.'

Earlier that day we were at a TAC workshop. I was just starting to learn about HIV and AIDS. I wasn't very interested but I'd just go because my friends were going. I would say, I don't feel like going, and they would say, 'We're coming to fetch you now.' So, I'd wait for them and we would go. I would just sit with my arms crossed during the workshops. I would listen, but in my mind I thought, HIV is not for us. HIV is in other countries, not in South Africa. It has nothing to do with me.

When she told me her status, I was in a dilemma. One part of me was saying, go out of the room, but this was my house I couldn't leave them alone. Another part of me was saying, just hug her.

My tears started to fall. I just hugged her and we cried.

After an hour, it was like the rain. Nombulelo started to disclose to me, 'Me too, my friend. I'm sorry to tell you this now. I know that I don't want to waste time. I don't want Narissa to disclose now and after a month later I disclose, because you'll ask why I didn't tell you then.'

'Ok, you're not dying anyway. You are my friend and we'll fight this together. Starting from today I'm telling you, I'm promising you I'll attend the workshops. You won't need to push me to go to the workshops I'll go to the workshops. Starting from today we'll fight this. We are friends and there is nothing that will break us.'

To me, it was like we are all positive, and we are all negative. There is no difference.

If I hit the street no one's telling me that there is a positive person there, and there's a negative person. We're beautiful, really hyperactive I could say, because if you go to the match, the match will be ours, the three of us.

People would say, Nombulelo and Narissa are there. We'd just sit in the back and they would keep on singing, they would keep on singing. We were very proud of it, because we were doing something that we loved to do.

Afterwards, I told myself, 'My friends are positive and that doesn't mean they're not my friends. They are my friends and, well, I have to go and know my status too.'

Before I didn't know anything, but now at least there was something that was telling me, go, go, go! I can support my friends. I didn't do it to please them. I did it because my heart was telling me to do it. I went to the workshops and went to the VCT. It was hectic because at that time it was like, it is your life you want to know about.

⁓

Later I had been involved in a car accident. I lost so much blood. I knew that I was negative, but it came to my mind that you don't only get HIV through sex. I was involved in a car accident, and I lost so much blood, and there was so much blood in that car, and everybody was bleeding, so I had to ask.

The guy who tested me said, 'Are you ready for this? Why are you doing this?'

I told him that 'I'm teaching people about HIV and AIDS. I tell them to get tested, to do their VCT. I'm not preaching. I just tell them to go and learn their status. We have to practice what we preach. I have to do what I'm telling other people to do. You must show up for yourself and then you can help other people.'

'Wow, I didn't expect that from you! You're still young and you just gave me the answer.'

He was really shocked.

'I'm ready for this. I came here to test so that I can know my status.'

'What if you're positive what will you do? What will you do? If I tell you now that you're positive what will you say? What is the first step that you will take?'

He kept on testing me in every way. And he said later, 'The results are positive.'

I laughed, and I said, 'Ok, can I go now?'

It was like, to me, I don't see HIV in the way other people see it. It was ok. I have a life after anyway. It doesn't matter what the results were. When I started to open the door, he said, 'Hey, come here. Sit down!'

I said, 'You're finished. What am I coming back here for?'

'No. Do you even want to know, to see the test itself, to be sure that you're positive or something?'

'You told me that I'm positive, you know my test, so what's the point?'

And then he showed me and said, 'I was told in the workshops that when this and this and this is like this, you're negative, when the signs are like this, you're positive.'

And I was like, 'But this shows that I'm negative. Why did you say I was positive?'

I sat down and said, 'What is it that you're telling me? I'm negative or positive? You already told me that I'm positive.'

Then he said, 'I wanted to make sure that you were ready. Now I know that you are ready. The test came out you're negative.'

I wish that I could have just... I don't know what I wanted to do with him!

---

Where does this thing take me? I tell myself, 'Keep doing it. This will help you one day and open your mind one day.'

There are times where I feel very hurt. Very, very hurt. I also have my own problems, family problems and all this stuff. There are times that I feel very hurt.

I've got this thing in my mind. I told myself if you keep on crying, things won't go right.

Things won't go the way they are supposed to go. I just tell myself, 'Ok, I have this problem, I will solve it. I will do anything. I will solve it.'

If someone is hurting me, even though the person doesn't realise they are hurting me, I just tell myself, I must distance myself from this person.

'The only thing that I'm doing, I'm not talking to you. I'll answer you if you ask me a question but I won't dig you. I won't. Because I've hurt already. The only thing that I don't want is to show how hurt I am.'

It's like, I'm this secretive person. I don't just go and say 'I'm hurt this and this happened.'

I don't, but I always ask myself, why not? Because people are coming to me and telling me their problems. Sometimes I would feel very sick because in my mind, there's my own problems, and other people's problems, and I don't have any space.

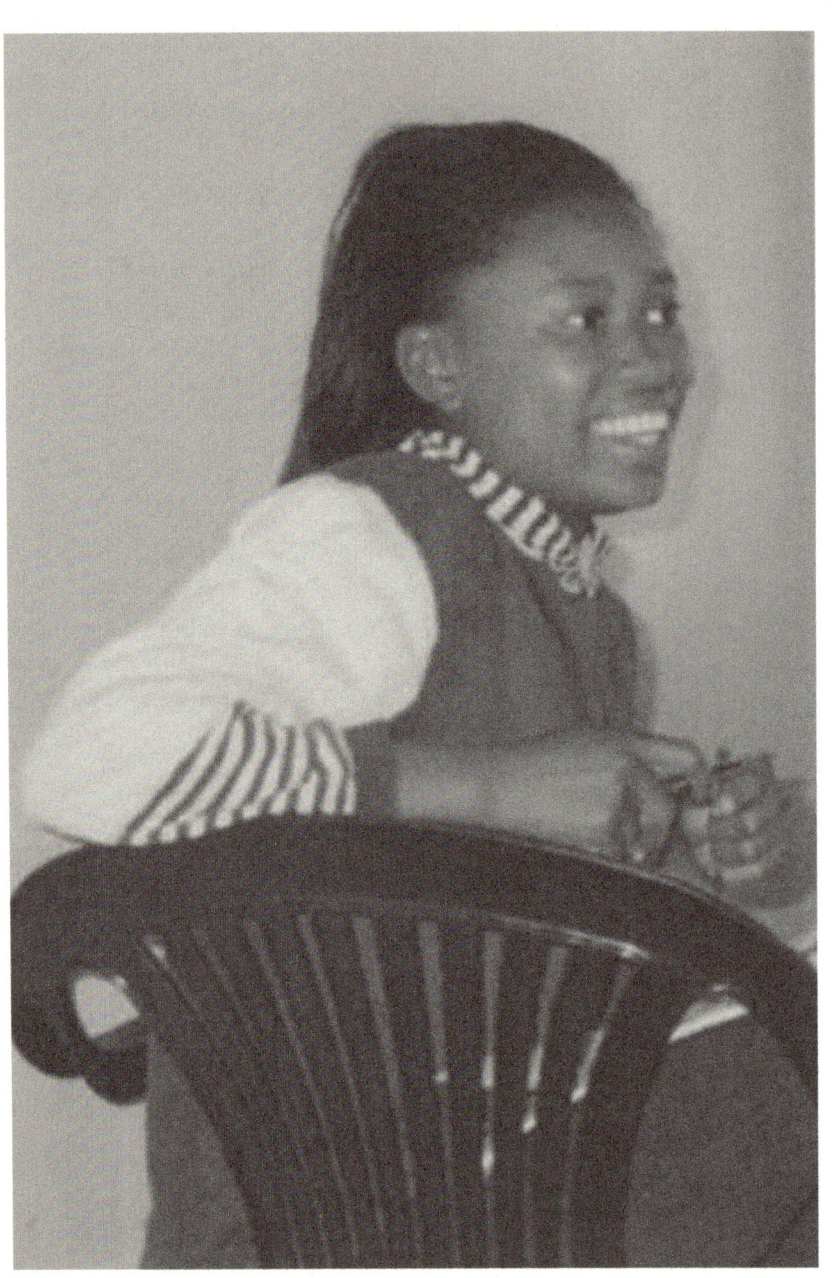

# 10

# Nosibusiso (Nosy) Mcunukeli

NOSIBUSISO, KNOWN AS NOSY, *has the spirit of a fighter. She is fearless in speaking her mind, sharp witted and passionate in everything she does. Raised in Khayelitsha, she has always seemed to us wise beyond her years. She is an advocate for women's rights and has been an HIV-prevention activist since her teenage years. Nosy was involved in the girls' participatory video* Street Fear *doing script writing and filming, and involved in the Khayelitsha-led video project in private schools* Facing the Truth *as well as in the writing and educational workshops. She has continued work as an activist and as an advocate for workers' rights as a shop steward, while also becoming a mother. Recently she has gone back to school to further her qualifications in wholesale and retail operations supervision.*

*Nosy always said that writing from a place of honesty and personal reflection had a deep impact on her self-growth. The* In My Life *writing workshops revealed an ability to express her innermost feelings and this has remained with her over the years. So, too, have the friendships that were built across cultures in an otherwise divided society. Nosy has committed herself to the lifelong journey of activism that she began as a young person, even amidst the many heartaches and hardships that she has had to face along her journey.*

# 2003

*Nosy at 17*
Excerpts from *In My Life*

I'm Nosibusiso Mcunukeli. I live in Site B, in Khayelitsha, in the city of Cape Town. I'm a 17-year-old girl in Grade 11 at Thembelihle Senior Secondary School. I live with my family. I love people who express themselves in every way that they can. I love conversations about things that concern me. I love shopping. I love joking and I love to smile a lot. I love my family, friends and especially myself. I love taking challenges. I also love making a good impression on people. I hate it when people see other people as inferior, and judge others by their clothes and all that stuff. I hate any kind of thing that doesn't bring goodness out in another person's life.

I remember the death of my older sister, what she died of, when and where. I also remember the death of my grandmother, who I loved dearly. I dream of achieving my goals in life. I dream about being an economist one day when I am old enough to handle anything.

I dream of being one of the most popular people on earth.

Readers – nothing is more important than yourself, knowing what you want, knowing what is the best thing for you in your life. Always be your first priority, and take challenges as challenges, or don't look at them otherwise. Always respect your own wishes.

It happened in my neighbourhood… It was 6:30pm, just when the *Bold and Beautiful* ended. The boy's mother asked him if he would go and buy sugar and potatoes and a packet of tea bags. He said, 'Yes I can, right after *Jam Alley*.'

His mother said, 'That's okay, I will only cook at 7 o'clock anyway.'

'Thanks Mom,' he said.

'What for?' his mother asked.

'Just about everything, but mostly for not yelling at me when I said I will go after *Jam Alley*.'

Then she said, 'You are welcome.' She gave him a hug.

When Jam Alley ended, he went out. As he went down the passage a drunk old man said to him, 'You better watch yourself son, there is a lot of violence outside there.'

When he stepped on the pavement there were thugs shooting at one another, and a shot hit him in the back of his neck. He fell on the road and a motor car hit him.

When another one hit him, this time it was a taxi. He went up into the sky. When he was just about fallen down another one hit him again. His mother heard the shots. She came running. She said, 'Please god, don't let it be my son.' When she saw it was her son she said, 'Ooh my god! Not my baby. Please it can't be.'

### In my neighbourhood

*My watch wakes me up, or the radio*
*train passing by*
*taxi, bus, motor car passing by*
*birds' song from the trees*
*smelling the fresh air*
*shoe-steps from people going to work.*
*laughs, talks*
*opening of the shop nearby*
*police talking or moving around with their cars*
*my neighbourhood late at night*
*juke box, especially on weekends*
*gun shots, cars non-stop*
*shouting of people, fights,*
*screaming of cats, dogs barking*
*police moving around*
*laughs*
*talks and steps of people*
*music, loud music*
*people having a while conversation.*
*screaming people.*
*people being beaten by lovers*

*telephones ringing non-stop sometimes*
*smashing of car doors*
*rudeness, especially on weekends*
*rude people trying to disturb us*
*because they are not asleep*
*highjacking of fidelity, of cars,*
*of people's money .*

*Sundays it becomes very quiet and very slow*
*people smoke dagga*
*go to church*
*everyone has something to do*
*always something to say*
*Sundays people cook, wear beautiful clothes,*
*it's not like Friday and Saturday*
*where everything is loud,*
*it's one of my favourite days*
*although I hate it sometimes because*
*when it is Sunday, tomorrow is Monday.*

*People in my neighbourhood*
*look like fools sometimes*
*when they act irrationally*
*fight, go around carrying guns, knives*
*not caring about the youngsters*
*there are few motivating things*
*even the police lack the spirit to motivate people*
*because they often work with the thugs we are*
*trying to get rid of*

*but for us teenagers*
*we don't let what is none of our concern*
*get in the way of doing*
*what we feel is right for us*
*we respect those who respect us.*

## When I'm Afraid

*It's like a part of me is being ripped from me*
*I feel like I'm dead when I'm alive*
*I've become very absent with myself*
*My stomach will tremble*
*and my heart will beat very fast*
*and my breathing becomes very wrong.*

*When I feel brave,*
*it's like I am in control of everything*
*I feel comfortable, hero-like*
*and I handle everything kindly and very fast*
*I become positive about things*
*it's where my self-confidence lies*
*and my dignity*
*I feel it in my mind and soul*

## THEY CAME TO TALK TO US

I was in a dance class. We were told about people with HIV coming to speak with us. We were dancing and were told to stop and go to our locker rooms to change. Around about 2:30 pm they came; four people, two boys and two girls. We didn't even know them. Our coach called them to him and they hugged. They told us to sit down and listen to them very carefully, but first to introduce themselves.

Then they told us that they were HIV positive. I didn't believe them, but they proved it to me with the tablets they were taking. I was shocked, but I didn't react at that point, because I was facing an internal conflict. I listened to them telling us how they got the virus. We listened and asked what we needed to ask and, at the end, I wanted a big hug from all of them. And we talked and laughed.

I was very impressed and very affected by them. Talking with them and gaining knowledge from them gave me a different kind of thinking. I felt greater. They made me realise that you have always to give the benefit of the doubt. I may see myself with a big problem without knowing that there are people with bigger problems than mine and mine to them is nothing. These people started for me the kind of difference that you yourself can ask for.

## WHAT PEOPLE THINK ABOUT HIV AND AIDS

'There is no cure. It is time for unmarried couples or teams to discover the importance of fidelity and the sacredness of chastity. So, we may as well reconcile ourselves with sexual morality.'

'People act as if HIV and AIDS is airborne. We are holding the solutions and answer to our own questions, the power to stop it, but still, still people are being stubborn, irresponsible and very unreal.'

'The time to act is now, not tomorrow, not two weeks after or before this day. Now. This thing is serious, works in mysterious ways, anonymous, famous, dangerous, it gets to people's lives.'

'Just because you have tested HIV positive, doesn't mean that you have AIDS. If you take care of yourself in a responsible and respectful way you'll be just fine. You can and may as well be living with HIV for many years before getting to AIDS itself. After you have been infected, you still have 10 to 15 years to live. If you eat properly and in a healthy way, exercise and eat your medicine or pills you'll be just okay.'

'Finding out that you are HIV positive must be very hectic, but don't let it be the death sentence for you, just don't let it be the end of the world. I know at first it will be very hard and very hurtful or disturbing but you may as well deal with the consequences of it.'

'After first hearing or knowing your HIV status you'll be bombarded by a whole lot of emotions like shock, sadness and denial, so it's important to go for counselling or just join a support group. If not, just tell a close or true friend of yours. Talk about your feelings and find ways to lead a happy and responsible lifestyle.'

## INTERVIEW WITH SINDISWA R. KHAYELITSHA, D SECTION, BY NOSIBUSISO

She said that at first the world seems to be coming down on you and you feel like you are falling apart. She felt like dying, knowing that she had to live the rest of her life HIV positive. She felt like god had turned his back on her. But she had a lot of health and counselling from family and friends. She knew that she was facing one of the biggest challenges in life. She has counselling, never misses or forgets to drink medicine. 'And I always get myself out of my need for someone to blame,' she said.

### INTERVIEW WITH BULELWA, BY NOSIBUSISO

She said that living with HIV is one of her biggest problems because at first people were rejecting her, calling her names, giving her judgemental looks. 'Looks that can just make you want to cry.' She couldn't believe that she was really, really HIV positive but the fact of the matter was that she was. She would look back, look at her life, her heart, and always find an empty space. But now all of that has changed. Letting herself fall apart was one of the biggest mistakes of her life. She said, 'The best way to get through it is to let those who can see that you are hurting and want to help, just let them do so. And adjust your reactions. Maybe, just maybe, they will be giving you exactly what you need and desire.'

# 2018

*Nosibusiso at 32*
Group discussion
Centre for the Book

I'm Nosibusiso, and I won't say I'm still the same person that I was 15 years ago. That would be weird. Like, back then I was naive, paranoid, and all of the above that you can mention. I was wild! I was out there.

But the main thing that always stood out to me was how I always opened up my mind to things and took them as a challenge. As I told you then, the project was a challenge to me. I needed something that would open my eyes at the time because I was 13 as an HIV activist with the TAC. I just started. I was just recruited at school. We had this project, and then we had the project at school. We had the kids in lower grades that we had to look after.

Coming here to the Centre for the Book, I would note that, OK, she's going through that, he's going through that and going through that. It made me think of ways I could implement education. If that one doesn't work then I'll use Mathew's idea, and if that one doesn't work, I'll use Thozzi's method. And because I have six methods that I can use to tackle one problem, okay, alright, I'm getting there. So, that's where it started.

I am kind of still a bookworm. I still read. I still write, a lot. I've got a lot of crap in my head right now. Even on my phone, and everything. My manager would ask me, 'Why didn't you write in the first place, because some of the stuff that you write, I don't know where the hell you get that from.' Sometimes, I'll be watching a movie and then I'll end up somewhere else, in another world thinking about other things. Then I'll just write.

I'm in my mind, writing something. I don't know where it comes from. I'll write, I'll write, I'll write. Then I'll see, no man, there's no more space to write, and I'll get a new writing book. I write in my book. I still have it. I still have those old notebooks that you gave us. They're still there. And some more of mine. Even though my parents were so against it.

My mother wanted a doctor in the house, she wanted police in the house, she wanted a teacher in the house, and guess what? I did commerce. I ended up being an accountant. Which was another thing that she never even knew that existed. I'm accountant and I'm an AIDS activist. When will I get time to, you know, be me, be free, to grow up?

I don't know why I didn't do theatre myself. I don't know why. But all the writing, I coached some young people through the years, even now, I still do. Some of them have published writing.

---

I'll talk about changes I've had, as it sums up everything.

The first one is my health.

When I was doing my second year in varsity, I got pregnant. I found out that I've got low blood pressure, and I had kidney failure at the same time. I was booked in for three months, because I was almost six months pregnant then. I had to stay in hospital until I finished the whole nine-month period, of which I didn't finish it, because there were more complications. On the eighth month, they had to do a caesarean and take my baby out. I was there for about a month longer. They were busy looking after my health. The child was discharged because, apparently, she was overweight anyway. And I was still as tiny as I was. Yeah.

The second change was my family. While I was doing Grade 12, my older sister died. My older sister got burned, then the other sister miscarried, and then my uncle died. From June, something happened, skip a month, July, something else, skip a month, all the way until December. My older sister's funeral was on the second of December. Right after we buried my uncle. He died on the second of September, on his daughter's birthday. While his daughter was being born, he was dying. It's been hell and back for my family. With my health, and my mom and dad are both diabetic.

There was a time in my life where I had to work and study at the same time. School was the only thing that kept me sane. Even though I only attended classes on Fridays and Mondays, the rest of the week, I would be drinking! I used to drink a lot. I think that's how I became pregnant as well. Because I was not paying attention. I wanted not to pay attention to most of the stuff that was happening around me.

Then work. I started at Cape Ads, from Cape Ads to the Refinery, from the Refinery to Caltex proper, and on to other places.

In all of these places I met people. I met different characters. I've dealt with things that are beyond my imagination and age. I've had older woman coming up to me because of the character that I have. I'm always talkative and lively, whenever I'm around. I want people to notice that I'm in the house.

People find it easy to talk to me, to share stuff, even though I was still young, because I was still in my 20s. There was a lot of stuff that I could, you know, relate to.

Especially at work, I would tell them most of the times, if your manager is unbearable, try your supervisor, or move up and step further, go straight to HR. When you get there, you must be weeping already. They can't tell you they're busy, because whatever call they are on right now, you are the emergency and you are at work. They have to deal. They must make time for you. I know 90% of the HRs, they want you to make an appointment. There's not time for you to make an appointment, you are at a breaking point.

Work has been like that for me. I've been elected as a shop steward which became my full-time job. In a way, it's been good and bad.

It's been bad, in a manner that at my workplace there is a lot of racism from the people that I work with, especially my managers. When you are a proud black woman, it brings up a lot of, I don't know, anger inside you? I don't have the right words to put it.

I've got people from Paarl, from many places all over, from the farms, who come to work here, and then guess what? The first thing they do when they see me, they speak Afrikaans. Then I give them a look. I don't even take it in a boardroom when I'm sitting in a management meeting. The moment they start speaking Afrikaans, I push my chair, I take my phone, I take my recording device, and I get out.

If they wanted me to be in THAT meeting, and to listen and hear what I have to say about MY department, they wouldn't have spoken Afrikaans. You get to be surrounded with such nonsense all the time, even at work in this day and age. After 1992 Mandela said 'no one shall be oppressed by another,' and he asked us to all be civil to one another. I don't see why there are still people who see the need to be that way. It's not being naïve or being silly, that is being rude... If there is one word that can put that under, then it is that. Because how I call it, you don't want to know.

I went to a multiracial school, right? And I was taught by Xhosa, Muslim, coloured and Afrikaner teachers.

I've had three important men in my life, who are not even in my family. My high school teachers: Mr Zita. He used to teach me guidance; Mr Fatella, that's the man who made me love maths; and Mr Carolas who was my accounting teacher. Those men, including my dad, have always been my fathers, all four of them. Whenever I needed someone to knock some sense into my head, or if I'm going off the line, straying, I knew they would be straight and narrow with me and not brush it off. They wouldn't care less how I feel about it. They would put it down on the table, like 'hey, wake up. I don't know which world you're living in, but if you go on like this, this and this, this is what's going to happen, and you're not going to come back to me.' So yeah, basically, it's been like that. They were great. In fact, they were fantastic, they were there for me.

⁓

Even I myself was shocked at the fact that I would actually be capable of murder. I don't want to lie, it was the first time ever I was that angry. Ever.

I think it had everything to do with the fact that there were a lot of things that were going wrong in my life at the time.

I didn't need the father of my kids to be putting a hand on me at that time. He had done it for a long time basically. It took a lot of things out of me while he was doing that. So, me being a martial art and a judo student, he didn't stand a chance at all that night.

That is why I'm saying, I didn't know that I was capable of murder. He ended up in the hospital! He ended up in the hospital, you know. He only slapped me once and then he choked me, and at the time I was eating, you know. I'm sitting on the couch and I'm eating.

That was the day I told him I wanted nothing to do with him. I was eating and I knew when I'm done, I'm taking my bags and I'm leaving. My bags were already packed. I packed them in the morning already before I went to work. I'm just going to leave my kids' stuff because I know whatever happens between me and him, it's got nothing to do with the kids. It's just ... I'm fed up. I can't put up with this nonsense anymore. He needs to grow up, and he's going to do it on his own. I'm not going to mother him. So, when he choked me, or strangled me, whatever he thought he was doing, I became ... I just fumed; you know?

I tried to look for something. I couldn't find anything that was close by. I got my phone. I had a P8 cell phone. If you can see, the Huawei P8 has got a silver thing on the side, it actually is like metal, because it doesn't scratch at all. I hit him with that and it broke his nose.

While he was concentrating on the nose, that's when I got the chance to see the fork. And then I stabbed him, three times, with the fork on his chest. By the time his sister walked into the door, there was already blood all over the house. He broke a broom trying to hit me. I jumped to the other side and then it hit the bulb, and then that's when I had one chance to hit him like there's no tomorrow. Because the moment he broke the broom, I told myself, you know, I'm born and raised from Eastern Cape, I will show him what I used to do when I used to go after the cows and the sheep! I'm going to beat him up! He's never going to hit another woman in his life.

And I moved. I mauled him. When my brother and my cousin came to fetch me, they saw the blood from the gate. There was already an ambulance, and police and everything. They thought it was mine. Because I had blood all over me. When the ambulance came, I was the first person they looked at, not him. And I was telling them, 'No, there's nothing wrong with me, except my throat, check him.'

At the time, I was calm as hell. That's the weirdest part. I wasn't angry. I wasn't angry, or, as angry, throwing things and all that. I was as calm as hell. Some way, somehow, my mind and my body were on another level. That is what I'm saying. I didn't know that I could be THAT angry. Because … I … did that. I remember each and every word. Like flashbacks. I remember. How I moved from where to where, got what, to do what. I KNOW all of that.

I'm not… I'm not evil. I'm not evil.

---

If you remember how things were, at school, even us as ladies, we were forced to join a certain gang, growing up. Because we went to a township school. So, it was either you were with the nerds, the roughnecks, there were even names. There was those who were in control of the school and then at some point they brought in politics into school. To try and get rid of all that, because it came to a point whereby when you at a certain school you can't go to a certain location in Khayelitsha, you must be working in other areas and all that stuff.

A lot of kids were dying during that time. To them, it was more pressure growing up. Even though, you know, you're not going to entertain it or whatever, because when you get home, and your mother hears that you're working in the streets, or you running things, from another mother in the street, you're getting a bang. I'm telling you. They'll beat you like there's no tomorrow. 'I never gave birth to a crook!' and they hit you.

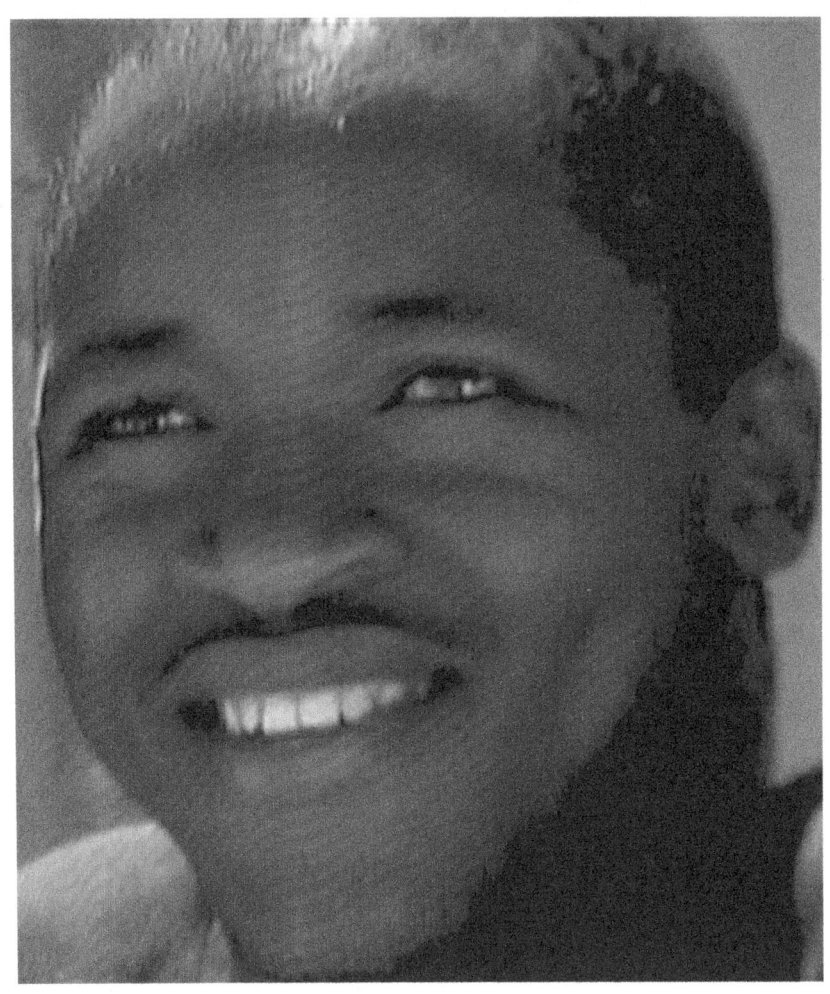
*Video still from* Fire & Hope, 2004

# 11

# Mphumzi Mphura Xokozela

ORIGINALLY FROM THE EASTERN *Cape, Mphumzi grew up in Khayelitsha. He was involved as a volunteer with the Treatment Action Campaign and was part of the School Representative Council alongside some of the other group members. After the workshops we did together, Mphumzi says he was propelled on a journey of activism and growth. He was actively involved in all our early workshops, writing and creative sessions as well as being soundman on the* Facing the Truth *participatory video and he was featured in the* Fire & Hope *documentary.*

*Mphumzi is the kind of person who always keeps the group positive and connected. From the very beginning of the workshops, Mphumzi showed himself to be a committed friend, and he was especially good at connecting those members who came from different communities and backgrounds. He has taken particular pleasure in nurturing and growing these friendships, continuing to learn, and staying open across cultural divides.*

*Like some of the others, studying beyond high school was not an option that was immediately open to Mphumzi, so after high school he went straight to work. After having children and getting married, Mphumzi moved to Port Elizabeth, but maintained close ties with the other group members. Recently, he moved back to Cape Town with his wife and children, and he continues to advocate for continuing creative educational work with young people today. He sees huge benefits of having worked as a young activist and talks about his appreciation for the network of close friends that resulted in our long-term work together. These days he hopes to go back to school and to continue his education, as he moves into the next phase of his life.*

# 2003

*Mphumzi at 19*
Excerpts from *In My Life*

My name is Mphumzi Xokozela. I'm currently staying in Khayelitsha and I attend Thembelihle Senior Secondary School. I am 19 years old.

Who am I? I am a Nigerian who is not quite used to the place he's in, who wants to smile, but the time has gone by. I remember being a very quiet boy in class. I remember my friends who I still miss a lot. I love going to cinemas, sharing ideas, listening to classical music, and my favourite food is pasta with cheese on top. I hate people who think of themselves before others and people who discriminate against people living with HIV and AIDS.

I dream of being someone who will work with people and meet new friends. I dream of seeing everyone equal, black or white, 'coloured' or African. Remember – it's important to know where you come from, so that you can know where you are going. And lastly – HIV is not out there, it's here, so if you are African you will support those who are positive, as I do.

### In my neighbourhood

*4am train going to the station,*
*people going to work, making a noise,*
*sound of cars and ambulances, police,*
*gun shots,*
*TVs, radios, people singing, juke box,*
*gun fire,*
*train after train,*
*buses, taxi hooter,*
*neighbours fighting over stupid things*
*smell of dead dogs, garbage, drains, meat, smoke.*
*Sundays everybody*
*preparing to go to church*
*on the road it's up and down*

> *even those who do not go to church,*
> *go to shebeens and watch soccer*
> *on the road it's up and down*
> *people go to the supermarket to buy groceries*
> *while other people are sitting at home*
> *watching TV, listening to radios*
> *and others are visiting,*
> *and me? always in meetings with my friends.*

## HOW HIV AND AIDS CAME INTO MY LIFE

I used to stay at home because almost everyone was involved in smoking or in gangs, and I did not want to get involved in that. Instead, I stayed at home and did nothing that was going to come between me and my mom. I felt good staying at home and I had fun reading books which I love, but it was very frustrating to be on my own.

Then one day my teacher told us: 'On Tuesday next week we will be having visitors at school. So please all wear uniform, and please whatever you do, ask as many questions as you can. It does not matter if you know the answer, just try to get him to explain.'

The day came and I was a little bit shy, but I helped to organise the chairs. The visitor spoke to us about HIV and AIDS and we asked questions as we promised, and it felt good to be able to communicate with other people and my fear that people or students were going to laugh at me was gone.

After that day I thought, 'Why should I sit at home and do nothing while people are dying?' So, I became involved at my school with the group called Abasha Phezulu. I feel good knowing that I'm there to educate and to help my friends and my community. I joined organisations like the Treatment Action Campaign, where I'm a volunteer. I'm happy because it's available to everyone.

But I'm still that Mphumzi that people know – and I'm happy, I hope.

### When I'm afraid

*I feel like I'm going to die*
*the first thing that is going to shake*
*is my body*
*and my stomach gives me that cramp*
*like I'm falling in something.*

*When I'm afraid I don't show it to people*
*but I can sense there is going to be something*
*wrong on this road or place*
*let me try another road,*
*maybe it will be better*

*When I feel brave, I feel good*
*because people rely on me*
*but there is still a little bit of shaking*
*and my heart pumps very fast*
*My eye does the twingle thing*
*and I get cold a lot.*
*I feel like shutting down.*

## WHAT PEOPLE IN MY NEIGHBOURHOOD SAY ABOUT HIV AND AIDS

Akhona Mayosi works at a lawyer's office as a receptionist. She is a Christian and she loves going to church. She loves people and is trying to pursue a career in Human Resources so that she would work around people. She says: 'I feel sad about the youth for not using condoms. I think everybody must use condoms or wait until they get married. People with HIV should not be discriminated against. They should be treated the same way those who are negative.'

Imkhitha Mofu says: 'I think that HIV and AIDS are not something to joke about. Some people think that HIV is not real, but they must know it's real. People have been told to be aware but they don't seem to listen. The other problem that people have is that they don't know that you cannot get infected by touching a person. I hate the fact that people don't even want to touch something that has been touched by an infected person. AIDS is real, people.'

# 2004

*Mphumzi at 22*
Interview for *Fire & Hope*
Khayelitsha

My name is Mphumzi. I'm 19 years old. I live in Khayelitsha. The work I've been doing I think has been making a change in some way, somehow.

If maybe I see a girl carrying a condom, it's not that she's expecting something, she just wants to be safe.

# 2006

*Mphumzi at 25*
Individual interview
Work site, Khayelitsha

My name is Mphumzi Xokozela, I live in Site B in Khayelitsha. I'll be turning 26 years old in September.

Since the last project I've been busy studying and everything, ups and downs. I lost my mom and everything, so, yeah, I know, but that happened. She passed on and then I started doing a service training here for about six months, learning about the machines I'm using. So, now I'm currently working, it's my first month here at Bumba Brick and Block. It's a black-owned company.

It's my first month but I can say for a normal person, it's a good starting job because, normally as a person you don't get to a company straight away. You go to the management. Normally you have to start from the bottom and then you have to get paid wages, but lucky for me I just got into the job and I started getting a salary and getting more responsible for my job. So, everything they put in about doing, I'm responsible for it. Even with the money.

Where I live in Site B I don't pay rent but I do help to buy food and everything. So, I'm going to help to buy food and everything and help when they need help. There only about seven of us living in the same house.

I left Iquayiya High School and then I went to False Bay College where I did business studies. I was supposed to continue this year, but unfortunately my mother passed away so, I couldn't go back financially. I'm going to do part time next year.

It was in the first month of January I lost my mother. She was in an old age home in Mitchells Plain. She had a few problems with her health, so I took her to the old age home to get better nursing than I did at home, because I had to go to school and everything. They supported her fine and everything. I have one brother. We're not getting along but we do talk. Jerome is my step-brother.

The project itself, Soft Cover, wow, I would say I gained more experience, got more open to people and being friendly to people and being recognised. You know everywhere you go people are like, 'I know you from somewhere' and it's like I've got this personality. They look at me and they see someone they can think of, people they see me and say wow. You know every time they see me, even for a year and they say you know what, the only time that I would know that AIDS exists or HIV exists is when people say you are dead because of HIV. If you are still living, it means that there's still hope. So, it's people like that that keep us going, that keep me going actually. Because you're being recognised, and because you know people and are able to travel.

The project made a huge impact 'cause now I have more opportunities because what I do have, that I can give out and say, you know, this is what I've done, this is what I've received. So, I can do this, I can do that. It's not like you get a job and you have to sit down and do your job. There are things that you can do in a job that your head prefers the opinions of, so that means do I have much information in my head I extend it to get out.

I think in terms of relationships, because I had a way of now approaching things. Normally, the way I used to, because you know the first time you just see a girl and you just approach her, but now it's like a question of, you look at a girl and you start thinking, ok I have to approach this person in a normal way. You have to talk and you have to take them out. So that's how I do things my own way, because I see the only way that you won't be able to get diseases and everything. You have to take your way, like you can think ok that's going to be like, it's going to suit you. Not for other people. At the end of the day, it's going to be you and you have to get responsible so. That's the only thing.

I think I've changed a lot.

I think I've changed in giving respect. Respect for people. Being able to communicate in a well-behaved way. You know, sometimes even if you're upset, you know, if I'm upset and the person is upset you don't have to go up [get angry]. Just lower down 'cause you're not gonna get anything afterward. It's like, just calm yourself down and say whatever. You can't talk to someone who's angry at this point, so I can just calm down. Nothing is going to get off me if I just shut up. And then the next day, I can ask that person, and say, 'Listen, what happened yesterday? Can we talk about it? You were angry and I was angry.' I think that's one of the things.

I haven't been involved in activism since I saw you. I left the TAC transmission campaign for personal reasons. I didn't like some of the members of the projects that were so involved. I think it's a question of as you grow, you start looking at what you're doing and you have to see improvement. If you don't see improvement it means there's something wrong. If you talk about what's wrong and then you don't get an answer for that – that makes you wonder why do you have to stick around? You see what you're doing is not going anywhere, so you have to look for something else new and develop that. If I have people who say, 'Listen, we are doing this, can you help us out', ok I can help you. But you have to say, where do you need help? Because everybody needs help at some point. I can give you a little information and give you places where you can go, but that's as far as it can go.

> I think I've changed a lot.

I'm not disappointed, I'm feeling actually great about it because you know, it's good to get someone who says listen I'm doing this, can you tell me how can I approach this. Because last year I had a police officer who wanted to know because she had a problem with a cousin, so she needed to ask me some questions, where can she go, what can she do, It's kind of things like that that motivates me. When people come to me and say, 'Listen, I know you're involved and you know this project so where can I get a reference to go to.' People can come to me and ask me, 'Of course he knows these things, he's been there, he's been involved' so it's not like a person when he gets to me is going to be like, 'um … do you know what can I go', 'No I don't', I'd be like, yeah you can go to this or if you go this, they're going to say this so you have to be like this.

The prevention projects and everything has affected my behaviour towards sexual intercourse and everything. I can say, even now, I'm still single. It's going to be the second year. It's an equation of even when I look, even if someone who likes me or if I get chicks … girls who like me will think that it's going to be the same as the previous relationship they were in. Now they come to you with it in mind. When she comes to you, she comes with a mind like ok, the man she had before, the experience that she had, she's going to bring it to me. Then from me she's not going to get the same treatment. She's going to get something different, much different from what she had. It's a question of how to handle yourself. Even today, the only thing I want to say to my friends is that's the point. That's the point of being in a relationship or all kind of relationships in your community. Because one day you're going to meet someone at the end of the day it's going to affect your marriage and everything. People are going to talk about you: 'you know this person was like this and that.' It's better to keep it down so you know whatever you're doing, you don't want to see someone in their marriage and be like I've been there, I've done something like this. You have to be cautious with everything you do, 'cause it's going to affect you at the end of the day.

In everything there are challenges because people get annoyed of using condoms. It goes back to you. What you want to do as a person that is supposed to use a condom. Do you want to use a condom, don't you want to use a condom? Because now it goes back to the

> In order to be appreciated you must appreciate yourself first

question of, I'm old enough. Someone will say, I'm old enough to have a baby, but I don't have one. Which I feel good about, because having a baby, that means more responsibilities. I don't really have responsibilities, which is good for me. I can just wake and see what I want to do so.

I've overcome some challenges, but there are still challenges. Even more challenges now that I'm working. When people challenge you into a relationship, I think it's a big challenge that I have to look at and see where do I want to go. If I'm gonna say, ok, to all the girls, ok they see me, this person is working now, he's buying clothes or … I know that they're gonna say wow, we can just get him easily. So, I know no one can get me like that, because I know what happens and everything. I've got a huge experience.

More challenges of girls wanting to be girlfriends of mine. I think that will be a challenge I'm going to have now.

It's a good challenge. But, at the end of the day it's going to destroy your reputation as a person. So, you have to look at it. Normally you have to understand the person who wants to be in a relationship with you. What is it for you in that relationship that you must go there? Because you can't get into a relationship if you're not getting anything out of it, only sex. It's going to end up messing up your reputation. You have to know, I'm going into this relationship because of this person. Knowing, learning, it's like a project. In a project you go because you love it and you want to learn more. At the end of the day, you're going to get something out of it. A relationship is also like that. You have to get in and understand the person, understand the family. That way you're going to get respect, which is something you must get, whatever you do. You must get respect. You must get respect, you must get appreciated. In order to be appreciated you must appreciate yourself first, so that's the one thing you need to do.

I know AIDS is out there but around me, all my friends I know they're actually safe because we talk about it. They know we are involved. I hope they do actually use condoms, whatever they use. I won't say I don't have a friend who was HIV positive. I've known now a couple have come to me and told me, 'Listen I'm like this so I want to do this. Where can I go?' Now you start a new friendship relationship as a person. Like, ok, we'll go check out a person, how you're doing and everything. So that's how basically I'm still involved with HIV and AIDS.

I think at this point, young people are focusing too much into sex and boyfriends. Mostly girls, young girls. Because they grow up now being able to do whatever they want to do. If you're 14, 15 and you are able to go out to a party, that means you got freedom, you can get involved, you can do whatever you want to do. I think that's a huge problem with teenagers and young girls, because they look at themselves as we are old enough so.

At this point, I don't see anything that can be done. People now are focusing too much on alcohol and that is the problem. People are getting raped after having drinks and everything. I think that's the only thing now that people are more involved in. They're more involved in alcohol, which is the one impact that is causing most problems now. I think the big problem is alcohol. I think it needs to be dealt with, in terms so people can learn to limit themselves using alcohol.

# 2019

*Mphumzi at 36*
Individual interview
Simon's Town

I got married. I've got three kids. I have an 18-year-old stepdaughter, who is mine. I've got an eight-year-old boy, and I've got a three-year-old, she just turned three in November. I've got a beautiful wife who always supports me in everything, every decision.

I actually had to make few adjustments in life, a few changes. I don't regret each decision that I made. I used to go parties and everything and go drinking. I had to stop drinking. It's been five years now I've not touched alcohol. It's one of those things. Now, family is the priority. If I want to do something, I'm normally just having a family braai at home, or we go out just to take the kids out.

I think the last time that we spoke in 2018, I had problems with work when you [Shannon] planned to come. I had to apply for leave, because they had to find someone to take my position for that time. I used to go around the Eastern Cape, and I had to apply for leave to get away for a few days.

Previously, the company I worked for before was a construction company that was making blocks. I was part of the management within the company. I was also part of the management in the company I worked before that, in the inspection department. Whenever I do something, I put my foot on it, no matter what. With great work there's good results. I resigned in 2018. After that, I had to help my wife with the kids in the house for the whole year.

At the beginning of this year, my wife and I spoke, and I thought I could come to Cape Town when I brought my daughter to Cape Town for school. I discussed with my wife about going back to school myself, because I didn't finish my matric. She found out more information and then I said, okay, let me just finish matric and see what I can do afterwards. So basically, that's what I'm doing now. I am just doing a part-time job to help out with this.

It's hard, but with patience I can do it. You know, when you want something, you have to work hard. You just adjust yourself, you put a few things away that you used to do. And then, you have to adjust to what you never learned. Like if we're doing maths, and I've never been a math person. I had to adjust and study those subjects that I never did. Basically, that's my way forward.

Hopefully, I make it and I can go to university next year. That's the goal. I'm thinking about going into HIV and AIDS nursing. That's one of the things. Hopefully, when I get my results, they will be good enough for me to go into HIV and AIDS management. Let's hope for the best.

Everything now has to involve my wife. We discuss it and come up with an agreement, so I don't decide for myself. That's married life. I should actually thank my wife because she's the one who always pushes me in everything, even though we don't always see eye to eye. She is the person who likes to say something, and then leave you to decide. I've got a supportive wife. Yeah, that's the best.

I think I gained a lot in my decision-making, in part because I made wise decisions about the people around me. My friends from this group, they were always talking, and we were always looking what each other was doing. We could see when someone was doing something positive. Yeah. And we were always talking and talking about stuff. I think that's the other thing.

What we did as young people really stayed with me. To be able to live my youth life the way I did, travelling and being busy with activities in my township. Back then we were able to change our fellow young people's mind, because we used to have groups where we would go out and just have a fun weekend, teaching them about HIV and AIDS.

Now, I still have a good way of talking to people. I like talking to kids and finding out what are their goals, and what are they doing. It's harder these days to be able to find people who can actually do that. Now everyone who gives another person a lift, it turns to something else.

Recently I had a boy, who is busy studying at a nearby college, come to me saying he wanted to shoot a movie. I asked him about how he would do it and the resources and everything. I suggested he go to schools and teach drama and work on the movies with those kids. If you give something back to the community, then you will be able to get support from the municipality, and then you will build your way up. He was interested in that.

I showed him some of my friends like KK, what he's doing. The boy was so amazed that KK is performing in such places. I told him, I understand this is the thing you want, you want to be there. First, you have to have a background, to be the way we are, by going into schools, doing drama in schools, then you can get there because you do have a brilliant mind. You just need to construct it into something positive for others.

I was given a chance, and that's what I'm happy about. There were so many people from TAC that could have been elected to be part of your project, but I was the one who was elected. That showed that there was something about me, of which I had to work hard to build myself and become who I am.

Last time I was here I saw Bridgette and Nosibusiso and KK. I went to visit them. I was constantly in contact with Bridgette while she was in and out of hospital and everything. Bridgette and I, we were really close. I learned a lot from her. We were quite close friends. I'm close with everyone, but she was closer. She was always trying to help me with everything.

It's so tragic. She had a heart problem.

She told me that she had to go for surgery, because she kept on having heart failure from time to time. She went to hospital and then she was fine and she says, ok, I'm out. One day we spoke right up around an hour. She was saying, this is the journey that I'm going through, and at some point, it is going to give up. I want you to understand. She was preparing me for the worst.

A few weeks just after she came out of surgery, there was a topic on Facebook about a girl who was killed at the post office. People were writing their stories, and Bridgette wrote that she was also a victim of abuse from her previous relationship. And I was like, what's going on? Because she never said anything. At the time of the relationship, I knew her. We were actually talking then. Then she was like, no, she suffered domestic abuse with a past boyfriend, but she managed to get out of it. There are some who don't. She finally spoke about it. I think that was also strong of her.

> Every day we spoke I think she was preparing me for the worst.

When she came back from surgery, we talked about it. She said she still had pain. She said, please do me this favour. I need you to be a spokesperson, as a friend, at the funeral if I happen to die. I said ok, I will do that.

Every day we spoke I think she was preparing me for the worst. Of which, I didn't see at that moment what was going on. We were talking just jokingly online, and we'll just talk about anything that comes to mind. We'll just talk about life. On the phone, WhatsApp, making voice notes. But at some point, I was like, no, I'm fine. I understand now. That the pain that she was feeling going in and out of hospital. Now she's resting at last, so at least I should be thankful to god.

Later, I received a call from Lindeka. It took her two or three weeks. I don't know, for some reason I knew. Lindeka never phoned me, so I just knew that something had happened. She phoned, and I said, 'Lindeka? Just get to the point.' And then she said, 'no, it's about Bridgette', and I just told her myself. Apparently, there were changes that were made about when she was to be buried. I was prepared to go. I was in the Eastern Cape so it was near me. But I had trips planned to come to Cape Town already. So, I couldn't make it to the funeral, so it is good that we can see her mother now.

I think that was one of the worst memories or tragedies that happened in my life. Yeah, I think so.

I'm thankful to god that she passed away in her sleep. When a person passes in her sleep, that's the best way to pass on.

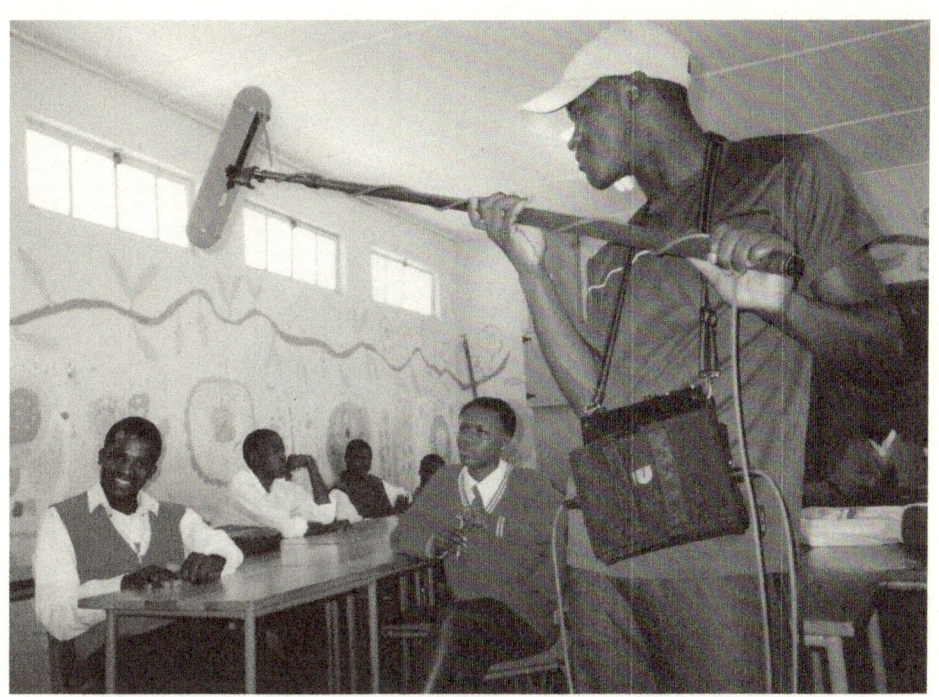

*Mphumzi does sound for the FAcing The Truth (FATT) project, 2004*

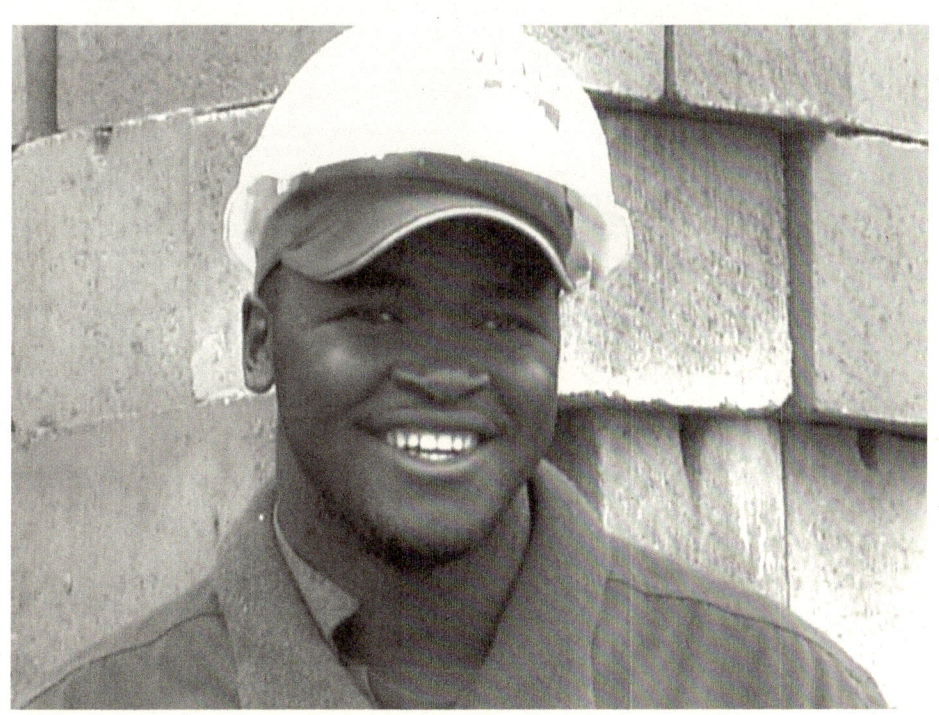

*Mphumzi interview at job site, 2006*

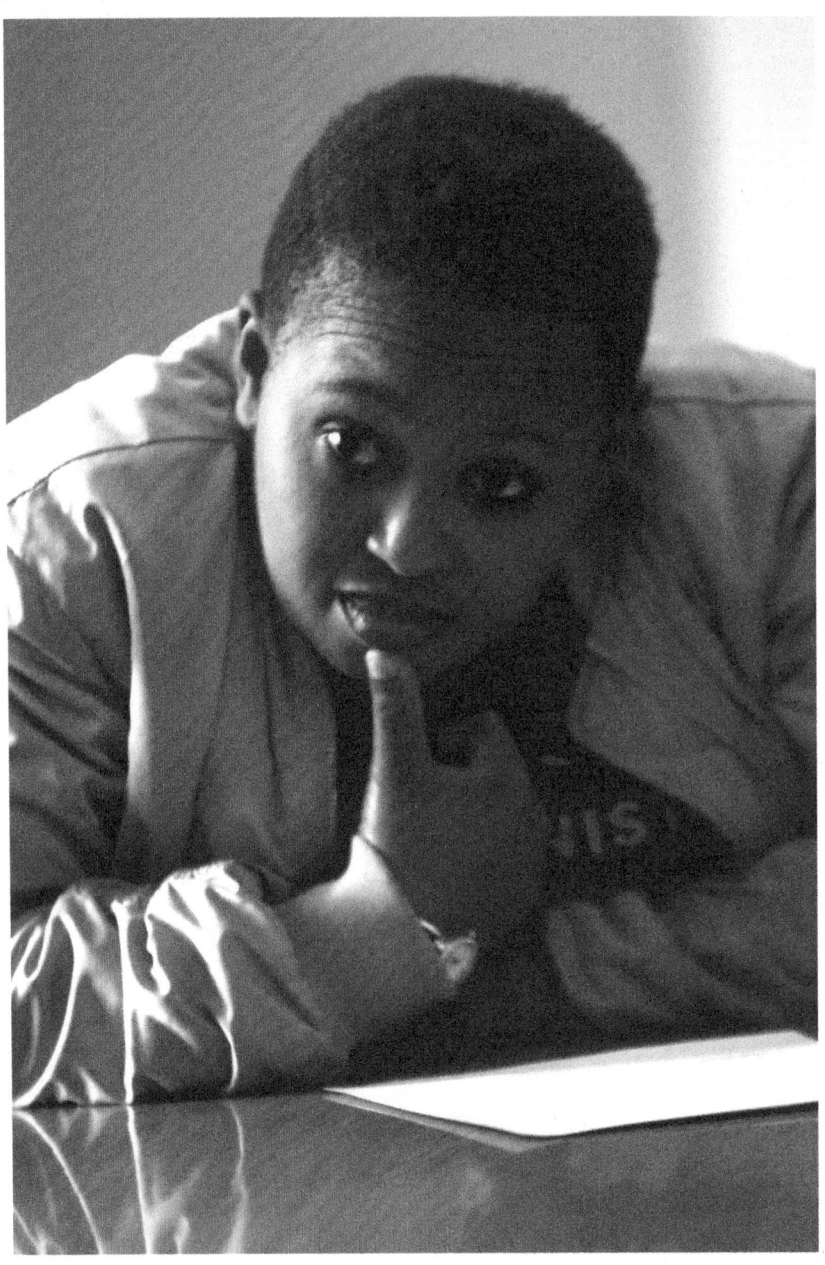

Photographer: Eugene Arries

# 12

# Bridgette Magqaza

*BRIDGETTE WASN'T PART OF THE original workshops in 2002–2004. However, she was close to many of the Khayelitsha activists from the Treatment Action Campaign who were part of the group. She said that she always felt vicariously part of things and over the years she became known to the group members. She joined us at the Centre for the Book in 2018 as part of one of the reflective process events and died the following year. She was very close to many of the group members who honour her memory here by including a short excerpt of her interview and writing in 2018–2019.*

## 2018

Group discussion
Centre for the Book

As far as I can recall, I was jealous of these people, especially when the book came out! They were like so exciting and there were pictures of them in this book and I was like, 'Ahhh my goodness, they have written something.' But you know those stories, I mean, I was so intrigued!

I was like, 'Is this what you have been doing all these weeks?'

In terms of coming and writing the stories, I wasn't involved. But I currently work in an emergency unit. All my life I've been involved with HIV.

I won't lie, it has affected me in so many ways in terms of family, friends, in terms of work. I've been involved in that. It has been quite interesting. It's still an interesting life, to know about the stories, and about the stigma that is involved around it.

You know, as much as you can say 15 years ago a lot has changed in terms of how the government is treating HIV and AIDS, in terms of getting treatment and everything, but in terms of the mentality you will be surprised how much you still have to change and convince them, especially with the male figures. I've been involved with many organisations when it comes to the HIV part, how it has affected people, our communities, and me myself, you know. Family-wise. You know, friends that I have lost to the disease.

It's quite interesting to be here. I'm looking forward to hearing more stories about other people because I'm saying, I was just a bystander outside. I've heard so many stories about 'Oh Bridgette you must come! Shannon this and this and this.'

Like I said, I've shared many stories with these people in terms of their lives. In terms of what they've gone through. What we have lost and what we have gained.

About two years back, 2016 or 2017, I was diagnosed with kidney failure. Both my kidneys failed.

And I've recently found out that I've also got cardiac failure. On the heart, one artery is enlarged. It's about 7-point-something of my left, which is bigger than my right. A normal person would have about 2.5, so I'm on 7 already and it's growing bigger and bigger.

They're busy discussing a transplant, they're dealing with that. So, I'm busy ... yeah.

Actually, I'm just talking about the negatives. There are a few negatives and then I'm going to go on to the positives.

The other thing is I'm removing my womb this week. They have to remove the womb, which was kind of a bummer because I think all my life, I wanted just one child. When you're growing up people ask you 'Bridgette, you are this age now, when are you going to have a child?' As if it's something that you don't want to have.

But, yeah. It was like... Ah [she shrugs].

I'm telling my grandmother every day, 'I'm going for a procedure', and she's like, 'Really? Do you have to do it?' I'm with this woman and I've been telling her all this time that I have to do it. Anyway, those are the kind of bummers.

And the last negative one, it's the abuse.

You know it's all in one place in my heart.

# 2019

## 7 September
## Last post by Bridgette on Facebook

Today I realised silence gets you nowhere, breaking silence means a lot to someone else.

[My former boyfriend] abused me and I woke up in ICU after three days with broken which the abuse didn't stop there. Men that abuse are employed by our govt and they are same people that promised to love us through everything. I have a sister that is not safe coz someone feels they have a right to take away to be a women. #NomeansNo.

*Bridgette died in her sleep on 20 September 2019.*

# 2019

## 21 September
## Post on Facebook by Mphumzi Mphura Xokozela

Just got a call from Cape Town that a best friend, sister activist, passed away last night. Two weeks back she shared her story of her ex-boyfriend who was abusive. When she was going in and out in Hospital before her operation, she said to me 'Mphumzi, when I depart please make sure you speak about me in my funeral'. For some reason she knew she wouldn't make it but when I spoke to her time to time, she was strong and that made me to have hope. Receiving a call just now telling me that she passed away in her bed made me cry a lot. Normally when she feels something, she speaks out, but this time she didn't. I know my friend you are in god's hands now. Knowing you has been a life saviour for me. We cried together, laughed together and those memories will forever be in my heart till I die. Rest in Peace Bridgette

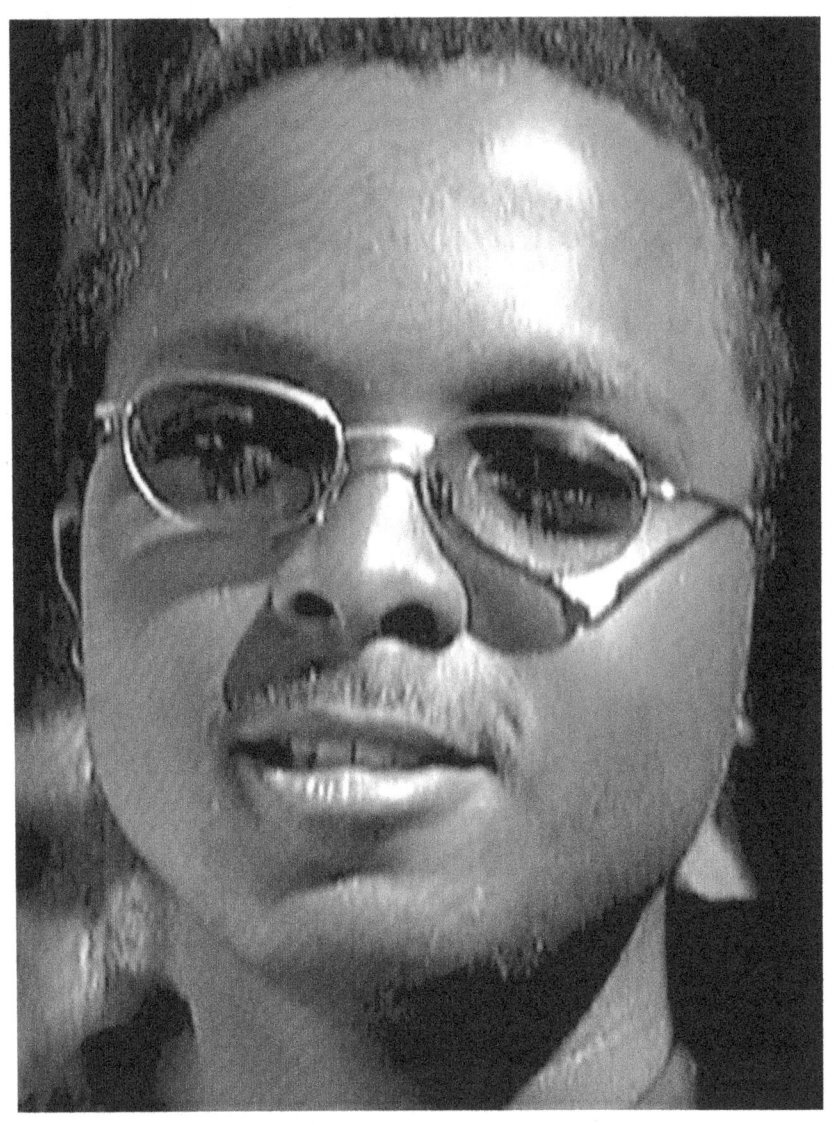

*Video still from* Fire & Hope, 2004

# 13

# Thozamile (Thozzi) Vanto

*Thozamile, known as Thozzi, is a soft-spoken, reflective person. Often, one needs to lean in to hear what he has to say, but what he says is often strongly stated. He is passionate to this day in his commitment to changing the conditions for young people in his community. As Thozzi writes in his story in* In My Life, *his experience with HIV and AIDS was very personal. A close friend disclosed her status to Thozzi, which prompted him to action and set him on a journey that would change his life. As a young person, he was an active member in his SRC and was involved in working throughout Khayelitsha as part of the Treatment Action Campaign. As he grew into adulthood things became more difficult. Work was hard to find, and social issues surrounded him. Nonetheless, he held on to his spirit and determination to change the conditions for the better in his community. After some setbacks and personal difficulties as a young man, he once again decided to turn things around. Thozzi has developed his spiritual side and explored work as a pastor, delving more deeply into a new aspect of community work.*

## 2003

**Thozzi at 19**
Excerpts from *In My life*

My name is Thozamile Vanto. I was born on 22 October 1981. My school is Rosebank College in Cape Town. I am doing a two-year course in business management. I live in Z section in Khayelitsha.

What I love the most is being with people around me and talking about issues that affect us like HIV and AIDS. I enjoy being in workshops, sharing ideas and experiences with other people.

What do I do with my life? I am a student, and also a volunteer at TAC. I love doing research and reading my books. My message is: HIV and AIDS is killing us. Please make a stand for your life and future – one condom, one love.

### IN MY NEIGHBOURHOOD

The first sound I hear in the morning is my small sister's voice, then after 10 minutes the radio, and then the TV, the noise of a kettle, the door of the bathroom, in and out, the sound of the water. My father's transport comes at 5am.

At night – crime, gunshots, people smoking, gangsters, people vandalising other people's property, fast cars. People drink a lot, go to shebeens 24 hours a day, drinking, fighting, stabbing one another, gun shots all night long. People go to parties, especially my big brother. He also loves playing music. When he is at home, he puts up the volume to the top.

In my neighbourhood, accidents and incidents, people lose their loved ones, people die in front of me, people shoot guns, carry knives in front of me. I have watched these things happening all these years. Drugs, stealing goods, cops go in and out chasing gangs, carrying guns. House breaking also happens around my street, vandalising, gunshots, people highjacking cars. The guys in my neighbourhood do not have a good future, to be honest, because they smoke dangerous drugs, like cocaine. Most of them even do house breaking and some carry guns.

On Sundays, some people go to church, some they just stay at home doing nothing, some they work, some go to watch rugby matches and soccer. I do my homework, cook, listen to sweet music, visit some friends, or my friends come to visit, and we socialise and talk about issues.

### MY MUM

My story is about how I lost my mum last year. The pain effect is in my heart. I was so shocked to hear the news. There was a silence the whole afternoon, the sky changed. For me it was a big shock. Even at TAC, they felt the pain too, they were there for me. I'm sorry I can't explain in words, because it is hard for me to talk about these. I hope you will understand.

My mum grew up in Retreat and was educated in Gugulethu. She got married and had two sons and one girl. From Gugulethu she moved to Khayelitsha, where she lived her life. She worked at GSH in the maternity ward, where she was a housekeeper for more than 20 years. She was a great example to her fellow workers. She was a hard worker and a motivator, and a down-to-earth person.

She gave me a lot. She taught me to believe in myself. She taught me the meaning of life and love, how to overcome my fears and the obstacles and barriers in life. She was a very good example of leadership to me, in terms of sharing work, caring, exploring ideas, openness, truth. She gave me a chance to be educated, and taught me how to cook, how to take care of myself. She always gave me the support I needed most. She told me I must appreciate something in life and accept life itself.

## MY STORY

I grew up in the township called Gugulethu in the 1980s. That time was during the apartheid era, and there was a lot of criminal activity in my life. We used to vandalise property, hit trucks, do high jackings. The police sometimes chased us. We used to carry tools to defend ourselves. I've done these things and played my role with gangsters.

I didn't stop my criminal activities when we moved away from Gugs and went to Khayelitsha. I continued to have street fights, and sometimes we stole goods.

Then something happened to change my life completely. My best friend told me that she was HIV-positive. I didn't believe her at first, because we used to joke around a lot of time, doing crazy stuff together. She was always joking with me. We were both in school. We spent our time studying, having fun, sharing ideas. We always joked a lot and made up stories, so it took me a whole year to believe her. But it was difficult for her to cope, and even though at that time I knew nothing about HIV and AIDS, the one thing I knew was to give her the support she needed.

It was a time of change, and something changed about me. She made me understand life and about HIV and AIDS, and other issues. Since then, my life changed completely. I quit lots of things and I took a big step in my life and quit being in a gang. She and I started an Action Committee at school. The whole school supported us. We did a lot of campaigning at school around using condoms, awareness about HIV and AIDS.

Since that day I never looked back again. I'm still supporting her all the way through giving her love, care, understanding, openness, acceptance. I understand there are new things around us, some for good some for bad, and sometimes we have to accept things in life as the way they are.

I dream of making this whole world a better place for all of us, one in which we have peace, respect and openness about our health condition, so that we can save a lot of people living with HIV and AIDS by providing them treatment and prevention earlier.

# 2004

*Thozzi at 20*
Interview for *Fire & Hope*
Khayelitsha

I got involved when my friend was being diagnosed with HIV and AIDS. I support her from day one until today, I'm still supporting her. She was my friend and is still my friend.

Many of the women are being raped. Some of them are being abused. But normally, if I meet many of the women who are being raped, I think HIV and AIDS affects us all.

I'm very, very inspired, especially with Mandla, because he has some new words for us every day.

# 2006

*Thozzi at 22*
Individual interview
Khayelitsha

My name is Thozzi Vanto, I live in Khayelitsha Z section and I'm 22 years old.

I've been working at Chicken Express. I was a griller. I was doing stocking sometimes. I was working for a year and two months. I just got retrenched. It's been quite hectic for me this year. It's been quite happy time and good moments for me and I've been working for a year.

Some of the hard times were when I had to leave work and find another job. That was a difficult part for me. The good times are when some of us have jobs and most of the time we're happy. Happy moments for us were when there were visits from our friends. Quite happy moments.

I have to find another job, still in the process. I was supporting myself, buying myself clothes. I was trying to support myself even at home, with my parents and my small sister.

Now, I'm struggling, but I'm still surviving. It's my father, my big brother, myself, and my small sister, are all living here.

I dropped out of school because of financial problems at home. My father asked us to. My small sister had to go to school, so I had to decide whether I would go to school or go to work. I decided to go to work, so my small sister would have a chance to further her education too.

I'm thinking to go back maybe next year, even just part time. I'm thinking of going back to school.

I finished Grade 12. In college, I did business management for three years. Before I finished my last exam, I decided to quit because of the financial problems at home. The following year, 2004 I went to work.

I was happy being part of the project we did together. First of all, it was an immense honour. Also, I would say, most parts were positive on me and my friends. It was some of my friends I recruited from writing books from the project, also it's been quite positive for me, positively to my work and my peers, and also to my friends. It created a lot of impact on me. It was quite an eye-opener for me, yeah, it was.

I'm kind and a nice person and I understand people. It created a healthy environment for me. And also, the project was close to my heart.

In terms of teenage pregnancy and STIs within our school and other schools, we gathered information to persuade people to live positive lives, and create a healthier environment in terms of communication. That way they could live better as a teenager.

Sometimes if I'm around, I visit clinics just to help those guys out in terms of facilitating. During the week, I go to LoveLife to assist them someway, somehow. Sometimes I do facilitation. I do pregnancy tests. I have those small tests. Sometimes I do even counselling with people I know, who live around this section. Just to make them feel like they're also involved. We live in the same area and I feel like they matter.

These days, some of the teachers don't want to participate in the projects. We have some principals, they have problems, but I think they just don't want to involve themselves to get aware. Teachers don't want to involve themselves or commit themselves to the project. I think that's the problem. We normally network and communicate better with those teachers who also worked with us at school, and did life skills and orientation skills.

It's not easy for us.

It's good to condomise and be aware on the contraceptives that we have. I use them myself so it's quite easy for us. I take two or three boxes of condoms from the clinic so I can distribute them at the shops or the containers, so that people can get them easier. Some people are afraid of taking them at the clinic, so I thought why can't I take a couple of boxes and redistribute them in our local shops? We have to help our communities.

> The project was close to my heart.

We have many orphaned children here, right across the street. There are a lot of them, like 80 or 90 kids. They're all in orphanages.

I think the projects are doing well, but we can't make you decide what to do at the end of the day. We can preach and preach, but at the end of the day you must decide on your own what is right for you and what is not right for you.

When you are alone with your boyfriend or girlfriend, only you decide. I might have preached to you and gave you information, gave you pamphlets and booklets, but only you decide what you do at home. It's your own choice and decision that you make.

We can do our best, but at the end of the day it's your own decision.

# 2018

*Thozzi at 32*
Individual interview
Khayelitsha

I'll be turning 33 years old on 22 October. Yeah, that's who I am.

I was 16 or 17 years old when we met. It was my youth at that time we met. Yeah, it was that long ago. Now I'm in my thirties, so it's been quite a long time.

At that time, I was in high school. We were doing projects: HIV projects with the TAC and other groups in the townships, LoveLife; community activism, and teaching school kids while I was also in my teens. I saw that advance in my youth.

What sticks with me the most is hanging out with my old peers, doing educational work and being an activist in the schools. Normally we travelled a lot through the schools. At that time there were 15 or 16 schools around Khayelitsha. We normally did the rounds of all the schools, supplying condoms, doing educational training and workshops also on the weekends.

I miss being around my peers the most. That was my high.

It changed me. I'm living a positive life. Even though I'm negative, I'm trying my best not to fall into the trap of infecting myself, or injecting myself, with lots of negative stuff along the way during my life. So, I've been living a positive life.

I have lost so many friends and family, and I lost my parents. It's been quite a big gap in my life.

Losing both my parents impacted me the most. It's been ... it's rough. There's nothing I can do, it's just the transformation of life. Sometimes you win, sometimes you lose. Sometimes god decides to take away something. You can always replace it with something else. That you can never change.

I've also been trying to decide to be, or not to be, a pastor. I have consulted my family and my friends. I consulted a prophet, and he said to me 'I am supposed to be a prophet, because I see things that happen before they happen in my life.' I told him, 'Yes, I know all those things, but I have fear of taking that responsibility.' My life has been conflicted with spiritual things after I lost my parents. I've been hearing or seeing things that are then happening in my life. There's a big transformation. The prophet also said to me that I was supposed to be elsewhere in life.

I have to accept and live life. I can't change whatever god decided to give me. It doesn't matter if you like it, it is your calling and you have to do it. You have to accept it at the end of the day. You can't always run away from it.

I want a permanent job, but when I had a permanent job for two years or three years I said, no, fuck this job, I don't want it anymore. The guys said to me; it's a spiritual thing, you can't run away from it. It's god's calling. God wants you to preach among the people. The guy told me this about a month ago, so I've been going to church, in and out. I've been busy, also taking responsibility at home. I can say my life is a journey, and it continues.

I would like to be preaching and healing people. Not a sangoma, but a Christian. The guy said, I can't allow myself to trap myself into being a sangoma. It's better if I accept god's way. I can receive more blessing from god. If I take the way of the sangoma, it's not in the god's way or the god's manner. Either way, it's up to me to decide which of them I'm supposed to choose at the end of the day. I'd much prefer the god's way. Because once in a while, if I see things, or if I see a thing that's wrong with you Shannon,

> the end of the day you must decide on your own what is right for you

I will come to you and say Shannon, and I see a, b, c and d with you. I've been trying to solve problems for the people that I meet.

Sometimes god sends me to people that I don't know, and I have to try to help them out. What scares me the most is saying to people, 'I can see that you are having this problem in your life', or 'You're having a problem with your mom'. I have to also supply the problem with a solution.

―

Mandla was a big part of my life. The philosophy the guy had impacted my life. You can see it in KK, you can see Lindeka, where we are. We don't have any scars or anything. Our life has been like a journey because of the philosophy that Mandla emphasised while we were growing up. We looked upon him as an adult, as someone who had experienced a long life. In our mentality, the kind of questions that Mandla asked were so advanced at the time. We never thought we could see ourselves as leaders or activists you know, even now. Mandla contributed along the way to us living a positive life. The organisations we worked with also helped us. They did a wonderful job along the way. You know, they contributed a lot.

I haven't seen Mandla for quite some time. I think 15 years ago was last time I saw him. He was at a lecture doing some IT work at a varsity. I miss him.

After high school I caught myself mixing with the wrong friends. I got arrested for stealing some gadgets. At that time, I didn't know they were stolen. Since I was young, I was so intrigued with gadgets of those times, because I never had a chance to have them. I was arrested and went to trial for a few months. The trial took a long, long, long time. At the time I was arrested, I was put in jail for 36 hours.

That was when the calling from god came into my life and said, 'You have to choose. If you make the right decision, I will get you free from this jail.' So, I chose the righteous way. I chose god. I went to trial for five or six years. At the end of the day, the judge never found me guilty. The judge said, I never understood and I was young, a juvenile. The judge understood. The intriguing part in that whole thing was the judge asked me, 'What do you want me to do for you?' I said to him: 'Set me free'. So, he did.

I was out of jail. All the charges were dropped against me.

It was at that time I saw that god really exists. I made a deal that I will live a positive life. I will never ever involve myself in wrong doings.

Choose life.

Once in a while you find yourself in your own bad habits because of your friends. I also fell into that trap. It was two or three months back, but I rose from my mistake. I never have ever had the chance to say sorry to that person. I'm still having a heavy heart and want to say: 'I'm sorry for what I did to you. I knew it was wrong.' I was advised just to let things be. Let things flow as they want to. Eventually I will meet them, and have my opportunity to say I was wrong. I admit I was wrong. I was the one who made that mistake. Can you please forgive me? I never ever have had that chance. It's not that heavy burden in my heart I have.

I also lost my parents. I lost my mom while I was still in my high school, then I lost my dad. My dad was sick. They said he had a heart attack at work. His colleagues came to my house to fetch me and take me to the port of Cape Town. He worked at the port for 35 years.

I found him lifeless. He was just like sleeping. I could not do anything. I could not even wake him up. It was quite hard to see your parent's lifeless body.

While I was growing up, it was hard having those gaps; not having parents. Not having guidance, not having a shoulder to cry on. Life has been like that for me. It's been hard.

There is a lot of responsibility since I have two kids. I also have to take care of that responsibility and still to take care of a home. Home is very important. I can go anywhere and everywhere in the world but the home is very important.

My kids, when they grow up, they must say: 'He was my father. I know that's my father's place or my grandfather's place.' They have to have that confidence to say, 'Yes, my dad did wrong. My dad is also good and bad in life.' It's better for them to pick up those good things when I'm always around them. I teach them, 'You have to do this. You have to do this.' They always ask, why are you saying I must choose this and not that? I have to convince them, sit down to them speak their own language. Just calm myself, and speak their language, so they can understand where you're coming from.

Most people say to me I am just like my father. It's quite huge to fill the big shoes of your parents, especially your father. When my father was still alive, you would say, this is Thozzi, regardless of my specs. He was just the way I am. I am the son of my father.

Life has been like that for me. It is in and out, in and out. I'm grateful to have people around me, my neighbours, the people I call my friends. I know god always supplies something at the end of the day for me.

I always hope that one day I will find a better job. I always hope my kids will do the same. I always hope that things will be better for everyone. I don't wish for anyone bad nor good, I wish for the best in their own abilities, and whatever god implanted in every one of us. That's my own view of things in life.

The programme that we had while we were teenagers was quite stressful sometimes, because we faced so many challenges. We studied school policies, and all the policies you have to study from the government. At that time, we were educators and facilitators. We forced government to supply us 800 sanitary towels, and like thousands of boxes of condoms. When I compare the time that we were in school and now, I think there's still a lack of understanding, especially when it comes to sanitary pads in schools. I find it very strange that the government is not supplying the kids. It's essential stuff. It's very intriguing.

I always say to these new kids: When we started, we demanded it from the government because we belong to them. We worked with government quite well at that time. I don't know what the breakdown means. Maybe they are knocking on wrong doors.

We wrote to the government from school. We said, we're going to force government to supply us with sanitary towels, condoms, doctors, social workers. It happened in my school. We never struggled with having sanitary towels in our school while I was there.

I don't know what happened, but something happened, something changed. Things changed. I do agree. Change is imminent. I do not understand the break down. It doesn't make sense for me. You need to just raise funds to bring essential things to school kids. Kids must demand from the government. They must supply. Because they are there in school in 365 days.

We understood at that time that we come from different backgrounds. We got donations from those who can help. In my school everything was there. You will think it's a model C school, or a school in town. It was a school in township that had resources. We took the teachers as our parents. We took our projects and educational purposes or educational tools as their material that we can prepare for students to go further in life. We took the negatives as our challenges. We went to each and every school. School to school to school, once or twice a week. Supplying materials and doing workshops out of our own pockets. Sometimes we called in to the local radio stations on Fridays just to say what we had to say.

When we were in high school, I was a supervisor for school representative council (SRC) and KK also was a head. It was easy for us to speak to the governing body of the school, to the parents, to the teachers of the school, to the government itself. It was easy for us, because we had that connection. I said to them, let's combine our own knowledge. It's better for us to have one head than having many heads. So, we had that combination.

We left TAC after our teenage days. I think TAC also collapsed. Mandla passed the torch to us. We also have to do the same to these young kids. But we were never given the platform. They say we are moaning and complaining about the truth. We always said to them, this is the truth. Things will change.

With the younger students, they can pass the torch when they are 18 to other people because after matric you can't do anything. It has to happen. The old activists will grow up. Some never had a chance to pass on the torch, to pass on their knowledge and their skills. Some of us were never given time to voice what we had to share.

I think kids now are facing a mounting task of understanding sex education. As we can see the statistics are too high, especially in Eastern Cape, and even Cape Town is too high. The number of pregnancies in school are high. You will find an 18-year-old with two kids still doing Grade 12. Is there any hope for that child? You can only pray for that child.

Today young people take everything they read or they see on TV as real as it gets. Meanwhile life is not like that. Life is difficult. Life always has challenges. Sometimes we need rain. When it rains, it will rain hail on you. You must know which way you are going and find the resources you need.

I think it's a misunderstanding or a miscommunication with today's young people because we never had opportunity to pass on the torch. We never had a platform to voice out our concerns.

Some organizations tried to recruit us about 10 years ago. Myself and KK. LoveLife and TAC tried to say to us we must come back and do the educational stuff. I said to them: Guys, listen up. These things won't change. The attitude that you have must change first. Change the attitude that you have. Amongst us. Don't do it for me. Don't do it for your own benefit. Just do it for the school kids. We told them these are the challenges we must face.

We went to TAC and we went to LoveLife, and said, guys let's face facts. Things have changed. We have grown up. These kids will think we are grandfathers. Let them teach their own peers. Let's recruit their own peers. Let's recruit those people who we know have problems in their homes. Those who look down on people. Because once that person that's been looked down upon by other people. Once you stand among the forefront of the rest of your own peers, your own peers will be surprised by the voice and the confidence that you have. We said to them.

> The old activists will grow up. Some never had a chance to pass on the torch, to pass on their knowledge and their skills.

It never happened.

I am a father who has two kids. What did they do with these projects? They employ parents to look after their own grandkids. Education-wise there's nothing. I promise you. You can go tomorrow, there's none whatsoever. There're million rand standing by doing nothing.

*Thozamile (Thozzi) Vanto*

I am disappointed. I am angry.

It is everyone for himself. If you took 20 cops from this site to search the homes of these high school kids, you will find knives, guns, pounders, and all of this harmful stuff. You'll never even find one pamphlet. You won't find it. You won't find a peer-educator, you won't find even an activist in one school. You won't find it. You will only find a social worker who is maybe too scared to speak.

---

I'm in a 'complication-ship' I can say. I might say I'm single or I might say I'm not single, but I'm having quite a complicated situation. I have someone in mind. It's just challenges that you have in any relationship.

I sometimes have my kids with me during the weekends. We share the responsibility of the kids, but I'm not on good terms with their mother. I have the chance to see my kids any time that I wish to do so.

Reflection on what has passed… I wish we can have another go at it one more time. Just one more time. Maybe we could change attitudes and change the people.

What we knew best was doing projects in schools. We excelled in schools. There's no doubt in my mind, even at the Centre for the Book. We do exceptionally in schools. If ever we were given that task again, we will do it once more.

There's always a will. There's always a way. There are always choices to make.

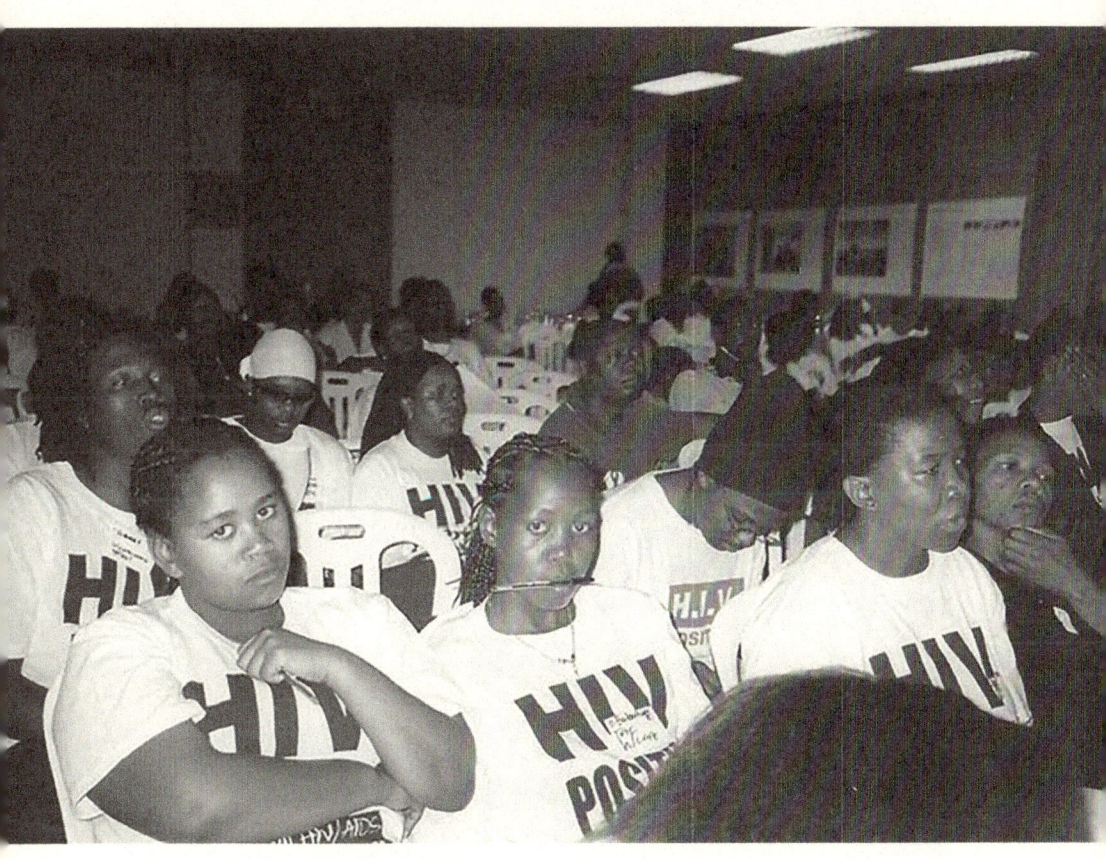
*Lindeka, Thozzi, and others at TAC training, 2002*

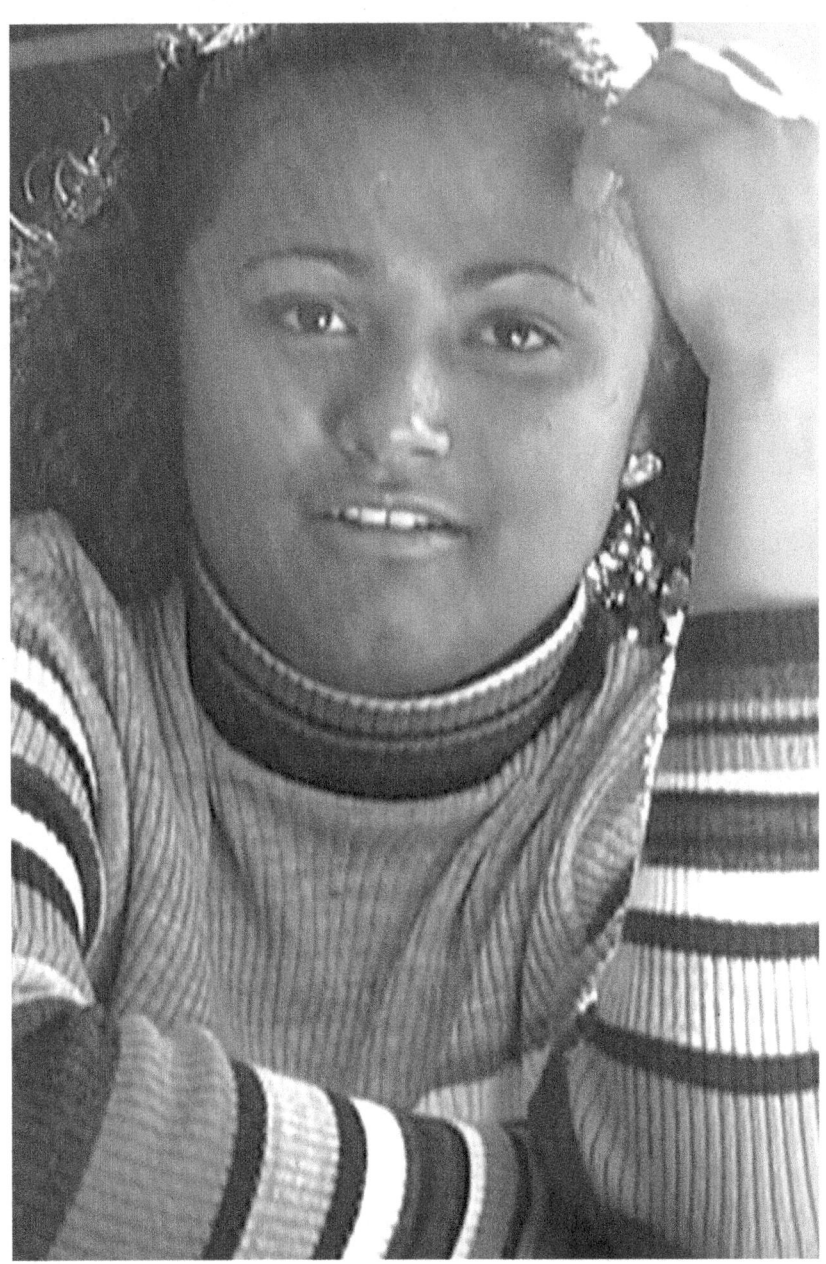
*Video still*, 2005

# 14

# Danlia Wiener

*When we met Danlia she was a smart, bubbly and articulate young woman with a drive to succeed. While she was part of the group for only the first couple of years, she nonetheless made quite an impact as a member of the Atlantis group that facilitated creative and writing workshop in high schools on HIV prevention. Back then, she dreamed of being a lawyer, before changing direction in her early years at university. Although her sights and ambitions changed as she grew up, she continues to be a vibrant and ambitious young woman. She is now a mother, and we caught up with her briefly as she reflected that her involvement with activism as a teenager is a role she has largely left behind as she has grown into adulthood.*

## 2006

*Danlia at 21*
Individual interview, with Kaylene
Atlantis

I'm Danlia. I recently turned 21, and I live in Atlantis. Last time I saw you I was done with matric, and then I went off to study law at the University of the Western Cape. Now I'm currently doing my second year.

What's happening in my life right now, you can call it a mission. I'm really looking for a boyfriend now, I'm not supposed to say this, but I am. I'm looking for a boyfriend, what else? One thing that I'm doing a lot these days is spending a lot of time with my friends. All these years, they've been important to me but now I feel, I've reached my twenties and this is when you really start discovering yourself. I just feel like there is no one else that I can learn better from how to be myself, who I am, than from my friends. I believe that the way people perceive you is not really who you are, but can add to who you become someday. So that's what I'm doing a lot. I'm spending a lot of time with my family and I'm just enjoying being 21.

Law school is not exactly what I thought it would be. I was very arrogant when I first started. I thought it would be so easy because a lot of people told me 'No, you just have to learn the work and then you'll know it.' But it isn't what people said it was. It's very, very difficult. It's not difficult as much as it's very demanding. You have to be very disciplined, and I'm not a very disciplined person, but I'm learning.

It's a lot of work but I'm coping.

I have a very active social life, but you know, when it comes to studies, like this year I learnt I have to be very dedicated. And you know I have a lot of friends, you know, like Kaylene, who supports me. So, a lot of friends that support me and encouraged me to work hard, so I'm lucky to have friends like them.

There is a hectic boy hunt going on. I've asked aunts to pray for me, I've asked uncles to pray for me, I've asked people in church to pray for me, I've asked friends to pray for me. Every day I come home and I'm like 'oh I met this nice guy'. We just want to know he's all proper, and if he's suitable, bring him home. But a lot of them don't want to come home with me. I don't know why. I think I scare them. I don't scare them, I intimidate them. They're intimidated by me.

You know that's the thing with me, like when I break up with guys or when things go sour in a relationship and we just decide to end it, I love remaining friends with them. The thing for me, what I'm scared about is, you know in a relationship you just share such a lot with somebody and when it ends, then you know, especially guys, they act like little two-year-olds and they tell their friends, she said this and that, 'she told me this about her,' and you know lots of lies. It's something that I don't want. What I share in my relationship should stay there, it's private. And that is why I choose to remain friends with them because I don't want people to talk about me behind my back.

The thing for me is, I've only had one boyfriend in my life I just want to know what it's like to be in a committed relationship, you know? I think I'd make a good girlfriend.

⁓

I definitely think being part of the projects we did together had lots of impact on my life. I always tell a lot of people who are surprised that I've done this, because I don't know if it's my personality, but they wouldn't think that I'd be part of something serious, you know like HIV and AIDS. What I always tell them is that if I didn't learn what I did back then, the decisions that I make today, decisions that I made perhaps a year ago or whatever, they wouldn't have been the same. I wouldn't have been as careful, so, definitely it had a lasting impact.

You know the one thing I learnt when we were doing the HIV/AIDS symposium and things is that it's not just about HIV/AIDS. It's about humanity, basic humanity. You know, how people care for each other. I think I'm more compassionate when it comes to things of serious nature like HIV/AIDS, illnesses or people's problems. I'm more compassionate. I'm more open to helping or listening. I think that's what people need.

What I learnt is also how to listen to other people's problems and help out. Also, it helped me decide on what I want to study. It made me more passionate about what I want to study, why I want to study it.

You know, the qualities that I learnt while doing it, I think those are qualities that I carried with me even till today. You know, compassion, and just having this hunger to learn more. Those are qualities that I took with me now.

It was a spark.

We did something beginning of last year where we spoke to the matriculants of the school that we attended. It was two high schools in Atlantis that we have. We did a workshop with them.

I told Mathew and Thozzi (they worked with me) that, it's funny how we thought we would come to the schools and bring the world across to them. But it's funny how much we took away from them, how much we learnt from them. A lot of the questions they asked us really struck a cord. We really didn't know what the answers were. It was called group discussions: what is your opinion, what do you think, what do you know about the subject? You know? So that was quite interesting for me.

There are always organisations that are involved in HIV/AIDS in Atlantis, but the thing about our community is that they don't make the people aware of it, you know. They don't reach out to youth and say you know here's these workshops, why don't you go here and see if you can help out? If you want to work on HIV and AIDS you have to do the research yourself, and you have to find out where those things are taking place. Which I think is very, very unfair.

I definitely imagine myself being involved in community work in the future! One thing that I want to work on is addiction: alcohol and drug abuse. It's something I really want to work on, 'cause it's something that I've experienced in my life personally. Someone close to me is a drug addict, so this is something I really want to work on.

What I want to do is either work with NICRO or SANCA, those are two organisations in South Africa that deal with the problem of drug abuse specifically. In two years after I graduate from university, I'm supposed to do my articles, but what I'm thinking of doing is going to NICRO and then doing community service or your community work with them. They recognise that in your articles. That something that I'm really considering.

I'm not seeing AIDS in my community that much, but I went for my first HIV test last month! I mean I was very, very scared, but I went and did it at campus. You know what the outcome's going to be, but I was still so surprised about how scared I was! Just sitting in the waiting room, waiting for an answer. The whole procedure was very exciting, because when I saw the blood, I was like 'Yup, they're taking my blood'. But waiting for the answer, waiting for the results from the test, it was very, very nerve wrecking. It was.

It's like your whole life flashes through you. When I was waiting for the results, I was thinking maybe I did get it that time, you know. All these thoughts go through your mind. It was just such a nerve-wracking experience, but when the result comes and you're so relieved. And one thing that I admire about those HIV tests is that they give the people pre-counselling and when they give you your result as well, they come and give you counselling as well. That's what I think is very, very good because you know you get a lot of people then they just go and they're like, 'okay I'm negative now, I'm just gonna go have unprotected sex now.' They're just so ignorant. But if you have counselling afterwards and they teach you more about the virus, and you're going to have second thoughts the next time you get 'in the moment'. You're going to have second thoughts. I think that's good.

I'm going to be honest with you. When you're young, you just want to experience a lot of things at one time, and when it becomes too much, you run scared. I think for the most part, being part of prevention projects changed my behaviour, but I'm not going to sit here and lie and say, 'Oh I'm a virgin and oh no, I have protected sex all the time, or whatever.'

You know, it's like, when you're in that moment and you think, 'Oh my word, well Danny if you're not gonna use a condom you're such a hypocrite because you worked on these things, you learnt about it.' If you're not going to do the right thing, what message are you sending out to the world, you know. I learnt about this. It's just going to be as ignorant as the people that upset you. You know what I'm saying?

When you're in that moment, it's just, you think twice. No, no let's just use the condom. But it's so hard when there's no condom to just say no. When we were viewing the videos and you'd see these girls and boys, saying 'It's hard to say no when you're in the moment.' I was thinking, what's so hard about saying no? When you experience it, it really is hard! It's like, I'm so angry right now. Why didn't you go to the pharmacy and get it! You know, but you just realise that you have to wait, unless you know that your partner and you have been tested and you're not sexually active, then it's fine...

This is my naughty box. This is my shirt from when I finished matric. Full of fluffy comments and things. And I have this, Kaylene, don't think I'm a freak! I've got this big bag of condoms. I'm collecting all of these condoms, but I'm not using them. My mom knows about it, but it's like every time I'm like, 'Oh mommy, you'll know when I'm sexually active...'

It started in Grade 9 with Bradley. Bradley's mom is a nurse at the hospital, so she brought him a load of condoms. Ever since then, I've been collecting condoms.

Something that I want to learn is how to put a condom on, I mean I know how, but I want to learn how to put it on the real 'thing'. I've never learned on the real 'thing' and that's not fair!

Something that I would definitely reiterate is that we're not saying abstain from sex. We are saying have sex but be responsible, protect yourself at all times. You know, because it's not just yourself that you're protecting but your future partners as well. That's a thing that is very, very important.

I don't think there was a better time for me to be part of the project than when I was. You know, when you, in your teens you are susceptible to bad influences and good influences as well, and you're just, you're so curious you want to learn about things.

I think I could be part of a project like this instead of being one of such a lot of youngsters who didn't know what was going on regarding the subjects that we covered and HIV and AIDS. I could really see what it's doing to the people, our community, our country, the world, you know as a whole. It makes me proud to think that I was part of a project like that. It really, really does.

Not only did I learn things but I can teach other people as well. Like I said earlier, my friends now and again we talk about sex and things and you know the thing that I admire is not only do we talk about sex, but we talk about if we used a condom and if we used protection. We really did learn. Not everyone is an empty shell! You didn't really know how you would act, but really we did learn and we kept it with us like all this time.

That's one thing that I'm really proud of.

> We are saying have sex but be responsible, protect yourself at all times.

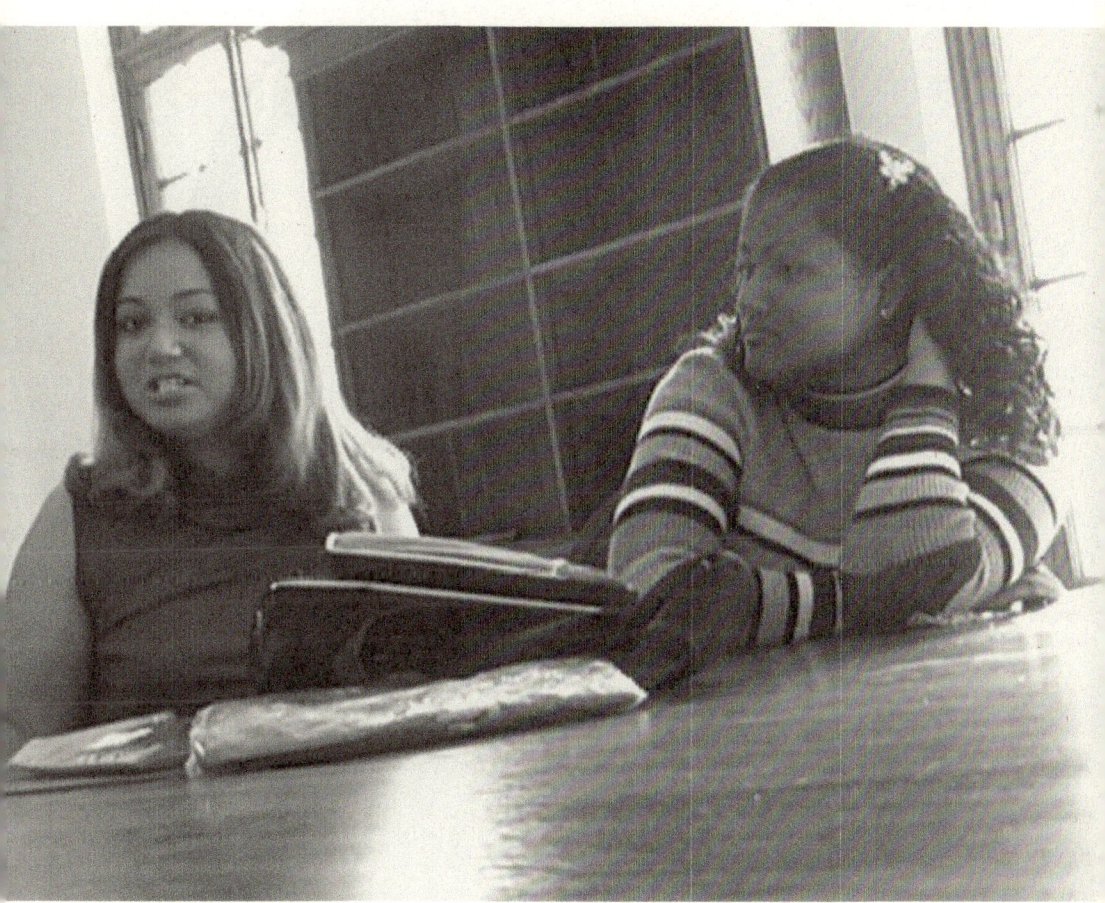

*Kaylene and Danlia at 'Soft Cover' workshops, 2002*

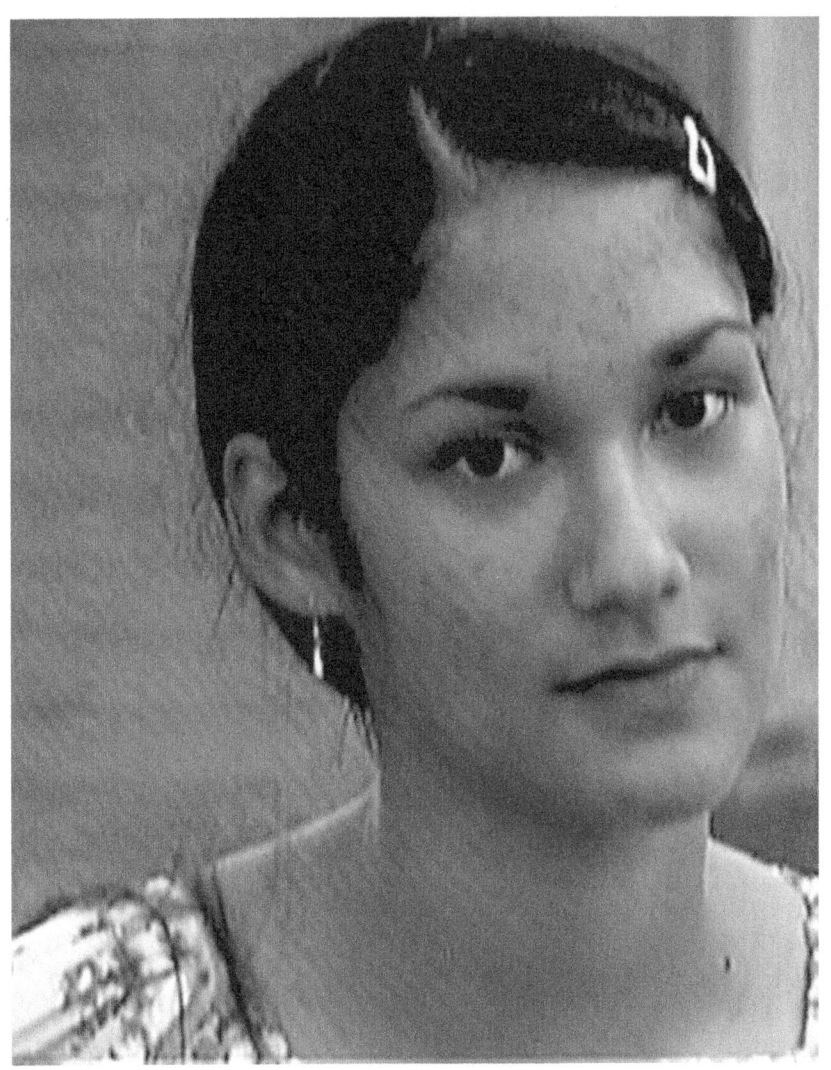

*Video still from* Fire & Hope, 2004

# 15

# Chinomy Jacobs

*SHY IN A LARGE GROUP, CHINOMY is chatty with an open one-on-one disposition. Kind and always very well organised, Chinomy talks about how she felt moved to be part of the group and was a consistent attendee for all the early workshops and events. She was a youth ambassador to Pretoria working towards HIV prevention, a memory she holds dear. Chinomy was part of the* Fire & Hope *video, and also took part in facilitating workshops in her own high school in Atlantis. From the early days, Chinomy involved her younger brother Morgan in educational activities, and had a strong belief that peer-to-peer teaching will have lasting and significant impacts. She studied at university and eventually took a job in the banking sector. Chinomy's activism as a student didn't carry through overtly when she became an adult. She was less active in the group events later in the project. However, she talks about how those early experiences taught her how to share knowledge with peers in the workplace today. This is a more subtle form of activism, but nonetheless one that she feels brings meaning to the work she does every day.*

## 2003

*Chinomy at 17*
Interview for *Fire & Hope*
Atlantis

The way I see AIDS now is different than I used to see it. I've met people that have HIV, which I didn't meet before, and they live a normal life like we do.

The challenges with HIV for girls, it's like there is like yes and no. Because even in a relationship with a guy, when they want to have sex or something the guys tend to say, 'Oh no, why use a condom?' Or 'why should we use a condom? We are in love with each other,' and all this.

Since males and females have equal rights, you have the right to your own opinion. The girl will take responsibility for carrying a condom on her.

Some of the girls would also think, 'Okay, the guy is a something, so he can do whatever. Whatever he says goes'.

You have to have self-confidence in yourself. If you have to say no, say it. Just be yourself.

# 2006

*Chinomy at 20*
Individual interview
Atlantis

My name is Chinomy Jacobs. I live in Atlantis, I'm 20 years of age.

I finished matric in 2003, and I started college in 2004. I studied financial management. I did that for a year and a half, N4-N6. I stopped in June, that was 2005, and then July I started my service at the bank. For 18 months I have to do my in-service. As soon as the 18 months are over, I have to go back to fill in an assessment, and I have to go back to get my diploma in financial management in N4-N6.

I am enjoying what I'm doing, working with numbers and the large sums of money. It's interesting. Every day is like a new day, new excitement.

At the moment, I'm living with my mother, my father and my brother. We're four in the house. I don't have any expenses. I don't believe in debt, so for me it's easier to live with my parents. I'm still single. I'm not married or anything, so I'm still under their roof. Part I'm saving, part spending, and part to my mother. And she can do whatever she wants to, mostly it goes into the house. I have to save further because I'm planning on buying a car soon. It will be easier for me to travel to work and where I want to go.

I'm not planning on moving any time soon either. I like it here.

Since I've been out of high school for about three years now, if I think back about the things we did, the projects and the booklets we made and the documentary we made. It actually makes you think. If I didn't take part in this project a couple years ago, I wouldn't know as much as I know now, or like at work, I wouldn't be able to answer the questions they asked. I wouldn't know what was going on.

I think it made a really big impact in what I bring in my life at the moment.

Before I didn't know anything about AIDS and HIV. Now, because I know about it and it impacted me, I'm more mature in that field. If I didn't know something, I could always go find out or phone Shannon. You know, find out.

It's been about two years since the last time we were together. Mathew and Danlia and I, we were called to do a workshop at high school and speak to the grades 11 and 12 about AIDS. We did a few workshops with them in the afternoon during the day, some ice breakers and stuff like that. They're at the age like we were, teenagers like 16 and 17 years old. It's still very strange to hear the jokes they make or what they think about AIDS, and all that. It was actually enjoyable. Afterwards, we all departed our separate ways because we were in college, studying, and some of us are working. Mathew went his own way. I went my own way studying.

At the moment I'm a bank teller at First National Bank in Tableview. I've worked there since July 4th, so for about a year. I've been permanent since for about two months now. At the moment life is just work and home. That's about it.

At work, every week we have meetings and they tell us, if you have something you want to talk about, you can bring it up. There was someone who actually mentioned the topic of AIDS. We had a broadcast on Tuesday, and our CEO of the First National Bank mentioned AIDS and the risks. He said to be careful, to keep the area clean and hygienic, you know the toilets and things.

It came up the next day in a meeting. I could actually share my knowledge and what I'd learned for the past couple years. I could share with them at work, and they were very interested in what I had to say. They didn't know what I did before I came there.

Afterwards, there were a lot of questions that came up and I could actually answer them. The myths about this and that. There are a lot of youngsters there, but most of them are married. It was from the youngsters that questions came. They wanted to know how long I'd been doing work around HIV and AIDS, why it started, and all that. When I went back to work on a Monday, there were a lot of questions I had to answer. I still enjoy talking about it, you know, and sharing what I have to say.

Now, it's not at school but at work where we can share our knowledge about what's happening and answer any questions.

Nowadays you have to be careful about anything. Like they show on TV, you have to get your partner tested. Of course, you have to get tested yourself, but you have to get your partner tested as well. I'd just mention to the person at the moment, you know, have you been tested? I've heard people say their partners might say, 'Why must I get tested? Don't you trust me?' I really think you must be careful, because you never know what the person's done before you.

People are not open about their status. It's very private and confidential. In other words, you wouldn't know. You would walk past the person and you wouldn't know they have AIDS or HIV. It's made me conscious that I should take note. Nowadays, there are more advertisements and stuff like that making people more aware of AIDS, especially in the community, like in the newspapers we get. I think now people are more aware than they used to be when I was young and when we started the whole project.

> I still enjoy being mother's and father's little girl.

At the moment I'm free and single. Still looking, but free and single. Since I've finished school, there actually hasn't been someone that I'm with.

There aren't many challenges for me at the moment, but there's probably challenges to come.

My brother is in matric this year. He used to come home and ask for help on his school work, like maybe he has to write an essay on women in South Africa. Then there would be stuff that I can relate to, help him with around HIV and AIDS. I have booklets I can show him and help him with that.

There still has been activism, it's been there.

We have development programmes every month at work and they ask you where you see yourself in five years. First of all, I don't want to become a branch manager. That's probably how high you can go in the branch, 'cause I'm in branch banking. I was an express teller which means we have about 5000 rand or less and no coins. They moved me over to bulk when I became permanent, which would be with any amounts of money. I'd like to go to foreign exchange to get to know the rates of the different countries and the notes, stuff like that.

I would like to start my own business in a couple of years, god willing. At least I have some knowledge of exchange rates and how things work. There were a couple ideas that came up but the implementing still has to come. We're still doing research on what we want to start. From there I would like to work for NedBank as a financial manager or something. I'll see from there.

Now because I'm permanent at my job, I feel more stable. Now I know what direction I'm going into with work, which I'm enjoying very much. Even though I get home late because I have to travel in the evening as well, I have to wait for the bus. Even when it's raining, you have to wait for the bus at the bus stop and arrive home late. You leave home in the dark, and you come home dark, because it's winter as well and it's cold.

I enjoy being at work, I enjoy being at home when my mother is at home. I still enjoy being mother's and father's little girl. It works, being everybody's little girl. Nothing more.

If we did the project now, I wouldn't do anything different. I'm very glad and that I took part in the project. I don't have any regrets in my life. Especially for knowledge gained, and meeting you, and everybody else. It's mostly for knowledge gained. What I would like is a reunion again!

I really liked talking about issues and the documentary *Fire & Hope* that we made. It's actually at work so it's going around. Everybody is watching it. I told them what we did, and they said I have to bring the video in so they could watch it. The girls I work with, from the manager to the supervisor, are all watching it.

We have a board at work, and I put condoms there. I had three ladies off for maternity leave so I thought to put the condoms there to show them, please use condoms, don't have more babies.

# 2011

*Chinomy at 25*
Individual interview
Salt Rock

At the moment, I'm 25 years of age and I still stay in Atlantis with my parents.

At the moment, I started a new job. I'm still getting the feel of things. I'm working at Eskom in finance. I like doing finance. I started a relationship and I'm very excited. Hobbies-wise, I like watching movies, relaxing on weekends. I'm not working weekends anymore. We just relax. I go out and with friends, socialise, clubbing now and then.

It was 10 years ago when we were together. For me, it had a positive impact on my life. The way South Africa is as a country today, there's a lot of ups and downs. If I did not have that knowledge that I have at the moment then who knows where I would have ended up. There are many people that even though it's all open now about AIDS and HIV and everybody knows about it, there are still people that are really negligent. I feel that I am very privileged to have done what I did in the course, to have learned what I have learned up until today. I've gained a lot of knowledge from that.

There were things that I didn't know, and after doing the project, I could see things in a different light. I feel that, like I said, it had a positive impact on my, and I'm actually glad that I do what I do now.

The friendships were important. People have a big impact in your life. If you don't have friends, you know, you feel like you're alone in the world and you just feel down.

All the friends that I've made from back then, I remember them, and I feel they also made an impact in my life. Even though we're not in contact much, or I hardly see anybody, but I remember, and that's the main point. Everybody that was there has a special effect, or a special meaning in how I am today.

My mom works at a disabled school, right? They're all disabled mentally, physically disabled kids. There are kids that are HIV positive. When she started there, she didn't know how to handle the kids who were HIV positive. I could enlighten her on how to handle the situation and approach them, because they ARE still kids, they are normal people. They can be treated like you treat everyone else. When it comes to them being sick, or not feeling well, how she should attend to it, and deal with it.

After this, I am planning on studying and finishing my degree. If I meet somebody in a couple of years, maybe start a family. Even in a couple of years' time, or 10 years' time, god willing.

I will be 10 years older obviously, but it doesn't mean that the knowledge that I've learned becomes less. I will always go forward with what I've learned and remember what I've learned. God willing, I'm hoping to be very successful, and still be the person that I am.

I was very shy, an introvert. After these 10 years have gone by, I became more open; open to suggestions, open to ideas, open minded. Not an extrovert, but open. I will speak out. I'm not that shy anymore. Taking chances or taking on challenges in other words. I think I've developed in this time to be a better person in the sense of being myself. Open more to knowledge.

There are so many kids that just go in life not knowing what they want. They are lost without direction, especially in the underprivileged communities.

I always wished that what we've learned could be shared. That a leader or someone could speak to a group of people, or go from home to home every year, to guide them, get them on the right path. With all the tik, and drugs and alcohol abuse, and all that going on in this moment, it's very sad to see where my generation is at the moment. It would be nice if there were people taking the initiative to go into places and try to help my generation. Not getting involved in alcohol abuse and drug abuse is a big challenge for my generation, especially drug abuse, because that can just get you way down. That is very, very detrimental to you. Fatal actually. I think it is the biggest challenge at the moment.

One of my fondest memories is when our group went to the Convention Centre in Pretoria and were with the LoveLife groundBREAKERs.[55] We went up on the podium and made human sculptures and we spoke to Kader Asmal, who was Minister of Education at that time. That stood out. It was like a big WOW at the time to me, and up till now, I still remember it.

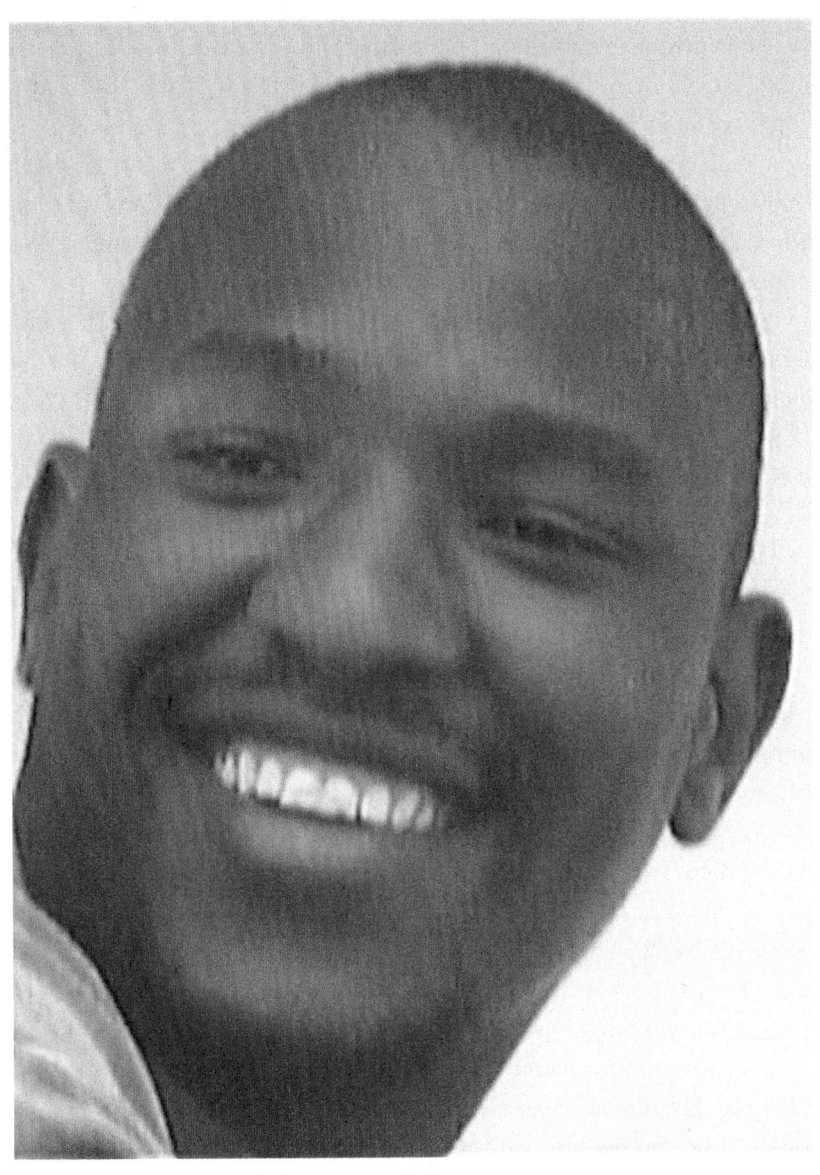

*Video still from* Fire & Hope, 2004

# 16

# Mandla Oliphant

MANDLA IS A COMMUNITY ACTIVIST, *facilitator and organiser based in Cape Town. He was intimately involved in the Treatment Action Campaign in its early days, as well as in many HIV and AIDS campaigns and educational initiatives in South Africa. Mandla was a key facilitator of the workshops and activities throughout the duration of the project from 2002 onwards. A long-time activist and community organiser, Mandla is also trained extensively in IT and in computer skills and education, and he opened one of the first cyber cafés in Khayelitsha. He has always been an inspiration to, and influence on, everyone who has crossed paths with him and is regarded as a mentor by many of the young people who participated in this project. Mandla was there every step of the way, in front and behind the camera, and in tracking everyone's life stories over the decades.*

## 2003

*Mandla at 26*
Interview for *Fire & Hope*
Khayelitsha

> *We've been reduced for 400 years*
> *To almost nothing.*
> *And all of that tragedy*
> *All of those inhumane acts,*
> *Violent acts, criminal acts,*
> *Against us.*

*Those shouldn't paralyse us as young people.*
*We need to be bold.*
*We need to be vigilant.*
*We need to be strong.*
*We must always believe that*
*We can make a difference.*
*If we can make a difference in our lives,*
*We can make a difference in our country.*

*We know we have been deprived of information*
*And that kind of stuff but*
*We mustn't let these things paralyse us.*
*We must walk tall and hope for the best.*

*'We are the miracle that god made,*
*To taste the bitter fruits of time.*
*We are precious.'*
*We must always believe that we can make a difference –*
*if we can make a difference in our lives,*
*we can make a difference in our communities*
*and in our country.*

# 2006

### Mandla at 29
Individual interview
Khayelitsha

My name is Mandla Oliphant. I live in Site B Khayelitsha. I'm renting a room in a house in Site B, R section. We are three in the house. The lady I'm renting from and my cousin. My cousin just started school again. He dropped out of school and he decided to come to Cape Town from the Eastern Cape. I'm helping him out with his schooling. He's doing electronic engineering in the Cape Town College.

Right now, I work here, at Khaynet Internet Café in Site B

Khayelitsha that I founded.[56] Ever since starting this business I've been working here, every day of my life. The business is an internet café, it serves the people of Khayelitsha. We do a lot of things here. We incorporate printing, photocopying, faxing and now we are going for the telephoning, the VoIP thing. We are hoping to implement that as soon as possible. We are also going to do small business support and volume printing or bulk printing.

In 2001, we approached the JDI Foundation. At that time, we were busy with the Soft Cover project in 2001–2002. I approached the JDI Foundation with the help of a friend, Raphaelle Cochran, who got me in touch with the JDI Foundation.

The JDI Foundation contacted me and I explained what I think this whole business thing is all about. We put together the business plan, just to jot down the ideas that I had. We had a meeting in January 2002, I think, and we discussed the business further and how the JDI Foundation could help out, and what is required from me. For my part, since I had nothing at that time other than time and commitment, I had to make a commitment that if they provided help, I would to be able to utilise it. I had minimum computer skills at that time. Working with the business plan we got donations for computers and furniture. We struggled for 18 months to get the premises, almost two years I think, trying to get the premises. In that time then I felt I might not be able to do it on my own, so I recruited Thembi and Vulani to work with me on the business in 2000. Since 2001 up until 2003, I have been working and getting the business up and running. In 2003, we finally got this space, this premises to work in. Before that we had to get operational capital, so we approached the Shuttleworth Foundation for that, and they gave us a R50 000 loan, of which we had to pay back very quickly. Loans are not very nice. After we got the loan, we started the business. We opened on 6 November 2003 and now it's July 2006. Since then, I've been under this roof every day, 12 hours a day.

## LOOKING BACK

Let me start with the Soft Cover project. Ideally, it has helped quite a number of things. One was to understand exactly what the project is all about and where it is going and what are the objectives, and where do I fit in into that: from learning all of those things and working with the Soft Cover project, implementing it fully and it became successful. I learned for the first time that I can do some really good work. It made me feel a little bit proud. Even though I've never said that to myself, that I've been proud, but honestly, I felt really good. I felt very good, not only for me but the people that I've been working with, the guys from Atlantis, from Khayelitsha, yourself and Claudia. Even for setting out on those different experiences made me feel good, really.

> I learned for the first time that I can do some really good work.

Following that, I've learned quite a lot of methods of how to implement different strategies with limited resources and that's what was important. It is the utilisation of limited resources to fulfil objectives, that was very good knowledge for me. I mean, I've been working with HIV and AIDS for a long time and somewhere along the line I was getting a little bit tired, because of the lack of innovation and creation around sending across the right message to the right people.

The Soft Cover project gave out a little bit of innovation, and some creation and creativity around sending out all of these sorts of messages to the relevant people. It's not a message for everybody, but for certain kind of groups of people, who'd enjoy reading books and poetry and everything that everybody has written. Maybe they will learn something from that. The experience of that is 100 per cent great. I mean I would do it again if you asked me to do it.

Our resources were limited and the message was for a certain group of people. It was not for everybody. In my mind at the time I thought, if we tell one person and this one person will tell another person, so it continues to grow. Since it was a research project, I think that's the only limitation and set back, because it was a research project. It was only meant to work for a certain period of time and it ceased to live and that's it. I think that's the only issue. If we had worked out another way of continuing the good work that the project had demonstrated, and the impact that it has on the people who were involved, maybe, just maybe we would have gotten to some great results from that.

Often, we do not take responsibility for our own creativity and innovation because we are disadvantaged. If one person has an idea, they don't know where to go, who to talk to, you know. Those kinds of things, somewhere along the line makes us rely mostly on other people rather than ourselves. I don't know how to correct that, but that is the way it is. Even if we have great ideas, we don't know where to begin with it.

Some of the things that I've learnt over the years in all the number of projects that I've been involved in is that, by ourselves we seem hopeless, we can't get things done, we have to wait for four years, we have to wait for you to come back and start rolling again. Perhaps we should take responsibility, more responsibility, awakening. The awareness is great but maybe we should take more responsibility. Get more involved in these kinds of things, I think.

I mean, I think my community work inspired all of this. If I hadn't worked with the schools, I wouldn't have noticed that there is a lot of information that is required that is missing. And not only information, but I wouldn't have learned that even they have challenges and problems. It doesn't help to give in and cry about them. If you're going to be a great activist, you better find a solution to the problems. That's some of the things that I have learned over the years being part of a number of projects.

There's a problem, provide a solution, or be in the process of finding a solution to that particular problem. That is what I have learned. All of this work that I am doing here at Khaynet, and all of this business is a result of all that work. If I hadn't gotten in contact with a community base, with a network, I wouldn't have been here right now. Basically, it is directly linked to that particular work. As a matter of fact, I approach the business the same way I've been approaching everything else. With activism.

I thought activism would work with business but unfortunately it doesn't. Activism requires action now! With business it takes a little time, you learn things as you go, but with activism it's now!

We have to just change the strategies at times. Take some of the business strategies, include those with the activism work, in terms of sustainability. Innovation and creativity have to come in. At the end of the day, it would not be such a great idea to create something that's going to die tomorrow it doesn't make such a great impact. If it's sustainable, it's ongoing and a lot of people are involved and it touches a lot of people's lives, then it helps to change behaviour. It gets people talking, it provokes debate and discussions. People see the reality for what it is. It becomes very great.

Khaynet is part of that process to me. To an extent that I'm thinking of ways to engage people in Khaynet, or have a separate programme that involves the kind of activist work that I've been doing previously. Talk a little bit more about the challenges that we are facing and how, collectively, all of us can come together in solving some of these problems that we are facing.

It is not only enough that people are coming and doing photocopies. I mean, that is not enough. There are big issues that need to be challenged. In order for those issues to come up, people need to talk. We need to find a way to let people talk about these things. We can't have a community that has a high number of women getting raped, domestic violence, high levels of crimes… I mean it is statistics in every proportion. How do you go around solving all of these problems? You know you have to find a mechanism that is going to work for everybody and help.

Let us help one another in every way that we can. The little knowledge that I have, perhaps, pass it on to someone else. It might not be useful here, it might be useful at home, who knows.

There was nothing to change in me, because I began with the change. Once I had changed everything else, I started to help other people to change. It brought quite a lot of new awareness into my eyes, and some things I wasn't aware of. Stuff that I didn't really know. I wasn't exactly sure until I had some other additional information about how certain things work. I wouldn't say entirely our project has changed or impacted me, but I have learned some information which was very important.

At that time, all people were saying was that to prevent HIV you need to use condoms. Just to say 'to prevent HIV you need to use condoms' is a very dangerous statement. You use condoms when you're having sex, but to prevent HIV you need some further knowledge. I think what I knew was to prevent HIV, you need to use condoms, but it's no longer about using condoms alone. You need information. You should not be in a state of panic when you are using a condom and it bursts or something like that. That's more or less what I have learned over the period of time learning from these projects and at the conferences that we've attended.

The unfortunate part is that young people are really oppressed. We are oppressed politically. We are oppressed economically. We are oppressed socially. I mean in all of these fields we basically are oppressed. As black people, I know that we are. Somewhere along the line, people found new ways of creating mediocrity, along the lines of living. Especially when it comes to young people, both men and women…

We are expected to be competent but there are a number of us who are uneducated, who drop out of school, who don't have access to universities, no access to jobs. All of those things. Yet, we all have access to alcohol and drugs. They are made available in the townships in large quantities. Those are the biggest challenges; not having access to education, not having access to work, not having access to tertiary education. How do people expect you to live then? I don't even want to start talking about unemployment and poverty. Basically, those are the biggest challenges that we're are facing every day of our lives.

If someone is not employed, that particular person is prone to either commit crime, or verify the crime, or find some other hobby. If you don't have anything to do then, you might end up raping people. Or, because you have all the time in the world you play pool, go to the shabeen, use your last rand on a couple of beers, then you remember that you have a friend in Harare, go visit your girlfriend and then you remember, oh, I have another one I can go to later. You'll continue rotating around. It continues to help HIV to spread.

I don't think once someone has drunk alcohol they are in their right mind. I don't think you can make the right decision. You can't drink alcohol and say, I want to make the right decision. Those kinds of things, they continue to create more problems. I know in Khayelitsha there is a lot of drinking that is happening because alcohol is made available very cheaply. Maybe it would be better to buy one beer for R100, maybe it would make a difference.

People are living in large families with only one grandmother earning R800 a month. You have to feed to seven people, or 12 people or 15 people. There are grandchildren, there are grandchildren's grandchildren. The influx continues to build around one particular person so it adds even more pressure. When you look at your peers you find out that they are five years ahead of you, and you are 10 years behind. More pressure. You don't want to be here. Definitely you don't want to be here. That's very scary.

I'm always here at Khaynet, so I'm not in touch with the real world. I mean I wake up in the morning and I come here and I sit in front of the computer. I work the whole day and I go home at night and go to sleep. I see things in the news, newspapers or someone happens to tell someone along the way. That this is how I get information around the community. Basically, I don't know much. Really, I don't know. Personally, over the years I've become someone absolutely different than I was before.

Being an activist was not enough.

I mean I needed employment. I was desperate for employment to avoid jail. I think, if you are not employed, your future is exactly jail. I wanted to avoid all of these things.

A journalist asked me in December last year, if I hadn't done Khaynet, where would I be. The honest answer was in jail or dead. It's either I'm in jail or I wouldn't be as conscious as I am. I would have committed suicide, because the pain is unbearable. You can't. It's unbearable.

I mean you can't print a CV today and go around to everybody, 'Please give me a job', and someone says 'You don't have what I need, try next door', and you are running around with a piece of paper and no one is interested. And you come home and you are sitting in bed and you cry. Because I can't drink alcohol. If I could, I would have drunk a lot of it. I would have drunk quite a bit.

The challenges are immense. Way beyond one person. It's not one person's job to solve all of it properly. I think we need to work together, all of us. I mean in fact we have initiated some stages in trying to solve some of these problems. I mean HIV is the biggest. HIV is very individualistic, it infects one person and infects one person, it infects thousands of other people, so all of these thousand need to learn about one thing: how to survive. How to survive the scourge of HIV and AIDS.

Then you have unemployment that contributes even further. You have people living in poverty. You have globalisation. You have politics. You have everything thrown at you and you are expected to cope with all of those things. It's a recipe for disaster. They push you to die.

Thank you. I mean really. I mean sometimes thank you doesn't really become sufficient, you know. Like, you wish you had a way of saying thank you to people. I think you have helped me beyond anything. As much as I think I am as strong as I am, I think I'm very strong, no I'm not. You have helped me to realise certain things about life and living. You might not be aware of that, but you have helped me quite a great deal. If it wasn't for you, I don't think I would have pulled out. I would have sunk further. It was going that way, it was, so you helped me. You reached out your hand and I grabbed it, and I was out. And for that, thank you very much. Grateful. If there is anything you would like me to do for you, I would do it in this instant, right now.

*Shannon: I mean, it goes both ways. You also, I think it's been so meaningful, I can't even express. Our relationship has meant a huge deal to me in my life as well. You've inspired me so much too. No, it's true. I mean, that's what's going to keep us friends, I hope, as well.*

# 2011

### Mandla at 34
Panel discussion
Salt Rock

At the time when we did the Soft Cover project there was a very big shift in South Africa: health, society, politics. There were a lot of things that were happening. It was very difficult to put one's foot down and understand exactly what was happening. I feel strongly that it's a good thing that it happened then, rather than if it had happened now. If it was happening now, I don't think you would find me here.

I think for me it came at a time when I needed to know who and what I am. And what I am going to be, with all of those things that were happening in the country. I had only just got out of school, I had my matric certificate. I thought I was very educated. I thought that I could really, really go somewhere. It turns out I was only certificated, not educated. I needed to start my education from the beginning. I had to start to learn to speak English, to be able to set goals and work on my personal development. I needed to have a job, have financial stability or economic stability.

I did not WANT to do politics. There was a very good chance that, had I said let me just join the ANC Youth League and go to parliament, then my life would be perfect. But I didn't do that, instead I felt strongly that, for my education to work, I needed to learn from different sources. I needed to tap into many different sources.

The Soft Cover project was just one of the things that I did first. It was one of the first to recognise me. Something that I didn't have... recognition. I was recognised. That's the first part; to be recognised. You know I was even given a title. 'Facilitator.' That's very big. Yeah, it was very big. So, I was a facilitator. With that, it looked like a job, at least now I didn't have to worry about where I am going to get a job, so that part was a little bit solved.

Then I started with the education part of it. It meant that I could go through tonnes of reading, tonnes of workshops, so as much as we were doing workshops, or facilitating workshops, I was also sitting there as a participant and learning about the very same things that KK and Kaylene and Eva were learning about. And to take those things, go home, deliberate a little bit. I was just like KK in a way.

I challenged everything. I would challenge anyone. To an extent that it became a little bit more dangerous to challenge everyone, so you kind of choose your battles. We interrogated a lot of things, so with the Soft Cover project, I got to learn a little bit about Canada. I got to learn a little bit about Shannon, and her thoughts and how that kind of ... you know ... I mean I come from Khayelitsha. I don't originate there. I happened to find myself there. When you're living in Khayelitsha, when a white person works there, it's hope. My life is going to get better. We hang onto that for dear life. That my life is going to change. We have never found that amongst ourselves. To the extent that I've lived there, I've only seen KK, maybe twice in five years.

From just being a girl that comes from Canada, we kind of learned quite a lot of things, and that she is as poor as we are [laughing]. And she did not leave. I work with many different people from America mostly, students, who do a lot of research, pack their bags and run for dear life. And I don't think she did that. She's still here. And to continue to want to work, and continue to develop our society. I mean, continue to try.

A friend of mine is a politician and told me that 'you know, chief, if you want to talk about change, you must be the change'. And of course, what he meant was, he needed to have all the things he wanted first. Then once he has all of them, then he would help show us how to get them. I mean in order for us to win the fight, and the battle with AIDS and HIV, we need sustainability. We need to earn money.

If you don't have money ... from my understanding money is used as a medium of exchange. It is some kind of power. If you don't have money, then it means you have to pay with your life and that is a very high price to pay. Something that we take for granted is to pay with your life. In an effort to try and help people not to pay with their lives, we have to integrate a skills development component so that people get developed.

In fact, that's what I'm working on, something that I'm trying actually. I'm working on three projects simultaneously and the one involves life orientation and leadership. I'm writing a movie, and the other one is health and wellness. In an effort to help in the community who have skills, I will be able to use those in order to generate work. And with the hope that we'll be able to create role models. Because some of the things that we don't have is role models. We don't have them, to such an extent that we have given up on role models.

# 2011

*Mandla at 34*
Individual interview
Salt Rock

Right now, I'm 34 years old, and I'm an IT specialist. I live in Khayelitsha. I've been here for the past 10 years. I did business for a few years.

I moved away from social movements. I closed a chapter with activism and politics and focused more on myself, I think. Doing business, empowering myself. Generally hopping around different circles, rather than activists and poets and those kinds of people. I have been more surrounded by the virtual world of the internet. I think I interact more with people there than I do in 'real' life.

I find it very difficult to connect, at a certain level, with peers and other people because we see the world differently. I don't know. I come from being an activist. I began life in Cape Town from an activist point of view. Fighting for something. When that journey was over, you kind of needed something to fall back on. So, the language kind of changed. And, even then, we were on a journey for different reasons.

After that, I went on to empower myself with technology skills. That came with its own territory and the painful reality of that is that I kind of disconnected. In a process of connecting, I disconnected myself from a lot of people. It is something I am beginning to realise. Like this year, is like, ok, I've lost quite a lot of people along the way. [laughs] I would want to know where they are and what they are up to. Generally, that is what I have been up to up till today. Technology.

I came to Cape Town from the Eastern Cape. The primary objective was to get a job. To work. And when you realise that that part is going to be very difficult because you are unskilled, you need to fit in somewhere, you know? I don't think that I chose to be an activist; it was kind of something I fell into. And it wasn't really in my blood. But when I saw what it is about, and how I felt about it, I kind of fell in love with it. Somewhere in between there, really, it kicks in. It's like, ok, you haven't really done what you came to do here, and the time is moving. Activism is good, but that's not what you eat at the end of the day. So, I think that's what, for me kicked in. I mean the reality of the matter is that I need money to live on. And activism is not going to give me this. I mean, not now.

We are fighting for the future, but I'm hungry now. I'm starving now. So, I needed a solution to that. I think, for me, the change started to happen there. It's like, now I'm empowered enough, I understand things and I understand, the vigour that I had to change things, that was not going to happen overnight.

It was kind of defeating really, when you actually see what you have been working hard for. It didn't make any difference. I mean, not much, just a very small difference, but you would have hoped that people would have understood things the way that you do, and change things the way you want things to change for all of us. Then it's kind of defeating to see, actually. Things are getting worse. All the knowledge, all the education, the workshops, kind of went to waste.

It is a drop in the ocean. I mean, you don't even want one person to be infected with HIV every day, and you are having a thousand. And that is not very good. I kind of faced reality. I mean, why should I really care, so much, about this? When everybody else, it seems, they don't really care. Maybe I'm missing something here. Maybe if I take a step back, I will perceive things differently. Or understand what the rest of everyone seems to understand that I'm missing.

> We are fighting for the future, but I'm hungry now. I'm starving now.

So yeah, I guess in the process of doing all of that, fiddling with all of that, I kind of said, ok well, activism, let me close this chapter for now, and work on this. Because this seems to be the one thing that is going to be mine. This is going to be the fruits of my labour. And if there are people that are going to benefit out of it, that will be a bonus. For me I think the chapter ended when I actually got to face the real reality. When it came to me, I had to choose.

Being involved in the Treatment Action Campaign, that wasn't my dream. I was supporting someone else's vision, someone else's dream. Someone else's dream came true, with all the hard work we put in. But that had to end somewhere. I think, generally, a lot of things came to my mind, and I kind of shifted into ... trying to find people who see things a little bit differently. People who were never involved, or who have never begun life as an activist. I mean, who did come to Cape Town to find a better life, but had never heard of the Treatment Action Campaign, and they are living.

I needed to find those kinds of people and understand how they make their life in that manner. How do they pursue their dreams without feeling guilty or terrible about the state in which our health system was in? I guess, those kinds of things.

I mean if you come to think of it, I mean, I think our lives begin differently. I mean, I think even with the project that we did. I think I went to it, not because it was a good project, or one of the best projects. It was a way out for me. It was a way out. It was a good way out in the sense that it brought material benefit to me. Because at the end of it, or my involvement with it, kind of helped me to live. So, in a way it was a way out, and maybe I felt a little bit good about it. When you actually get appreciated, and rewarded for the hard work that you do, then simply a thank you. I think that what my involvement has been, if I look at it right now, it's kind of, you came along, and I think, if you were black, I don't think we would be where we are right now. I don't think so. Because, the mentality here is, it would have been, 'Okay, you are just one of us anyway, so you aren't really going to change anything'. But because you happened to come from another country and you showed interest, for me, literally, that was a way out. That was the way out. I think that the friendship came later. So, you became an employer, you became bread and butter. Certainly.

> We are building yards; we are building houses. We aren't building friendships.

I mean, there are many things that we got out of the work that we did. Lots and lots and lots of things. But for one person, and that person is me, maybe I had a different vision. I subscribed to the vision of the project because I had a vision. Maybe not the vision of the project, but an ambition, or a goal. That goal was really to get out of the situation, as terrible as it was. To get out of it. To get out of activism. To *live* a little bit. But how am I going to do that? You know? So, you came along, and we worked together. I think the friendship part, I think it came a little bit later in life. In the beginning it really was about work. It was about work; it was about accomplishing the project and its goals. I didn't even know what was going to happen after the project was finished. I mean, even the youth symposium, I didn't even know what was going to happen after that. I knew this was going to happen, but I didn't know what would happen after that. It was a big surprise when we moved on, and we kept in touch, and we continued talking along the years.

The one thing that stands out the most out of everything that we did, I think it is the connections that we have built, and the ability to trust each other in everything we did. The encouragement, and, I mean, we differ in many different ways, but we managed, in a way, to build ourselves to become a unit, or a circle. And keeping in touch, something that I really rarely do. I mean trying to find people; I don't have time for that. I got to learn quite a lot, quite a lot of things. One of the lessons that came out of there is that, as much as for me it was about the employment, then, it kind of pointed to how it's not always going to be about employment. Life can be about ... it cannot be about only that. Sometimes, we just have to do things because it is the right thing to do.

Whether what happens to the future of what we did, time will tell us. As things stand now, it turns out to be an awesome thing, because, here we are. We may have lost some people along the way. We may have upset people along the way, but the bottom line is here we are. And that says a lot about the character of the people, who we are.

You know, I was talking to a friend of mine recently and we were going through the Freedom Charter. Right there at the bottom it says that 'there shall be friendship'. I have never heard anyone in this country talk about friendship. It is there. It's part of the declaration. There should be... There is going to be friendship. We are talking about wealth, we are talking about peace, we are talking about democracy, we are talking about all these things, and no one is saying anything about friendship. Maybe that is the problem.

We aren't building friendships. We are building yards; we are building houses. We aren't building friendships. Maybe, I don't know, maybe we need to re-look into the Freedom Charter and start to work on that one element. That there must be, there should be, friendships. I mean what kind of person can we be if we don't build friendships? It's going to be terrible.

I think the project came at a time when everybody was looking for something to fall back to, you know. I mean, we have had this big problem with unemployment, with HIV and AIDS, with the politics of Thabo Mbeki and his government, with our prices, with education. I mean everything was really in chaos, and still is. Everyone was looking for somewhere to belong. I think one of the strengths of the project was that ability to give us a place where we can belong. Secondly, it brought different people from different backgrounds. Something that is very rare. People coming from different areas. But not only that, but they got excited about doing the project. I mean, I remember the Sundays and Saturdays travelling back and forth, waiting for people from Atlantis, and then the excitement of everyone when people see each other. I mean that was pretty awesome. But we lost people and we did not follow up on that.

At some point we want to catch up on this, and see how far it went. Did we make something out of the workshops that we received? Did we make something out of the writings that we learned? Did the people that we interacted with there, did we make something, did we build contacts? Did we build relationships? Did we build a network? What exactly did we do with all that information that was made available? I think that is something that we did not do.

Because of the excitement, we kind of ran with things without even thinking. I mean we felt so good about ourselves, and so invincible, to an extent that we forgot about all the realities of the world. We wanted to rush. We wanted to change things. We wanted to test the new knowledge, the new ideas that we had. I think that the one weakness that we had, I mean that we are having, is not being able to build on that momentum. Keeping us a little bit together. We should have built a bridge between Atlantis and Khayelitsha and Rondebosch and Mitchell's Plain. We should have done that. We should have helped each other even more in many different ways, rather than being faced with the same kind of reality every day and so that we can't see others as being different. They are people from Atlantis or Rondebosch, so that they would know things differently. We have a different culture; they have a different culture. Maybe if we had built a network of support, I mean we had the knowledge, we had been given the workshops, and we shared the experience, but we did not have a support system that was going with us as we continued the journey towards the future. I think some of the nitty gritty of the project was that.

# 2019

*Mandla at 42*
Individual interview
Simon's Town

Quite early on, I think when I got invited to participate in projects, I got invited because I was involved with the HIV/AIDS struggle and activism. If I was employed and working at that time, there's no doubt in my mind that I would never have been into activism. My focus really would have been on my job. That's where my life would have been. That's the reason that I joined the HIV/AIDS struggle in the first place: because I had time. That said, it was something that was constructed by other people. It was their mission, their vision. They knew where it was going. Whereas I didn't. I was just a part of it. If the Treatment Action Campaign (TAC) had closed their office [in Khayelitsha] that year or the following year, then I would have moved on to something else, because it wasn't really mine. I was part of the struggle, which wasn't my struggle. It wasn't my mission. It wasn't my vision.

The challenge even with this research was exactly the same at the beginning. So, the people in it, they were in it because they got invited to be in it. It didn't come naturally to them. They didn't make it.

I mean, I think KK and others learned and saw a greater potential than I did at the beginning too. I mean, because he came up with the Facing the Truth project on his own. And then, with your help, we managed to bring that to life. The opportunity existed right there, but we didn't have the money to go beyond that. And with comrades in the TAC, even the HIV struggle within the Treatment Action Campaign itself kind of evolved and changed.

At first, people who were HIV positive wanted to fight for treatment because they needed it, not because they wanted to, but they needed to. When hope showed up and it was clear that treatment was expensive, people said, let's fight for it. For them, it wasn't a matter of wanting to fight, it was a matter of needing to. I need this. Over time, within the organisation itself, there was a shift. Because HIV and AIDS, and being HIV positive, took centre stage. For those that were HIV positive it opened up a lot of opportunities.

I spoke to a comrade who is HIV positive and went on to do a PhD. The opportunity opened up for her to understand public health through living with HIV. She lived with HIV on a daily basis, and so she knew what it was like, and it opened up a whole lot of opportunities for her to actually continue that journey in a deeper way. She has a different influence now. It's at the policy and government level, which is different than people who are picketing or protesting on the street level. The struggle for HIV has dramatically shifted. We are no longer fighting only HIV; this shift is towards saying 'we are here to fight for a better public health care for all'. So, if you are HIV positive, we are fighting for you. So, come and fight, together.

The fact that HIV treatment is available in some public ways is a very big achievement.

I was there and I think what was never actually clear was that normally a project has a start date and end date. Once things start, it ends. It's a project, it's supposed to end. There's normally no continuity beyond the end date. Evaluation and assessments, that's like a day or two. Lessons learned then done. In fact, I didn't even know what was going to happen to it. Actually, I have never asked myself or anybody else, not even you. What's going to happen to it? You collected all of the data, what are you going to do with it? Where did it end up? I had no idea. I don't think there was a requirement on my part to actually know. I was part of the journey, but it wasn't my mission. It wasn't my vision.

I was in *Fire & Hope* because I was an activist. This story resonated with the work that we were doing. Secondly, a lot of people came into this country, interviewing, taking photographs, writing stories. I don't think I have ever looked at it beyond what it was – storytelling and a project. Then we are done.

There was nothing in it that says this is going to be a life journey. But somehow it continued. I mean, it continues to evolve and morph into different things. Somewhere along the line I became involved more deeply.

It wasn't planned. It was someone coming from overseas, coming to Africa, to do something. I mean, that has been what has actually been happening ever since I've been in the Treatment Action Campaign. Lots of people coming from overseas. We tell them what we do, how we are doing it, and then they work out how it fits into their visit. And then they take a couple of volunteers. I mean there was photography. That guy, Gideon Mendel, I believe he still does that to this day, has a showcase in New York showcasing what 2003 looked like, what the stories were around HIV. Now we see a whole new set of stories. I don't think even the people who participated in those photo exhibitions knew about that, maybe some of them have passed away a long time ago. If you were to ask them now, do they actually even know what was done? What is it about? They wouldn't. They wouldn't know.

Looking back, the same way that we fought HIV, discrimination against HIV, we should have worked harder on gender-based violence as well. But we never actually identified that. A lot of effort went into fighting discrimination against gays, lesbians. Wherever we were, gays and lesbians and their rights, they were there. But gender-based violence – we have never included that as part of our struggle. Which we should have focused on more.

I mean it's interesting. When you said reflection I kind of look back at how we looked at things. And then ask oneself very hard questions. If it wasn't that struggle, what else could we have done? Where would the journey have taken us?

I mean, I never thought about all this.

It changes, it changes life, it's a life-changing project. This has been a life-changing project.

I was asked about what I consider my failures a couple of years ago. I've never looked at my life as having failures, but maybe a lesser version of failure would be a setback, when things are not really going the way that you really want. That's basically my whole life. My whole life has been a very big setback.

Maybe a smaller way to say that would be ... things haven't really worked out the way that I want things to work out.

*Shannon: That's pretty huge thing what you just said – 'My whole life has been a setback.' What do you mean by that?*

Mandla: I spend a lot of my time thinking. Sometimes I look through the lens of other people's lives, to look at my own. I wonder: who made them, and who made me? Which factory produced me? Which engineers designed this? That is exactly where I want to be, but what do I have to do to get here, when others, they just get there? The factory that produced me, I guess, that's where the faults were made in a way. I guess that's what I mean. I'm saying, it's quite a very big setback.

I would have loved to be a little bit further along in life. More financially secure. Enjoying living life, but I haven't actually done that. I haven't done that. I've been mopping up problems; problems that aren't even mine. The 'black tax' that everybody is talking about, that sort of thing. That is what I've been spending my time mopping up. I guess that's a pretty big setback. We'll take one step forward, and then you have to pull up other people and move them forward as well. I guess that's what a setback really is.

We are sitting back, watching other people's lives move on at your expense.

Why I didn't drink is a million-dollar question. I think it would have been a very nice escape, to become an alcoholic. I know the problems. I'm dealing with them, day in and day out. That's what I'm fighting. So yeah, I guess it's part of life. I mean, what would I have been without the setbacks? What would I talk about?

When I was asked about my failures, I think it started way back when I was in the church choir. I mean, if you can't make it in the church choir as a musician, then you're out. I was reflecting on this with my psychologist a couple of years ago. I thought I was doing it, you know, singing through the roof, because I was really literally looking at the ceiling. I was singing, and I didn't realize that the song had ended like five minutes ago. Everyone was listening to me. Finally, when I was done, the conductor said, 'Well, that's enough now', and people laughed. They laughed, and they clapped, and they laughed.

> I've been mopping up problems; problems that aren't even mine.

I didn't make it into the church choir. I was like, okay, this is a very big failure. All of the musicians that I know started their music careers in a church choir. I carried that failure for a while. I kind of wondered, why didn't I make it? This thing is free. I didn't need to learn anything. It's simple. Why can't I do it? Why didn't I make it?

I guess if you're talking about setbacks, that's a real one for me. Not to make it into the choir. I thought that I was really good. [laughs] I really thought that, but I was out of sync, completely out of sync. I wasn't actually carrying the note.

If you move life forward, I think, considering where we come from, and how long we've been walking, I think to be healthy, to be strong, to be independent in thought, to be able to hope and dream for a better tomorrow; that's a very big reward in life. I mean, everything else in life is needed when it's needed.

There are some things, though, that you always need, like hope. You have to be hopeful, even when situations are not. That only applies to my life, I can't be hopeful about other people's lives. I'm only hopeful about mine.

It's a huge accomplishment to be alive today. By the end of 1998, there were about 15 of us left from my matric class. Last year when I went home, we tried to get a reunion together, and I found out actually eight of the people that I went to school with were dead. In that matric class, eight are gone. There's a very small number left. I was like, okay, who's next if everyone else is gone? I guess it kind of adds to the accomplishment list, that you managed to live this long, when people have died 15 or 20 years ago. That's a very big accomplishment, I mean, in this country which we're living in.

To live through to democracy, to live through AIDS, to watch the World Cup, and, and now the latest victory with the Springboks. Those are very good and hopeful things.

On a more personal level, I'm much more skilled, much wiser, than I was a long time ago. That's a very good thing and is in the list of things I am proud of. And in my interactions with you [Shannon], that our relationships still exists to this day, to some level of mystery... That's a very big accomplishment.

I ran into a friend of mine who was looking for me, and she bumped into the link for *Fire & Hope*. She didn't see the video, but she saw a document about *Fire & Hope*, and my name was on it. I've never googled my name. I never look for myself on the internet, because I'm not there. So, that was very good. I guess it's a huge victory.

The fact that we are here today is a very big victory. I mean, despite our minor setbacks for the day, we are here. And I see that Mphumzi is well, and all the weight I lost, he gained. [laughs ]It's a very good list. I'm an entrepreneur. I'm an adventurer. I'm a hiker. And yeah, I think it's been good.

We are here. We are in the final days now. As we are moving forward, our every step counts. We are on the clock. We have to nurture relationships. We have to love people more, actually, intentionally now. And honestly. We can't be postponing things to tomorrow, because you may not be here tomorrow. We have to be sure that whatever we are doing now, it's meaningful, and it's genuine and truthful. That important.

When you step out of high school, you're confronted with HIV, then you think this is the worst that it can get, so, you need to position yourself to be strong. But, it's only the worst as far as HIV is concerned. Worse is still coming.

Now we are fighting battles that we shouldn't be. I mean, how hard is it to be a human being? How hard is it? It's the simplest thing in the world, but it seems to be the hardest thing to be a human being and live well with other human beings.

In some of the workshops that I attend, many speak about issues of gender-based violence. The people that annoy me the most are these so-called experts. Those people are really annoying. We went to the 'Brothers for All' conference. It's all men. And people sit there and say the reason that men and boys behave the way that we do is because we didn't have role models when we were growing up. This is nonsense.

> We have to love people more, actually, intentionally now.

Kids today know Lionel Messi. I mean, he came to South Africa only twice, but they know him. And he's a role model. Every kid that kicks a ball wants to be Lionel Messi. So, they know him. Where does this notion come from, that we don't have role models? It makes no sense.

And then the second thing, that we didn't grow up with fathers. There is no guarantee in life that we are supposed to grow with fathers, or mothers. Mothers can die at childbirth, so you will grow without one. There is no guarantee in life that you're supposed to have parents growing up. It's just incidental, that you have one, you should be grateful that you actually have one. If you don't have any, you have nothing to regret.

You only know you are ready, when ready is required. You are ready as far as a situation is demanding that you become ready. Then you have no choice, but to be ready.

Now we are fighting battles for identity, economy, finance. We want to live in a peaceful world. Violence free. All of these things.

People keep on pointing the fingers in the wrong place. Whereas, it's people. It's not animals. There's nothing in our biology, there's no gene in your system that is specifically tailored towards violence. There's nothing there. You can't go to genetics. You can't look at DNA to find out why someone would do or act in a certain. You do things because they benefit you. Why would you waste energy on something that doesn't benefit you? If violence benefits your development. That's my understanding. Historically that is what war was for. No one would send anyone to war unless it benefited them. That is the world that we live in.

The world requires us to think, quite a lot, about a lot. You can't think about just one thing. I mean, cultures and traditions are fading into the background, and new ones are emerging. People want to hang on to their old ways, but the old ways are fading. They feel we have no place in this new world. They are floundering. I mean, it is what it is. The world is what it is. I guess we're doing the best that we can with the best that we have.

*Shannon: Maybe we can do better. One of the questions that we're left with was, what difference does it make? Being part of activism as a young person, being a leader and a facilitator like you were in our projects, but also in the TAC, and being involved in AIDS activism? When you look back on that, what do you feel remains? What difference do you feel like that has made in your life?*

Mandla: Basically, if you didn't become involved in anything, whether it's activism, going to church, or playing sports, then you are basically standing nowhere. Your options are quite limited. Then, anyone who gives you something that's appealing, you take it. That's the lesson that you learn quite early on.

Standing for something, even sometimes for things you don't fully understand, is far better than not standing for something at all.

Because now, you will fall for anything, you will take up anything, just to fill that need to fit in, because you are fitting nowhere.

I think activism gives you hope. That you're standing up for something.

We had this conversation many years ago. One of the most difficult things about being a young person in South Africa is not the sleeping part, it is the waking up part. Going to sleep is okay. I mean, you don't have to worry about anything. But once the morning comes, what are you going to wake up to? What are you going to do? What are you doing, today? That's the hardest part.

If you're involved, you can get excited about things. You can't wait for tomorrow so that you can get to be some way. It lessens the anxiety and the frustration of watching the clock, watching every minute pass by, realising that time is moving forward, but you're standing still. You're not going anywhere, and tomorrow doesn't look great either.

Activism gives you the oomph that you need actually – 'I'm involved in something, and it's changing my life and it's changing my worldview.' It doesn't matter the reasons why you're doing it; it's the fact that you decided to do it. That's something that is actually good for me.

Sometimes it's difficult to measure impact. I worked quite a lot in a variety of projects where project managers have a headache trying to figure out impact. One ingredient doesn't necessarily mean that, in the end, that's what created the impact. Usually, it's a combination of lots and lots of factors that create an impact. You can't claim that you are the only one, you are one of many variables that creates a positive impact.

With positive impact and positive results, it takes time, as opposed to the negative ones. If you're going to use drugs, that's quite immediate, and the negative impact will be immediate. If you're doing something that's positive that's changing someone's life, including your own, you don't usually feel that immediately. You don't see it immediately. You see it over time.

The reaction of the group just now when they saw *Fire & Hope* after they hadn't seen it in a very long time was interesting. It kind of makes people panic, like, whoa, did I do that? Is that me? I think that's the wonderful thing about things that are positive. You don't get to see the impact immediately. It's only after a while, when you look back, and you kind of say, oh, that actually had an impact.

I think that's what activism does. It's hard work. And you are up against people who don't care about what you're trying to do. In fact, they're doing everything in their power to make sure that your voice is drowned out, and that no one hears you. We have had to go through all of that. Even at the end, still people don't see it.

We fought. We joined the Treatment Action Campaign to fight HIV, create awareness, fight stigma. We did that for six years. Did it make a difference? Was it worth it? I mean, shouldn't we have just spent our time doing something else? What we know for a fact in life is, if we didn't do anything, then it would be worse. These things may not be better, but they are certainly not worse. There would be no treatment to talk about. There would be no prevention to talk about. There would still be a whole lot of people who died, and those got killed simply because someone suspected that they had HIV and AIDS. So, things would have been worse.

> You only know you are ready, when ready is required.

With activism, because the results are not immediate, it can be harder to see. It would be a nice thing if it was as impactful as other things. Like you do something now and people change right now. It would be very nice. But, unfortunately, activism is a lifelong journey.

It's a journey of struggle. One struggle, feeding into another, and another feeding into another. One generation handing over to another, and another one takes over, and then gives it to yet another.

Many people, many years ago, never dreamed that they would ever get to graduate or go to university. People fought for that. Today, in fact, the future for anyone who wants to go to university is that the doors of learning are open. Money will no longer be the issue, because government is making funding available for anyone who's qualified to go to university. That struggle took a lot of people to fight. It took many years. Actually, it took nearly 26 years to fight and, by 2030, we'll have everyone going to university, graduating. Then that struggle will be over.

Then we'll continue to fight, another issue will show up. New generations grow up, new struggles. A whole lot of different activists are required in different sectors of our society. I mean, there are people now who are fighting to standardise infrastructure in schools to make sure children have toilets. There are people fighting to make sure that Khayelitsha has trains. There are people on the ground who are fighting to make sure that Khayelitsha is safe for anyone who wants to live there. So, we have a lot of activists doing a whole lot of work in many different quarters of South Africa. When you pick up the newspaper, you read about what people are doing. That's all you do, you read about what they're doing. You don't see what they're actually doing, until much, much later.

In fact, the people who are fighting the struggle, they never benefit from it. It's always the next generation.

*Shannon: Do you feel pride about all the people's lives you've touched? I mean, you've been such an influence to so many young people over time, in so many ways.*

Mandla: I mean, they should be proud. I think they should be the ones who were getting inspired. They are the ones getting something out of all this experience.

*Shannon: But you have given so much of yourself, to so many people over the years. I think you should feel proud of that. I just want to underline that for you.*

Mandla: My psychologist asked me, in the last page of my autobiography, who would be on the thank you list. I think it's usually either in the front of the autobiography or it's the last words. She asked, what would your last words would be? Who would you thank? Who would be on that list?

Off the top of my head, of course, I would thank my grandmother. I think my grandmother, and grandfather, in that order. Then I would thank my mother, and then my father, even though I've never actually met him. Then I would thank my sister, my cousins, the extended family, from the family side of things. Once that part is sorted, of course I would thank the comrades from the Treatment Action Campaign, I will thank them.

Then the utmost, then, will go to you. The utmost thanks, it will have to go to you [Shannon]. Hence, I said, we have to set up your legacy project in this country, so that generations to come know that you were here.

I mean, I guess in the same way that I touch other people's lives, then you touched mine and others.

Maybe you contributed to that, in some way, me becoming the way that I am. Considering I've never been overseas, so I don't know what life is like overseas. I've looked at that life through you. I mean, how you live your life; you're an activist.

Basically, what that means is we're no different. What's happening overseas, what's happening here. We are human beings. You get affected. My thank yous, my utmost thank you, then, will go to you, will go to Claudia, will go to the university.

And then, people that I know as friends. Then that would be that would be it. I mean, I don't have a long list of people to thank. It will end right there.

I mean, it's a wonderful time to be alive.

# PART THREE

*Endings?*

# 17

# This is not the last chapter

IN MANY WAYS, THIS IS A BOOK with no ending as much as it has been a project with no ending.

Just a few days before the beginning of 2020 and the outbreaks of COVID-19, Mandla, Shannon, Claudia, Mathew, Nosibusiso, Lindeka, Mphumzi and Khayalethu gathered for a weekend in an Airbnb in Simon's Town just outside Cape Town and a few kilometres down the road from where Khayelitsha meets the sea. All had managed to extricate themselves from families and work for a check-in, a revisiting of the project, a connecting up, and a looking ahead. Bridgette, a friend and activist who had been close to our work and present for recent gatherings, had died suddenly a few months earlier, so it was also a time of collective mourning.

The gathering was meant to be a round-up of sorts and to mark an inflection point in the last 18 years of work together. We couldn't have foreseen that Covid would delay the completion of our book and lead to our doing some further check-ins for another two years through to 2022.

Yet, this was our last in-person session. It was a crucial one, both in relation to being an important moment in time, but also since it was a way to mark an ending to this phase of the journey. In many ways, it felt as though we were setting a stage or film set, finding a location, developing something of a script in relation to how it could be organised to make the most of our time together, and, of course, involving all the many key actors. It even included a cameraperson, Linda, being on site with us for the entire weekend.

In amongst the working sessions were many interludes with lots of chatter and laughter over the weekend, catching up, deciding what we would eat, lots of running down to the local Pick n Pay to get more supplies, lots of food preparation and questions like, 'Who's going to braai?'

If this were a play unfolding, its scenes would have included a series of vignettes or episodes capturing what we felt as we brought the past and present into conversation.

## SCENE ONE: VIEWING AND REVIEWING

With drinks in hand and conversation bubbling, we arranged ourselves, in the fading afternoon sun, on couches and arm chairs in front of the large screen. Shannon hooked up the computer, and switched on the TV to play the short documentary *Fire & Hope*, made fifteen years earlier. The room was quiet as the early 2000s South African hip-hop on the soundtrack set the opening scenes in motion.

It was, of course, not a first screening for anyone, but it was the first time in many years that we had viewed the film as a group. Everyone watched *Fire & Hope* with rapt attention. In some ways it felt like we were all watching it for the very first time. Linda, the cameraperson, captured instances of delight and deep concentration on our faces. The film was like a time machine taking us back to another time and place and to another iteration of our previous selves. There were smiles and laughter, and a slight sense of loss as well. Our group was shrinking, bit by bit, in part now because of the various needs and demands of life, in part as people had moved away, or lost touch. After the screening we took some time to talk about the viewing experience as a group and to explore out loud some of what we felt.

KK told everyone that he had been hesitant to come when Mandla first told him about having been invited. He was emphatic that while the issue of HIV and AIDS was so urgent back then, these days being infected with HIV had become a chronic illness, more like diabetes. Issues about antiretrovirals were less urgent as treatment had become more widespread and accessible. Forever a talented actor with a real stage presence, KK held the floor, asking what good revisiting would do, when there were now such stark issues like violence and poverty gripping the country. Everyone turned to KK, now standing, as he expounded on the daily realities where graduates couldn't get jobs, where there were high levels of corruption, with black outs caused by load shedding and a range of other issues. He had moved on.

Hadn't we all, really, and wasn't that part of the point? As we reflected together about where we had come from and where we were now, in a very real sense, KK identified precisely how the terrain of struggle had shifted, and how even the ways we might have come together then might not work now.

The conversation continued. Mphumzi remarked:

> I think what KK is saying, is now there's a new struggle, which is no longer the same as the one we were fighting before. It's not a continuance. The continuance that you have now is that he can write in the Memory Book, so that anyone can read it when the book is finished.

Discussion continued on the shifts we'd made and how much each of us had our own version of the story of our time together. It was another way of reiterating what Lindeka had said so long ago, 'This is my story and I am the narrator of the story.'

Mandla continued,

> Maybe what was absent from our invitation was that what we are doing here is around what is happening now, and what we're doing now. I mean, the journey has been for about 18 years and we have lost quite a number of people. We didn't see this coming. We didn't even know that by 2019 we would have actually lost some people.

We sat thinking about all of this. There was a heaviness to the moment as we discussed what it meant to be together now, at this age, in these times and with these losses. Mathew and Lindeka chimed in.

Mathew said,

Whatever it is we are doing, we're like a family. We've got a very interesting dynamic. It's interesting to actually notice the complexity. A couple of days ago, I actually had a panic attack. I was checking with my psychologist and asking, why am I having a panic attack? And it made me realize how much we take stock of exactly what we're doing in our lives when we are together.

It's not everyone that gets this opportunity to sit around with friends, that have been through so much over many years, and we make time to take stock, to look at what is what: What is going on now? Where are you now, and how do you feel about that? That is something I love. It makes sense. It's just a different dynamic for this family. You don't find it just anywhere.

Lindeka added:

Yeah, I think even in telling our stories, even informing you guys how far we are now, it's also a journey of self-discovery. You know? Nobody asks you these questions. How do you feel about something, what are your reflections? Normally, you don't even think about it. Not until someone comes to ask you, how do you feel about this? What are your reflections about this?

Mathew then said:

It was like the thirst has been placed there, that thirst, and that need to explore, the need to know why. Because you have gotten a taste for it. If a few years go by and you don't check back in with yourself, you do feel that vacancy. You can take stock, enjoy each other's company, and then just see how this journey that we've taken together has developed us. How things change and how we change. And how we change but stay the same and stay the same but change.

## SCENE 2: WE REALISED OURSELVES IN TELLING THESE STORIES

Sunlight streams through the rooms in the early morning. Seen through the window, the coastal waters lap the shore. It's a tranquil scene, far away from everyone's daily lives. We sit around a big dining room table and finish our breakfast together.

The Memory Books that we had created for each member of the group came out again. As we discussed in Chapter 3, an idea about how to work with memory at this phase of the project was to design a method through a tactile experience of the visual and written history of our work together. The idea was to create individual booklets, including photographs and transcripts, spanning the past 18 years. Each Memory Book contained transcripts, photos and video stills, poetry and other materials related to what we'd collected during that time. Prompts were added and blank spaces allowed participants to write directly into the booklets or to draw if they were so inspired. The books were meant to both elicit memory, and to gather current reflections.

Everyone has a chance to flip through the pages, and then write or draw. There is momentary confusion at the beginning: 'Oh, this is just about me?' and a sudden recognition that everyone's book was different. Some people exchange books at certain points to see what some else's book looks like.

Each person was given a clean version to keep, and passed over to us copies with their writings and drawings. Discussion continued as we worked and reflected together.

Shannon: It's interesting to see how we've changed, and see oneself over time. When I was looking at all the Memory Books and the interview transcripts, I was sometimes embarrassed by my own questions. Or, feeling the different emotions that we felt at different periods of time, I see the hopefulness and the naivety now, which I didn't see back then.

Lindeka: Another thing I don't think you realise is that culturally for us, we're not a people that express emotions. Especially for men also in our culture. You don't really talk about what you're feeling and stuff like that. This was a platform for us to express those deep inner feelings that you wouldn't just tell anyone. Things that you wouldn't even want somebody to know. Somehow it just comes out, especially in the writing exercises. You'll find yourself writing about something that you didn't even think about before, just putting it all down on paper. Things that you wouldn't normally say in conversation.

I think all our daily lives is just about skimming off the top, no one really going deep... I heard someone say the other day that even when you ask someone 'how are you' you don't expect them to tell you how they are. You would get more than you bargained for if they actually told you how they feel!

KK: You never ask them how they really feel, like never.

Lindeka: Yeah, I think this was a great platform for us to go deep. That's why I say: we realised ourselves also in telling these stories.

Mphumzi: I think I would say one thing about coming together 18 years later. It's about friendship... Because I will tell you, if I go to KK's house, there are no boundaries. I go to the kitchen, make myself food. We made friends. Yes, some of us knew each other before but because of what we did we became stronger than what we were before. For myself, I would say, I am thankful. It's one of those questions that, as I think about the book, we have to reflect years back. I would say, I myself can thank everyone who's here, and who's been part of my life. I was able to see things differently. I was able to change my lifestyle.

We managed to live our lives, and we like talk to each other. I remember when Bridgette started getting sick, we lost contact and then started talking again. I remember the phone call I received from Lindeka telling me Bridgette had passed. Bridgette was preparing me every step of the way. Yeah, so that's what I'm saying. This friendship. This proof.

KK: We were friends before.

Mphumzi: Yes, we were friends before but after we did *Fire & Hope*, our friendships became stronger.

KK: True, and we had to find Danlia, Kaylene, Chinomy, Andrew Fisher, Nazeema, Nosibusiso, Khayaletu Mofu, Thokozela, Lindeka, what-what ... [KK ends mid-sentence, pauses, and then continues] But now we are old. I was old even back then. It's not only that I'm short! I can't do otherwise.

Laugher erupts all around. KK always has everyone entertained. Finally, Mathew sums up the spirit of this scene,

I love you guys and so it's always nice to check in with everyone. This is adding to my life. To have this quality of relationship in anyone's life is a blessing.

### SCENE 3: THE LAST SUPPER

It is the end of the weekend. Everyone has packed up. We take pictures together during the windy morning, with the blue sky above us and the cool waters of the Cape behind us. There are hugs goodbye and promises to keep in touch. The cars are full and everyone sets off homewards.

After all that remembering and reflecting, Mandla, Shannon and Claudia are left alone for a quiet last dinner together. There has been a lot to process and a lot of energy keeping things going, listening, and recognising how emotionally challenging this time together has been for everyone.

This time, Mandla takes centre stage. His words are provocative. 'There was nothing in it that says this is going to be a life journey. But somehow it continued. I mean, it continues to evolve and morph into different things. Somewhere along the line I became involved more deeply.' While Mandla is talking specifically about how he came to be involved in HIV and AIDS activism, and by extension involved in the Soft Cover project initiated 18 years earlier, his reference to not knowing that this was going to be a 'life journey' acts like a collective mirror for the three of us on how we continued working together, what we thought we were doing, and what the significance of this work might be.

We three have such different lives. Mandla has become an IT specialist and is now also a runner, Shannon is a filmmaker and now teaches film as an associate professor at a Canadian university, Claudia is a professor who runs multiple major research projects around the world on visual methodologies and educational initiatives.

Scene Three is a life journey. Ironically, we started writing a version of this book in 2006, long before the life journey truly began, and even had quite a few draft chapters prepared, but we could never finish it. The project never seemed quite finished enough for us to write about. Yet, here we are and we still don't know if it ever will end.

As we sat together and chatted during that last supper, we felt a range of emotions. What does it mean to close this chapter? What remains? These are not the early days of wild optimism about changing the world, but a much more sober sense of taking steps forward, day by day and, on some days, taking steps backwards. We have a sense that this journey, a life journey, will never be over. Little did we know then that it would be the last time we'd see each other for another few years.

## TWO YEARS LATER: ACROSS PANDEMICS

The fieldwork for the stories explored in *In My Life* started in 2002 in the middle of the AIDS pandemic. Most of the young people who worked on this project had already been engaged either in their schools or in community-level activism with the Treatment Action Campaign. It was a time for taking to the streets to advocate for massive social change in health policy in ways that were reminiscent of the 1976 Soweto uprising.

The last in-person gathering of the group took place in late December 2019 just weeks before the world would see a new pandemic as a result of the coronavirus. By March 2020 there would be lockdowns around the world. At that last in-person gathering, one of the key topics that participants returned to was how to pay forward what they had learned as young people. How could they give some of this back? They wanted to do something for young people today.

As we now know, for months and months into the COVID-19 pandemic in South Africa in 2020, the idea of taking action on any cause was challenging, and as documented in an analysis of what we termed 'ethnography at a distance' with activist work with girls and young women, could run the risk of doing more harm than good.[57] This was particularly the case in rural South Africa in relation to elevated rates of domestic violence.

As we complete this book of collective voices 'at a distance' in June 2022, through WhatsApp, Facebook, Skype and email 20 years on from the 'Getting the Word Out' symposium of 2002, 'disrupted lives' has become the new dominant narrative for so many young people.[58] COVID-19 has had a devastating impact on them in so many different ways. The double and triple intersecting pandemics of HIV, gender-based violence and racism have exacerbated health inequities, co-existing with increasing poverty, food insecurity and a bleak picture of unemployment. As Dudu Hlatshwayo writes, we have 'a heartbreaking 65.5% youth unemployment rate' as the June 16th Youth Day of 2022 comes around.[59]

For youth activists and researchers both then and now, this multi-pandemic analysis can be taken as a cautionary tale about the unforeseen nature of the world in which we live. As KK so passionately highlights, the focus of the activism can change as we saw in the student protests as part of the #FeesMustFall movement in South African universities and in the Annual Silent Protests over the last 10 years at various universities as a protest against the silence around rape and sexual violence. More than anything we think it can also be taken as a compelling argument for using longitudinal study approaches to socially engaged research.

# Notes

[1] Njabulo S. Ndebele, 'The rediscovery of the ordinary: Some new writings in South Africa', *Journal of Southern African Studies* 12 (1986): 143–157.

[2] As Shannon Walsh has written elsewhere, friendship in South Africa is always also complicated by race. The history of friendship is tied up with racial segregation, Indian indenture, Indigenous genocide and settler colonialism. Liberal modes of settler colonialism often operated through discourses of affection that made it more difficult to notice this simultaneous codified racial difference, white supremacy and anti-blackness. Nonetheless, the project of thinking politically about friendship is also a way to consider both practices that resist structures of oppression and those that enable them: intimacies and complicities. In this project, we want to think about how friendship, however precarious, created and disrupted ways young people related to themselves and others during the AIDS crisis. For further discussion around friendship and its complications see the edited collection by Shannon Walsh & Jon Soske, *Ties that Bind: Race and the Politics of Friendship in South Africa*, Wits University Press, 2016.

[3] Ndebele, 'The rediscovery of the ordinary', p. 156.

[4] Stacy Hardy & Lesego Rampolokeng. 'Bound to violence: Scratching beginnings and endings with Lesego Rampolokeng', in *Ties that Bind: Race and the Politics of Friendship in South Africa*, edited by Shannon Walsh & Jon Soske, Wits University Press, 2016, pp. 48–69.

[5] Ndebele, 'The rediscovery of the ordinary', p. 153.

[6] Richard Iton, *In Search of the Black Fantastic: Politics and Popular Culture in the Post-Civil Rights Era*, Oxford University Press, 2008, p. 8.

[7] Fanon called for a revolution of consciousness amongst black people in order to break from the dis-alienation caused by the racist and colonial gaze. See Mabogo More, 'Albert Lithuli, Steve Biko, and Nelson Mandela: The philosophical basis of their thought and practice', in *A Companion to African Philosophy*, edited by Kwasi Wiredu, Blackwell Publishing, 2004, pp. 207–215.

[8] See Ahmed Veriava & Prishani Naidoo, 'Remembering Biko for the here and now', in *Biko Lives!: Contesting the Legacies of Steve Biko*, edited by Andile Mngxitama, Amanda Alexander & Nigel Gibson, Palgrave Macmillan, 2008, pp. 233–251.

[9] Veriava & Naidoo, 'Remembering Biko for the here and now', pp. 233–253.

[10] Gramsci coined the term 'subaltern' to indicate non-elites, or the dominated classes. Scholars such as Gayatri Chakravorty Spivak, Ranajit Guha, Partha Chatterjee, Edward Said and others explored how subaltern narratives 'from below' can activate political and social change. Vinay Bahl criticised the theoretical lean of the Subaltern Studies group towards writing better histories and abandoning engaged working-class struggles and the real locations of oppression (*What Went Wrong With 'History From Below': Reinstating Human Agency as Human Creativity*, KP Bagchi & Company, 2005).

[11] Activist ethnography locates knowledge and learning within the experience of social movements and spaces of struggle, rather than only from the academy. David Graeber urges the reciprocity of theory and practice – allowing practice to infuse how we 'do' theory (*Fragments of an Anarchist Anthropology*, Prickly Paradigm Press, 2004). Theory developed in movements is based on practical, real-world concerns, but also offers nuanced engagements with the project of transformation. See also Douglas Bevington & Chris Dixon, 'Movement-relevant theory: Rethinking social movement scholarship and activism', *Social Movement Studies* 4, 2005, pp. 185–208.

Likewise, Dorothy E. Smith developed the idea of Institutional Ethnography to explore the social construction of power through a close attention to everyday practices. Her sociology for people went on to influence political activist ethnography (PAE), which linked everyday experience with knowledge developed through, and by, social movements and activists, including the contradictions that only become apparent through being implicated ourselves. Other critical references include: Aziz Choudry, 'Transnational activist coalition politics and the de/colonization of pedagogies of mobilization: Learning from anti-neoliberal Indigenous movement articulations', *International Education* 37, 2007, pp. 96–112; Aziz Choudry, *Learning Activism: The Intellectual Life of Contemporary Social Movements*, University of Toronto Press, 2015; Caelie Frampton, Gary Kinsman, A.K. Thompson & Kate Tilleczek. 'Social movements/social research: Towards political activist ethnography', in *Sociology for Changing the World: Social Movements/Social Research*, Fernwood Publishing, 2006, pp. 1–17; Dorothy E. Smith, *The Everyday World as Problematic: A Feminist Sociology*, University of Toronto Press, 1987; Dorothy E. Smith. *Institutional Ethnography: A Sociology for People*, Rowman Altamira, 2005; Shannon Walsh. 'The dilemma of objectivity: Challenges for activist research in the academy', in *Political Activist Ethnography: Studies in the Social Relations of Struggle*, edited by Agnieszka Doll, Laura Bisaillon & Kevin Walby, Athabasca University Press, in press.

[12] Shannon Walsh, 'Ethnography-in-motion: Neoliberalism and the shack dwellers movement in South Africa', in *Education, Participatory Action Research and Social Change*, edited by Steve Jordan & Dip Kapoor, Palgrave Macmillan, 2009, pp. 181–193.

[13] Visual and arts-based research methods have a long history of being used by

scholars interested in social change, where data is not only collected, but can dynamically re-enter the social sphere to transform it. In this type of work, research can, and does, create positive change. See Claudia Mitchell, *Doing Visual Research*, SAGE Publications, 2011.

[14] Walsh coined the term 'ethnography-in-motion' during her doctoral research. See Shannon Walsh, 'Ethnography-in-motion: Neoliberalism and the shack dwellers movement in South Africa', PhD dissertation, Concordia University, 2009. The term evolved from ideas related to critical pedagogy and conscientisation, which imagines education as a means of challenging domination, and creating contexts for political and social transformation. Critical pedagogy allows teachers and students to work together to tease out oppression in their daily lives and work together towards a liberatory practice. Freire called the development of critical consciousness conscientization. Others, such as bell hooks, Henry Giroux, Joe L. Kincheloe and Peter McLaren, have gone on to develop on Friere's pedagogical approach to include issues on race, globalization, feminism and other aspects of oppression. See Walsh, 'Ethnography-in-motion', pp. 181–193.

[15] Ndebele, 'The rediscovery of the ordinary', p. 154.

[16] James Ferguson, *Global Shadows: Africa in the Neoliberal World Order*, Duke University Press, 2006, p. 67.

[17] Longitudinal research is not without critique and also not without its own tensions. KK's anger highlights the potentially vexed relationships in this work. We have been grateful to review the work of a number of scholars who have written reflexively about some of what might be described as the politics and ethics of qualitative longitudinal research: Sue Cannon, 'Reflections on fieldwork in stressful situations', in *Studies in Qualitative Methodology: Learning about Fieldwork* edited by Robert Burgess, JAI Press, 1992, pp. 147–182; Elaine Batty, 'Sorry to say goodbye: The dilemmas of letting go in longitudinal research', *Qualitative Research* 20, 2020, pp. 784–799; Zachary Morrison, David Gregory & Steven Thibodeau, '"Thanks for using me": An exploration of exit strategy in qualitative research', *International Journal of Qualitative Methods* 11, 2012, pp. 416–427. At the same time other researchers have written about the significance of building and sustaining relationships in qualitative longitudinal work: Carolyn Ellis, 'Telling secrets, revealing lives: Relational ethics in research with intimate others', *Qualitative Inquiry* 13, 2007, pp. 3–29; Gallmeier P. Charles, 'Leaving, revisiting, and staying in touch: Neglected issues in field research', in *Fieldwork: An Inside View of Qualitative Research* edited by William B. Shaffir & Robert A. Stebbins, Sage, 1991, pp. 224–231; Sevasti-Melissa Nolas, Christos Varvantakis & Vinnarasan Aruldoss, 'Political activism across the life course', *Contemporary Social Science* 12, 2017, pp. 1–12; Leila J. Rupp & Verta Taylor, 'Going back and giving back: The ethics of staying in the field', *Qualitative Sociology* 34, 2011, pp. 483–496; Roberta Rehner Iversen, 'Getting out in ethnography: A seldom-told story', *Qualitative Social Work* 8, 2009, pp. 9–26.

[18] Laurent Dubois, 'Man's darkest hours: Maleness, travel, and anthropology', in *Women Writing Culture* edited by Ruth Behar & Deborah A. Gordon, University of California Press, 1995, p. 313.

[19] See Nancy Scheper-Hughes, 'The primacy of the ethical: Propositions for a militant anthropology', *Current Anthropology* 36, 1995, pp. 409–440.

[20] In an important move, the TAC brought global attention to a major court case in which pharmaceutical companies were attempting to block cheap access to AIDS medications. The Pharmaceutical Manufacturers Association (PMA) took the South African government to court in 1998 to contest an amendment to an Act put forward in South African parliament that would make essential medicines more affordable. The PMA, made up of about 40 major pharmaceutical corporations, contested the Act, saying that it violated the international patent laws contained in the TRIPS agreement. Once the case was on its way to court in 2001 TAC asked for permission to join as *amicus curiae* (friend of the court). TAC used the case to mobilise civil society and bring global attention to the issues, and the case was eventually withdrawn. It was an important win and, by 2003, the South African government announced that it would begin an antiretroviral (ARV) rollout throughout South Africa. Widely believed to be the result of both internal and external pressure on the Mbeki government, the rollout intended to make ARVs accessible throughout the country to those in need.

[21] The project 'Investigating social change in action: Reading adolescence as (more than) a literary space in South African young adult fiction' was funded by Social Sciences and Humanities Research Council of Canada (SSHRC) and led by Claudia Mitchell. The findings from this project framed a follow-up study, also led by Claudia, 'Sick of AIDS: South African youth cultures, communication and sexuality' as well as another project led by June Larkin at the University of Toronto 'Gendering HIV/AIDS and youth in Canada and South Africa', both funded by SSHRC.

[22] See Claudia Mitchell & Ann Smith, '"Sick of AIDS": Life, literacy and South African youth', *Culture, Health & Sexuality: An International Journal for Research, Intervention and Care* 5, 2003, pp. 513–522.

[23] See also Rob Lowe, *Love Life*, Simon & Schuster, 2015.

[24] See for example, Nancy Lesko, 'Talking about sex: The discourses of LoveLife peer educators in South Africa', *International Journal of Inclusive Education* 11, 2007, pp. 519–533.

[25] Catherine Campbell's *Letting Them Die: How HIV Prevention Programmes Fail* (Indiana University Press, 2003) remains one of the few books that provided context for understanding the lives of young people, and the high rates of infection in young people, during this era of AIDS research.

[26] See Kylie Thomas, *Impossible Mourning: HIV/AIDS and Visuality After Apartheid*, Wits University Press, 2013.

[27] See Ann Cvetkovich, 'Video, AIDS and Activism', in *Art, Activism, and Oppositionality: Essays from Afterimage*, edited by Grant H. Kester, Duke University Press, 1996, p. 196. Marilyn Martin's ground-breaking chapter,

'HIV/AIDS in South Africa: Can the visual arts make a difference?', in *AIDS and South Africa: The Social Expression of a Pandemic*, edited by Kylie D. Kauffman & David L. Lindauer, Palgrave Macmillan, 2004, pp. 120–135 remains a cornerstone in this work.

[28] For example, see the video *Work Your Body*, New York City Gay Men's Health Crisis, 1989.

[29] Douglas Crimp, *AIDS: Cultural Analysis, Cultural Activism*, MIT Press, 1988.

[30] Jackson Davidow, 'Viral visions: Art, activism, and epidemiology in the global AIDS pandemic', PhD dissertation, Massachusetts Institute of Technology, 2019.

[31] We would argue that this work had a major influence on initiatives in HIV and teacher education in South Africa. See Ken Harley, Naydene De Lange, David Donald, Claudia Mitchell, Relebohile Moletsane, Jean Stuart, Linda Theron, Tessa Welsh & Lesley Wood, 'Piloting of HIV Module in Teacher Education Faculties in the Higher Education Institutions in South Africa'. Report prepared for Higher Education South Africa HEAIDS Programme. Pretoria, South Africa: HEAIDS, 2010. It also influenced how Comprehensive Sex Education and Sexual Health and Reproductive Health Rights education evolved later in the 2000s and beyond in South Africa and in sub-Saharan Africa more broadly.

[32] Bren Neale, 'Foreword', in *Young Lives and Imagined Futures: Insights from Archived Data*, edited by Mandy Winterton, Graham Crow & Bethany Morgan-Brett, University of Leeds Press, 2010, pp. 4–7.

[33] Johnny Saldaña. *Longitudinal Qualitative Research: Analyzing Change Through Time*, Rowman Altamira, 2003; Bren Neale, *Qualitative Longitudinal Research: Research Methods*, Bloomsbury Publishing, 2019. Several key texts stand out in this but most specifically Saldaña's (2003) book and Neale's (2019) book as part of the Timescapes series. Neale writes about the 'temporal turn' afforded by longitudinal research. It is humbling to read all the steps in Neale's book that we missed as a result of landing into longitudinal work rather than planning it from the beginning. At the same time, there are many aspects of what Neale describes that do not apply (e.g., keeping participants engaged over time, tracing participants and so on). Neale also talks about ways of building relationships as a feature of longitudinal research. She is right, of course, that such points are critical. In our case, the longitudinal nature of the project is a result or outcome of being engaged and building relationships.

[34] Claudia Mitchell, 'Fire + Hope Up: On revisiting the process of revisiting a literacy-for-social action project', in *Learning and Literacy over Time: Longitudinal Perspectives* edited by Julian Sefton-Greene & Jennifer Rowsell, Routledge, 2014, pp. 32–45.

[35] We were delighted to come across Singer's book on the Up series: Bennett Singer, *42 Up:'Give Me the Child until He Is Seven, and I Will Show You the Man'*, The New Press, 1999. The book includes an introduction by director

Michael Apted. The book itself was inspiring in affirming our decision to draw so fully on the conversations with the Soft Cover participants found in this book. While the Up series follows a more linear Q&A format than ours does, it still shows, we think, the power of the direct words of the participants in a transcript format as opposed to a format that is narrated and explicitly curated by the researcher.

[36] Joe Coscarelli, 'What happens now to Michael Apted's lifelong project 'Up'?'. Accessed 14 January 2021. https://www.nytimes.com/2021/01/14/movies/michael-apted-up-series-future.html.

[37] Mitchell, 'Fire + Hope Up', p. 32.

[38] Mitchell, 'Fire + Hope Up', pp. 32–45.

[39] Neale, 'Foreword to *Young Lives and Imagined Futures: Insights from Archived Data. Timescapes Working Paper*, pp. 4–7.

[40] For more detail on some of processes and challenges of working with transcripts in publications, see Haleh Raissadat, 'Participatory visual researchers reflect on youth-led policy dialogue', PhD dissertation, McGill University, 2021.

[41] See Judith Lütge Coullie, 'The memory box project: Ethical considerations of memory work amongst AIDS orphans in South Africa', *Current Writing* 30, 2018, pp. 182–95; and Vasquez, Gioconda. 'Body perceptions of HIV and AIDS: The memory box project', *CSSR Working Paper*, 64, 2004.

[42] Thanks to Trish Everett for the incredible work in helping bring together all this material, and the graphic design work of Lan Yan in bringing the Memory Books to life visually.

[43] See Neale, *Qualitative Longitudinal Research: Research Methods*.

[44] One of the participants in the film *63 Up* references the director, perhaps left in by the Michael Apted, as a way to signal his positionality. Now in middle age, many of the subjects are frustrated about how they have been portrayed over the years. They point out that Apted arrives for a week every seven years and, from a week's worth of footage, their lives are then summarised in mere minutes. (www.theglobeandmail.com/arts/television/56-up-a-celebration-of-ordinary-life/article14830996/)

[45] Claudia has written about personal relationships and research in a number of publications. See in particular the following: Claudia Mitchell, 'What difference can this make to our teaching?', in *Academic Autoethnographies: Inside Teaching in Higher Education*, edited by Daisy Pillay, Inbanathan Naicker & Kathleen Pithouse-Morgan. Basingstoke: Springer, 2016, pp. 175–190; and Claudia Mitchell & Fatima S. Khan. 'Jackie and me, Jackie and us', in *Polyvocal Professional Learning through Self-Study Research*, edited by Kathleen Pithouse-Morgan & Anastasia Samaras, Sense Press, 2015, pp. 75–91.

[46] Cited in Shannon Walsh, 'We grew as we grew: Visual methods, social change and collective learning over time', *South African Journal of Education* 32, 2012, pp. 406–415.

[47] See Mandla's chapter in this book.

48 Longitudinal studies are often used in fields such as medicine, psychology and sociology to look at otherwise hidden causal relationships. Longitudinal assessment also poses problems around memory, perception, and autobiography.

49 This project was monitored half way through by the Michael O'Connor from the Canadian International Development Agency (CIDA). He visited South Africa and interviewed staff at the Centre for the Book as well as some of the youth and produced a qualitative evaluation.

50 Soft Cover was a partnership between McGill University and the Centre for the Book in Cape Town. It was funded through CIDA/CHIR's HIV AND AIDS Small Grants fund, Phase II.

51 See Mark Schoofs, 'Apathy, lack of funds imperils AIDS prevention', *The Village Voice*, 12 July 2000.

52 Mandla Oliphant, Abigail Dreyer, Shannon Walsh and Claudia Mitchell spoke on a panel and hosted a working-group session, 'Building bridges: Community vision, youth, and AIDS' at the 'Sex & Secrecy' conference in Johannesburg. The conference was sponsored by the International Association for the Study of Sexuality, Culture and Society, and hosted by the Wits Institute for Social and Economic Research (WISER), the Gay and Lesbian Archives of South Africa, and the Graduate School for the Humanities and Social Sciences, Faculty of Humanities, WITS, Johannesburg, 22–25 June 2003.

53 In 2004 the workshops and videos in Atlantis and Khayelitsha were funded by AWID and FQRSC. Shannon Walsh wrote about this for her master's research, 'The ground beneath me: Creative vision, youth and HIV/AIDS', MA thesis, Concordia University, 2004, as well as in various articles and chapters noted in the related publications in the Appendix to this book.

54 We had T-shirts made which read 'Each one, teach one' as part of the 'Getting the word out' symposium.

55 Established in 2001, the groundBREAKER programme was one of the most well respected and successful youth peer-to-peer education programmes around HIV prevention in South Africa: https://lovelife.org.za/en/groundbreakers/.

56 Mandla's cybercafé business Khaynet was opened in 2003 in the Sanlam shopping centre next to the Khayelitsha commuter train station. The café offered internet access, printing and other office services. Khaynet was written about in the local press, and also by Steve Song. 'Looking for Possible Village Telco Entrepreneurs in Khayelitsha', https://manypossibilities.net/2008/04/looking-for-entrepreneurs/cybercafé business, accessed 16 April 2008.

57 Claudia Mitchell, Relebohile Moletsane & Darshan Daryanani, 'The ethics of risk research in the time of COVID-19: Ethnography at a distance in privileging the well-being of girls and young women in the context of gender-based violence in rural South Africa', in *Critical Studies in Risk and Uncertainty*, edited by Patrick Brown & Jens O. Zinn, Palgrave Macmillan, 2022, pp. 295–321.

⁵⁸ Here we are referring to the virtual conference 'Disrupted lives: Pandemic policies and youth wellbeing', McGill University, Montreal, 7–14 June 2022.
⁵⁹ Dudu Hlatshwayo. 'Are we being the leaders that our youth deserve?', https://mg.co.za/opinion/2022-06-07-are-we-being-the-leaders-that-our-youth-deserve/, accessed 7 June 2022.

# Publications Related to the Project

## BOOKS

Schuster, A. (ed). (2003). *In My Life: Youth Stories and Poems about HIV and AIDS*. Centre for the Book, 2003.

## ARTICLES AND CHAPTERS

Kumar, N., Larkin, J., & Mitchell, C. 'Gender, youth, and HIV risk'. *Canadian Woman Studies/Les Cahiers de la Femme*, 21, 2, (2001), 35–43.

Larkin, J., & Mitchell, C. (2004). Gendering HIV/AIDS prevention: Situating Canadian youth in a transitional world. *Women's Health and Urban Life: An International and Interdisciplinary Journal*, 3(2), 62–83.

Larkin, J., Andrews, A., & Mitchell, C. (2006). Guy talk: Contesting masculinities in HIV prevention education with Canadian youth. *Sex Education: Sexuality, Society and Learning*, 6(3), 207–221.

Mitchell, C. (2004). Youth participation, Health, Education and HIV/AIDS. Creating Spaces for Youth Participation, 15, 22–38.

Mitchell, C. (2006). In My Life: Youth Stories and Poems on HIV/AIDS: Towards a new literacy in the age of AIDS. *Changing English: Studies in Culture and Education*, 13(3), 355–368.

Mitchell, C. (2012). 'This has nothing to do with us—or does it?' Youth as knowledge producers in addressing HIV and AIDS in a Canadian preservice program'. In F. J. Benson & C. Riches (eds), *Engaging in Conversation about Ideas in Teacher Education*. New York, NY: Peter Lang, pp. 83–92.

Mitchell, C. (2014). 'Fire+Hope up: On revisiting the process of revisiting a literacy-for-social action project'. In J. Sefton-Greene & J. Rowsell (eds), *Learning and literacy over time: Longitudinal perspectives*. New York, NY: Routledge, pp. 32–45.

Mitchell, C., & Smith, A. (2001). Changing the picture: Youth, gender and HIV/AIDS prevention campaigns in South Africa. *Canadian Woman Studies/Les Cahiers de la Femme*, 21(2), 56–61.

Mitchell, C., & Smith, A. (2003). 'Sick of AIDS': Life, literacy and South

African youth. *Culture, Health & Sexuality: An International Journal for Research, Intervention and Care*, 5(6), 513–522.

Mitchell, C., Reid-Walsh, J., & Pithouse, K. (2004). 'And what are you reading, Miss? Oh, it is only a website'. The new media and the pedagogical possibilities of digital culture as a South African 'teens guide' to HIV/AIDS and STDs. *Convergence*, 10 (1), 80–92.

Mitchell, C., Stuart, J., De Lange, N., Moletsane, R., Buthelezi, T., Larkin, J., & Flicker, S. (2010). 'What difference does this make? Studying South African youth as knowledge producers in the age of AIDS'. In C. Higgins & B. Norton (eds), *Language and HIV/AIDS Toronto, ON: Multilingual Matters*, pp. 214–232.

Mitchell, C., Walsh, S., & Larkin, J. (2004). Visualizing the politics of innocence in the age of AIDS. *Sex Education: Sexuality, Society and Learning*, 4(1), 35–47.

Mitchell, C., Walsh, S., Moletsane, L. (2007). Speaking for ourselves: Visual arts-based methodologies in working with young people to address gender violence in F. Leach, C. Mitchell (Eds.) *Combating Gender Violence in and around Schools*. London: Trentham Press.

Walsh, S. (2007). Power, Race and Agency: Facing the Truth with Visual Methodologies, in N. De Lange, J. Stuart (eds.) *Putting People in the Picture: Visual methodologies for social change*. Netherlands: Sense Books.

Walsh, S., & Mitchell, C. (2006). 'I'm too young to die': HIV, masculinity, danger and desire in urban South Africa. *Gender & Development*, 14(1), 57–68.

Walsh, S. and C. Mitchell, (2008). I'm too young to die: HIV, masculinity, danger and desire in urban South Africa. In Welbourn, A., with J. Hoare (eds), *HIV and AIDS*. Oxford: Oxfam.

Walsh, S., Mitchell, C., & Smith, A. (2002). The Soft Cover project: Youth participation in HIV/AIDS interventions. *Agenda: Empowering Women for Gender Equity*, 17(53), 106–112.

## THESES

Walsh, S. 'The Ground Beneath Me': Creative Vision, Youth and AIDS, MA thesis, Concordia University, 2004.

Walsh, S. 'Ethnography-in-Motion: Neoliberalism and health in Durban's shack Settlements'. PhD Thesis, McGill University, 2009.

# VIDEOS

*Fire & Hope*, DV, 15 minutes. (2004). Directed by Shannon Walsh, Produced by Claudia Mitchell & Shannon Walsh.

*Youth and Creativity: The Centre for the Book*, DV, 15 minutes. (2003). Produced by the Centre for the Book.

*Facing the Truth (FATT)*, DV, 10 minutes. (2005). Directed by Ann Themba Dipa, KK Mofu, Lindeka Ridwa, Mphumzi Tokozela, Nosibusiso Mcunukeli, Produced by Shannon Walsh.

*Street Fear*, DV, 6 min. (2004). Directed by Ann Themba Dipa, Chinomy Jacobs, Lindeka Ridwa, Nadia Brown, Nosibusiso Mcunukeli, Wendy Tapleni, Produced by Shannon Walsh.

# Index

#FeesMustFall uprisings 14, 301
13th International AIDS Conference 15
  'Breaking the Silence'
*14 Up* 20
*21 Up* 20
*28 Up* 20
*35 Up* 20
*42 Up* 1
*63 Up* 20, 26

**A**

Abstinence-Be-Faithful-Condomize 16
Achmat, Zackie 176, 180
ACT UP (North America) 17
activism 18, 25, 30–31, 38, 42, 68,
  102, 108, 124, 139–140, 146, 153,
  158, 159, 197, 211, 217, 247,
  255, 258, 267, 273, 274–276, 279,
  285–287, 299, 301
  AIDS 17–18, 38, 279, 285–287,
    299
  commitment to 115
  community 237, 300
  cultural 17
  political 19
  social 24
  workshops 146
activist/s 3, 7, 9, 11, 18, 25, 39, 40,
  44, 49, 53, 89, 90, 98, 151, 160,
  175, 180, 192, 211, 229, 237, 239,
  242–244, 267–268, 270, 274–275,
  280, 287–289, 293, 300–301
  agenda 16
  AIDS *see* HIV/AIDS (below)
  community 263

cultural 39
ethnography 6
ethnography-in-motion 6–8
HIV/AIDS 3, 6, 7, 37, 39, 40, 49,
  116, 123, 128, 197, 203–204
Khayelitsha 227
political 109
school 237
teen/youth 9, 18, 19, 24
work in schools 23
AIDS and HIV/AIDS 14–18, 21, 24,
  27, 28, 31, 38, 45, 54, 55, 66–67,
  71, 84–85, 89–91, 93–94, 97,
  99–100, 102–106, 116–118, 119,
  121–123, 128, 140–143, 152, 160,
  175–180, 186–187, 190–194, 202,
  204, 212–216, 219–222, 228,
  231–232, 234, 249–250, 252, 255,
  257–258, 260, 263, 266, 270, 273,
  277, 279, 283, 285, 287, 294, 299,
  300
activism *see* activism, AIDS
activist/s *see* activist/s, AIDS
awareness activities 23
awareness initiative 24
campaigns 42–43, 263
cultural activism 17
denialism 16
discrimination around 17
education apathy 38
fight against 17
infections 97
messages 38
movement in South Africa 18
pandemic 8, 14–18, 89

313

people living with 39
political context 39, 45
prevention 37, 44
-related illnesses 4
safe sex, practising 21
sexual health 19
social context 39
vulnerability of youth 38
workshops 40–42, 66
writing project/s 44, 46
youth-led approach to
    prevention 37
alcohol 62, 92, 94, 116, 123, 125–126,
    129, 162, 176, 220, 250, 269, 270
    abuse 125, 250, 261
alcoholic/s 56, 282
ANC Youth League 272
Ann *see* Dipa, Ann Thendeka
anti-apartheid movement 14
anxiety 168, 286
    issues 156
    management of 167
    medication 82
apartheid 145, 148, 179, 233
    end of 14
artistic expression 17, 18
arts 47, 77, 78
    activism 38
    AIDS activism 38
    exposure to 164
    In townships 108
    love for 164
    theatre 11
    working with 151
    youth culture 38
arts-based
    educational approach 16
    educational workshops 3, 37
    HIV&AIDS awareness
        initiative 24
    international health project 37
    prevention projects 22
    productions 21
    visual and literary arts project 37
    work with youth on HIV and
        AIDS 21
    workshop 25
    youth engagement 21
ARVs 27, 129, 190
Asmal, Kader 261
Atlantis 9, 23, 43, 53, 54, 56, 57, 58,
    61, 63, 65, 68, 71, 72, 76, 77, 85,
    86, 106, 139, 140, 142–144, 154,
    247, 249, 255–256, 258, 266, 278
    gangsterism in 56
    HIV/AIDS in 250
    Secondary School vii, 44, 46, 140
    *Voices from Atlantis* 23, 43, 46, 51
autoethnographic reflexivity 30

B
Bambanani Women's Group 18
    *Long Life: Positive HIV Stories* 18
Biko, Steve 6–7, 179
Black Consciousness Movement 6–7
body shame issues 126
*Boyhood* 27
'Breaking the Silence' (XIII
    International AIDS conference) 15,
    16
Bridgette *see* Magqaza, Bridgette
Bush Radio 16

C
Canadian Society for International
    Health Initiative 37
Celebration of Youth Creativity 40
Centre for the Book 20, 37, 39, 40,
    44, 47, 68, 77, 99, 103–106, 115,
    124, 175, 181, 192, 203–204, 227,
    244
Centre for Visual Methodologies for
    Social Change (UKZN) vii, 47
    (*See also* visual methodologies.)
Chinomy *see* Jacobs, Chinomy
Claudia *see* Mitchell, Claudia
coming out (as gay) 124, 139, 153,
    165, 169
community work 32, 67, 72, 75, 143,
    231, 250, 267

community worker/s 39, 40, 44, 74, 184
Comprehensive Sex Education 306
Conference on HIV/AIDS and the Education Sector: An Education Coalition Against HIV/AIDS 40
COVID-19 11, 48, 80–81, 84, 85, 293, 300–301
    communications 48
    lockdown 80
    pandemic 300–301
    patients 81

D
dance 17, 40, 140, 144, 155–157, 167
    ballroom dancing 139, 144
    class 155, 201
    competition/s 170
    floor 167
    hip-hop/Hip Hop 38, 64, 155–156, 294
    instructor/s 140, 155, 156
    partner/s 156–157
    school 144
    studio 154, 155, 167, 170
    types of 144, 156
dancing *see* dance
Danlia *see* Wiener, Danlia
Department of Social Development 67
depression 82, 130
Dipa, Ann Thembeka 23, 42, 87, 173, 175–196
    poem/s 179–180
documentary/ies 10, 24, 42, 53, 74, 89, 100, 105, 113, 139, 150–151, 211, 257, 259, 294
    AIDS 43
    *Facing the Truth (FATT)* (*see the main entry for "Facing the Truth (FATT)".)*
    film/s 9, 42, 105
    *Fire & Hope* (*see "Fire & Hope* documentary")
    interview/s 3
    presentation 105

drag 150–154, 157–159, 170 (*See also* Johannes, Mathew.)
    community 139–140
    persona 139, 150–151
    queen 151
DramAide 16
Dreyer, Abigail 37, 40
drug abuse 78, 130, 250, 261
drug lords 73

E
ethnography 7, 300
    political activist 6
    institutional
ethnography-in-motion 6–8, 20, 22, 26
Eva *see* Mathew/Eva

F
*FAcing the Truth (FATT)* 23, 43, 45, 89, 100, 115, 128, 175, 183, 197, 211, 225–226, 279
*Fire & Hope* documentary 23, 24, 27, 29, 42–48, 53, 54, 76, 89–91, 97, 105, 128, 129, 139, 142, 168, 211, 215, 234, 255, 259, 263, 280, 283, 286, 294, 298
Fisher, Andrew 11, 298
friendship 4, 5, 8, 10–12, 13, 30, 75, 169, 219, 276-277, 298

G
GAAP *see* Gendering Adolescent AIDS Prevention (GAAP) project vii, viii
gangsterism 54, 56, 92, 129, 171
Gcaza, Nomonde 178–180, 184
    educating others about HIV and AIDS 178
Gendering Adolescent AIDS Prevention (GAAP) project vii, viii
Getting the Word Out symposium 19, 37, 44, 115, 301
*Glitterboys & Ganglands* 139, 150–151
graffiti 38–39
Grassy Park 65
graphic novels 38

group work 45, 67, 68, 72
Gugulethu 40, 108, 233

## H
hand-made books 39-4
Hardy, Stacy 4
'Healing Words' workshops 46
HIV and AIDS unit (Nelson Mandela University) 47
HIV-positive 39, 41, 191, 233
    discrimination 14
    people 14, 39
    status 41, 126, 180
HIV prevention workshops 46
HIV/AIDS *see* 'AIDS and HIV/AIDS'
homophobia 158

## I
*In My Life* 3, 23, 25, 27–28, 97, 100, 105, 110–111, 115, 116, 122, 126, 128, 129, 231, 300
    excerpts from 198–203, 212–215
    *Youth Stories and Poems on HIV/AIDS* 24, 40–41, 44, 49, 97
    writing workshop/s 48, 197
International AIDS conference *(Breaking the Silence)*, 13th 15, 16

## J
Jacobs, Chinomy 11, 46, 47, 87, 173, 255–262
    activism 255
Johannes, Mathew 11, 23, 32, 46–48, 57, 68–70, 75, 85, 126, 129, 139–174, 204, 249, 257, 293. 295–296, 299
    Matthew/Eva Torez 47, 75, 139, 150, 160
Johnson, Nkosi 93, 176, 178, 180
    death 176
Joka, Lindeka Cynthia Rwida 25, 45–48, 87, 115–137, 173, 223–224, 239, 245, 293, 295–296, 298

## K
Kaylene *see* Schroeder, Kaylene

Khayalethu (KK) *see* Mofu, Khayalethu (KK)
Khayelitsha 9, 23–25, 40, 43, 44–45, 65, 89, 90, 96–97, 101, 102, 107, 110, 116, 122, 211, 212, 279, 293
    activists 227
    inequalities of township life 89
    making Khayelitsha safe 288
    site B 96
    video project
    worksite in 215
Khayelitsha West 96
    High rate of HIV and AIDS infections 97
Khaynet 197
Kwela Books 40

## L
Leclerc-Madlala, Suzanne 39
Lehlongwa, Thabo 39
Lewin, Thandi 37
Lindeka *see* Joka, Lindeka Cynthia Rwida
Long Life: Positive HIV Stories 18
LoveLife 16, 128, 236, 237, 243. 261
    groundBREAKERs 261

## M
Magqaza, Bridgette 11, 47, 115, 123, 125, 137, 222–224, 227–230, 293, 298
    death 11, 229
Mahlatsi, Teboho 39
Makhukhanye Art Room 90
Malan, Robin 39
Mandla *see* Oliphant, Mandla
Manenberg 65
Mathew/Eva *see* Johannes, Mathew
Mbeki, Thabo 277
    denialism 16
    government 14
McGill University Participatory Cultures Lab 47
Mcunukeli, Nosibusiso (Nosy) 11, 45–48, 197–210, 222, 293, 298

attitude towards HIV and
  AIDS 202
interview with Bulelwa 203
interview with Sindiswa
  Khayelitsha 202–203
Khayelitsha-led video project 197
poem 199
Meeran, Naseema 11
Memory Books viii, 20, 28–29, 48,
  166, 168, 295, 297
Memory Box/es 28
  project 18, 39
Men in Partners 98
Mhlope, Gcina 39
Mitchell, Claudia 12, 15, 16, 22, 23,
  30, 37, 42, 44, 46–47, 48, 96,
  266, 289, 293, 299
Mitchells Plain 65, 216, 278
Modisane, Jerry 6
Mofu, Khayalethu (KK) 9, 11, 23–25,
  45, 47–48, 89–114, 293, 298
Mphura *see* Xokozela, Mphura
Muizenburg gathering 45

N
Names Memorial Quilt Project 38
Ndebele, Njabulo 3, 5, 8
Neale, Bren 26, 28
Nelson Mandela University HIV and
  AIDS unit 47
*Night and Day* 90
Nosibusiso (Nosy) *see* Mcunukeli,
  Nosibusiso (Nosy)
Nova Park 65

O
Oliphant, Mandla 5, 6, 8, 12, 24,
  30–32, 37, 45–46, 47–48, 65, 99,
  110, 113,115, 173, 234, 239, 242,
  263–289, 293, 294–295, 299

P
pandemic/s 8, 11, 170, 300–301
  COVID-19 300
  gender-based violence 301
  global 84

HIV/AIDS 8, 14–18, 38, 89, 300,
  301
impacts of the 18
racism 301
symposiums 16
participant-led research 8, 10
Participatory Cultures Lab (McGill
  University) 47
peer-to-peer interventions 23
Pityana, Barney 6
post-apartheid 4, 5
  context 8
  era 18
  experiences 4
  South Africa 5

Q
qualitative longitudinal research 20,
  26, 29

R
reflexive revisiting studies 20
relationship/s 29, 30, 43, 57, 59, 97,
  101, 111, 124–127, 142, 147,
  157, 159, 167, 168, 169, 171, 183,
  216, 218–220, 223, 244, 248–249,
  256, 260, 271, 278, 283, 284, 299
  abusive 74
  calibre of 169
  key elements in 147
  long-term 157
  open 111, 142
  personal 26
  sex within 66
  under-studied component/s of 26
  with God 59
researcher/participant divide 8–13
Rhode, Robin 37
Rice, Dammon 37
Rondebosch 278

S
Salt Rock conference 47, 152, 153,
  260–261, 271–278
  panel 99–102, 150–152
Schroeder, Kaylene 9, 11, 46–47, 53–

Index    317

88, 247, 248, 251, 253, 272, 298
Schuster, Anne 40
self-exploration 165
Sello-Duiker, Kabelo ("K") vii, 4, 39
*Seven Up* 20–21
sexual health 17, 19, 32
Shannon *see* Walsh, Shannon
Simon's Town 20, 48, 166–172, 220–224, 279–280, 293
social engagement 8, 33
social movement/s 7, 14, 273
social work 53, 58, 70, 71, 76, 78, 83
social worker 53, 61, 67–70, 72–73, 78, 79–80, 85, 241, 244
Soft Cover project 23, 24, 40, 42, 44, 46, 66, 69, 71, 77. 100, 101, 102, 153, 154, 169, 265–266, 271, 272, 299
Soul City 16
South African National Gallery 18
STDs 55, 98
Stemmel, Clinton viii, 41
Steps for the Future 16
stories 3–8, 11, 18, 20, 23, 24, 28, 29, 31, 33, 39, 46, 48–49, 89, 103, 105, 106, 128, 153, 184, 223, 227–228, 233, 280, 281, 296–299, 300
   content warning 49
   everyday 6–8
   life 4, 9, 263
   personal 28
   poems and 46
   transcript- 28
   writing 280
storytelling 3–12, 280
*Street Fear* 23, 43, 46, 87, 115, 122, 128, 130, 175, 197
Studio Good Life 155
Subaltern Studies group (Asia) 7
symposium/s 16, 19, 37, 39, 44, 69, 99, 115, 187, 301
   Getting the Word Out *see* Getting the Word Out symposium
   HIV/AIDS 249
   Salt Rock (2011) 30

youth 276

T
TAC *see* Treatment Action Campaign.
teacher/s 3, 6, 10, 32, 42, 43, 63, 102, 104–105, 141, 145, 156, 169, 178, 182, 184, 204, 206, 213, 236, 242
   high school 206
   dance 156
*The Champion* 90
*They Died* 258, 277
Thozamile (Thozzi) *see* Vanto, Thozamile (Thozzi)
transcripts vii, 27–29, 44–45, 48–49, 297
transgender people 152, 158
transphobia 158
Treatment Action Campaign (TAC) 9, 14, 16, 31, 37, 89, 99, 105, 109, 115, 121, 128–129, 180, 211, 213, 227, 239, 263, 275, 279, 280, 285, 287, 288, 300
trust 29, 56, 147, 156, 258, 277

U
University of the Western Cape: Public Health Unit 40

V
Vanto, Thozamile (Thozzi) 24, 45, 115, 204, 231–246, 249
Voices from Atlantis workshops 46
Voluntary Counselling and Testing (VCT) 189
visual cultural production 38
   animé 38
   graffiti 38–39
   graphic novels 38
   hip-hop 38, 56, 155-156, 294
   hip-hop stars 56
   music videos 38
   street fashion 38
visual methodologies 32, 299
visual methods 7, 32
*Voices from Atlantis* 23, 43, 46, 51

## W

Walsh, Shannon 8, 9–10, 12, 23–24, 26–30, 37, 43–48, 65, 81–83, 85, 87, 96–98, 99, 108–111, 128, 164, 168, 173, 220, 228, 238–239, 257, 271, 272, 281, 283, 285, 288, 293, 294, 297, 299
Wiener, Danlia 11, 46, 85, 87, 146, 247–252
World AIDS Day 57–58, 143
working with transcripts 28
 (*See also* "transcripts".)
workshop/s vii–viii, 9, 16, 23, 30, 37, 43, 48, 53, 57, 62–63, 65, 89, 106, 113, 114, 115, 123, 128, 139, 140, 142, 143, 145-147, 151, 164, 173, 175, 177, 181–182, 191–195, 197, 211, 227, 232, 237, 250, 253–254, 255, 257, 263, 272, 275, 278, 284
  AIDS 66–67
  arts-based educational 3, 37
  creative 16, 39
  facilitated 46
  hands-on 47
  Healing Words (HIV prevention) 46
  poetry vii
  sexuality 47
  Soft Cover 44, 46, 113, 114
  video 46
  writing vii, 23, 40–42, 48, 197

## X

Xokozela, Mphura 5, 11, 25, 45, 47–48, 115, 173–174, 211–226, 229, 283, 293, 295, 298

## Y

Yellow Men 110
Youth Declaration on HIV/AIDS 40
youth engagement 15, 21